Advances in AI for Health and Medical Applications

Advances in AI for Health and Medical Applications

Editors

Sidong Liu
Cristián Castillo Olea
Shlomo Berkovsky

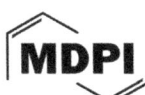

Basel • Beijing • Wuhan • Barcelona • Belgrade • Novi Sad • Cluj • Manchester

Editors
Sidong Liu
Macquarie University
Sydney
Australia

Cristián Castillo Olea
Autonomous University of
Baja California
Mexicali
Mexico

Shlomo Berkovsky
Macquarie University
Sydney
Australia

Editorial Office
MDPI
St. Alban-Anlage 66
4052 Basel, Switzerland

This is a reprint of articles from the Special Issue published online in the open access journal *Information* (ISSN 2078-2489) (available at: https://www.mdpi.com/journal/information/special_issues/AI4health_medical_applications).

For citation purposes, cite each article independently as indicated on the article page online and as indicated below:

Lastname, A.A.; Lastname, B.B. Article Title. *Journal Name* **Year**, *Volume Number*, Page Range.

ISBN 978-3-7258-0367-5 (Hbk)
ISBN 978-3-7258-0368-2 (PDF)
doi.org/10.3390/books978-3-7258-0368-2

© 2024 by the authors. Articles in this book are Open Access and distributed under the Creative Commons Attribution (CC BY) license. The book as a whole is distributed by MDPI under the terms and conditions of the Creative Commons Attribution-NonCommercial-NoDerivs (CC BY-NC-ND) license.

Contents

Sidong Liu, Cristián Castillo-Olea and Shlomo Berkovsky
Emerging Applications and Translational Challenges for AI in Healthcare
Reprinted from: *Information* **2024**, *15*, 90, doi:10.3390/info15020090 1

Ornela Bardhi, Daniel Sierra-Sosa, Begonya Garcia-Zapirain and Luis Bujanda
Deep Learning Models for Colorectal Polyps
Reprinted from: *Information* **2021**, *12*, 245, doi:10.3390/info12060245 5

You-Zhen Feng, Sidong Liu, Zhong-Yuan Cheng, Juan C. Quiroz, Dana Rezazadegan, Ping-Kang Chen, et al.
Severity Assessment and Progression Prediction of COVID-19 Patients Based on the LesionEncoder Framework and Chest CT
Reprinted from: *Information* **2021**, *12*, 471, doi:10.3390/info12110471 18

Cristián Castillo-Olea, Roberto Conte-Galván, Clemente Zuñiga, Alexandra Siono, Angelica Huerta, Ornela Bardhi and Eric Ortiz
Early Stage Identification of COVID-19 Patients in Mexico Using Machine Learning: A Case Study for the Tijuana General Hospital
Reprinted from: *Information* **2021**, *12*, 490, doi:10.3390/info12120490 32

Antonella Cingolani, Konstantina Kostopoulou, Alice Luraschi, Aristodemos Pnevmatikakis, Silvia Lamonica, Sofoklis Kyriazakos, et al.
HIV Patients' Tracer for Clinical Assistance and Research during the COVID-19 Epidemic (INTERFACE): A Paradigm for Chronic Conditions
Reprinted from: *Information* **2022**, *13*, 76, doi:10.3390/info13020076 51

Ruyi Qu and Zhifeng Xiao
An Attentive Multi-Modal CNN for Brain Tumor Radiogenomic Classification
Reprinted from: *Information* **2022**, *13*, 124, doi:10.3390/info13030124 68

Fawad Taj, Michel C. A. Klein and Aart Van Halteren
Motivating Machines: The Potential of Modeling Motivation as MoA for Behavior Change Systems
Reprinted from: *Information* **2022**, *13*, 258, doi:10.3390/info13050258 82

Abdullah Ahmed, Jayroop Ramesh, Sandipan Ganguly, Raafat Aburukba, Assim Sagahyroon, Assim Sagahyroon and Fadi Aloul
Investigating the Feasibility of Assessing Depression Severity and Valence-Arousal with Wearable Sensors Using Discrete Wavelet Transforms and Machine Learning
Reprinted from: *Information* **2022**, *13*, 406, doi:10.3390/info13090406 96

Huiquan Zhou, Hao Luo, Kevin Ka-Lun Lau, Xingxing Qian, Chao Ren and Puihing Chau
Predicting Emergency Department Utilization among Older Hong Kong Population in Hot Season: A Machine Learning Approach
Reprinted from: *Information* **2022**, *13*, 410, doi:10.3390/info13090410 107

Hai Van Pham, Cu Kim Long, Phan Hung Khanh and Ha Quoc Trung
A Fuzzy Knowledge Graph Pairs-Based Application for Classification in Decision Making: Case Study of Preeclampsia Signs
Reprinted from: *Information* **2023**, *14*, 104, doi:10.3390/info14020104 122

Sohini Roychowdhury
NUMSnet: Nested-U Multi-Class Segmentation Network for 3D Medical Image Stacks
Reprinted from: *Information* **2023**, *14*, 333, doi:10.3390/info14060333 142

Md. Jamal Uddin, Md. Martuza Ahamad, Md. Nesarul Hoque, Md. Abul Ala Walid, Sakifa Aktar, Naif Alotaibi, et al.
A Comparison of Machine Learning Techniques for the Detection of Type-2 Diabetes Mellitus: Experiences from Bangladesh
Reprinted from: *Information* **2023**, *14*, 376, doi:10.3390/info14070376 . . . . **165**

Lenni Dianna Putri, Ermi Girsang, I Nyoman Ehrich Lister, Hsiang Tsung Kung, Evizal Abdul Kadir and Sri Listia Rosa
Public Health Implications for Effective Community Interventions Based on Hospital Patient Data Analysis Using Deep Learning Technology in Indonesia
Reprinted from: *Information* **2024**, *15*, 41, doi:10.3390/info15010041 . . . . **184**

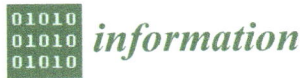 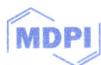

Editorial

Emerging Applications and Translational Challenges for AI in Healthcare

Sidong Liu [1,*], Cristián Castillo-Olea [2,3] and Shlomo Berkovsky [1]

[1] Centre for Health Informatics, Macquarie University, Sydney 2113, Australia; shlomo.berkovsky@mq.edu.au
[2] School of Medicine and Psychology, Autonomous University of Baja California, Mexicali 21100, Mexico; castillo.cristian@uabc.edu.mx
[3] Faculty of Engineering, La Salle University, México City 06140, Mexico
* Correspondence: sidong.liu@mq.edu.au

The past decade has witnessed an explosive growth in the development and use of artificial intelligence (AI) across diverse fields. While the precise trajectory of AI's evolution is complex and multi-faceted, it is discernible that it has been shaped by several key, interconnected technological trends, including the paradigm shift to generative AI [1,2], the emergence of foundation models [3], and the rise of human-centred AI approaches [4], along with incremental improvements in AI generalisability and explainability [5], data transparency and privacy [6], automated AI [7], and edge AI [8], among others.

Healthcare is no exception. In fact, AI is at the forefront of driving pivotal changes in the healthcare sector, opening up innovative and enhanced methods of care delivery. It holds the potential to have profound impacts on contemporary healthcare challenges. By leveraging AI, we can uncover patterns within vast clinical datasets and develop sophisticated computational reasoning methods that support human decision making.

This editorial accompanies the Special Issue titled "Advances in AI for Health and Medical Applications", which endeavours to spotlight the cutting-edge developments of AI in the healthcare and medical fields. This Special Issue proudly features twelve manuscripts that have been meticulously selected for publication, encompassing a diverse array of original research and review articles. Detailed below are the contributions (contributions 1–12), which span from theoretical frameworks to practical applications, addressing everything from diagnosis and treatment to healthcare management and public health.

The advancements in AI from a technical perspective have been noteworthy. For instance, Roychowdhury introduced an innovative Nested-U Multi-Class Segmentation Network (NUMSnet) model for the semantic segmentation of 3D medical image stacks, and it outperformed the state-of-the-art U-Net models. In contrast, Taj et al. made an important contribution to the theorical framework by demonstrating how to generate and maintain motivation. Their work advances the personalisation and adaptivity of digital interventions through behaviour change techniques, thereby assisting designers in making their mechanism of action more explicit.

Several studies have highlighted novel uses of AI methods to improve disease screening and diagnosis. For instance, Qu and Xiao incorporated the attention mechanism into a multimodal Convolution Neural Network (CNN) model to predict the O^6-methylguanine DNA methyltransferase (MGMT) promoter methylation status, a crucial biomarker for predicting chemotherapy response in brain tumour patients. Bardihi et al. reviewed the latest research on the use of deep learning to enhance colorectal polyp detection, providing a comparative analysis of various algorithms across multiple datasets. Furthermore, Uddin et al. conducted an extensive comparison of machine learning algorithms for the detection of type 2 diabetes, pinpointing specific features indicative of the disease. This work holds potential for the effective identification of individuals at risk of diabetes, ensuring timely intervention and patient care.

Citation: Liu, S.; Castillo-Olea, C.; Berkovsky, S. Emerging Applications and Translational Challenges for AI in Healthcare. *Information* **2024**, *15*, 90. https://doi.org/10.3390/info15020090

Received: 25 January 2024
Accepted: 26 January 2024
Published: 6 February 2024

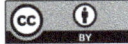

Copyright: © 2024 by the authors. Licensee MDPI, Basel, Switzerland. This article is an open access article distributed under the terms and conditions of the Creative Commons Attribution (CC BY) license (https://creativecommons.org/licenses/by/4.0/).

In recent years, COVID-19 has precipitated a profound shift in the digital landscape, revolutionising numerous facets of daily life, with healthcare being the most significantly impacted. To assist the care management of COVID-19 patients, Feng et al. utilised deep learning to detect and segment lung lesions from chest CT scans, thereby automating the assessment and prediction of patient severity and assisting in patient triage. Conversely, Castillo-Olea et al. applied machine learning to pinpoint the significant early-stage variables in COVID-19 patients. The pandemic has made it clear that hospital resources are finite and face substantial challenges in crisis situations such as COVID-19. This underscores the difficulties in the healthcare management of vulnerable patients due to their risk of infection. For example, managing patients infected with HIV during the pandemic was particularly challenging. To address such challenges, Cingolani et al. introduced an innovative e-Clinical platform, driven by a machine learning system capable of predicting HIV-related alerts. This platform facilitates remote patient management, carefully considering the real needs of patients and ensuring vigilant monitoring of the crucial aspects of care for people living with HIV/AIDS (PLWH) to maintain an adequate standard of care.

The work by Zhou et al. is particularly noteworthy for its exploration into the correlation between temperature fluctuations and emergency department (ED) visitations. They innovatively employed a machine learning model to predict daily ED attendance rates. The development of AI-based analytics tools also opens up new avenues for public health research, facilitating a more nuanced comprehension of public health issues and fostering the design of targeted prevention strategies, enhanced models of healthcare delivery, and community engagement initiatives. Building upon this foundation, Putri et al. utilised various data analytics methods, including machine learning, to discern patterns, trends, and associations within health data.

Encouraging results have been reported, suggesting that AI has become so powerful that it outreasons human experts in areas such as radiology [9] and ophthalmology [10]. Although clinical specialties such as radiology might not disappear, they will certainly be heavily transformed, and clinicians will play a major new role in the time of AI [11]. Pham et al. illustrated a novel application by integrating fuzzy inference techniques based on knowledge graph pairs with clinicians' preferences in decision making. This integration has proven to be effective in the detection of preeclampsia signs, showcasing the potential of augmented AI in clinical diagnosis.

Advancements in sensor technology have been a catalyst for the widespread integration of AI into a plethora of everyday activities. Within the healthcare sector, smart Activities of Daily Living (ADL) monitoring systems and wearable sensor devices that are equipped with AI microchips can effectively assist patients with chronic conditions and disabilities in self-management. Ahmed et al. explored the feasibility of accessing depression severity and valence arousal with wearable sensors, revealing that machine learning combined with a multimodal analysis of signals from wearable devices can effectively identify and forecast individual patterns of depression.

We have also seen emerging applications of generative AI and multimodal models within the healthcare domain. A prime example is Med-PaLM M [12], a proof-of-concept multimodal generalist biomedical AI system conceptualised by Google Research and Google DeepMind. This system boasts remarkable flexibility in encoding and interpreting a wide range of biomedical data, encompassing clinical language, imaging, and genomics. To probe its capabilities and limitations, Med-PaLM M was benchmarked against radiologists in the creation of chest X-ray reports. When reviewing 246 retrospective chest X-rays, clinicians showed a preference for the reports generated by Med-PaLM M in approximately 40.50% of cases when compared directly with those produced by human radiologists, indicating significant progress towards its application in clinical settings.

The integration of AI into every facet of healthcare and medicine is poised to become commonplace. However, the path to embedding clinical AI into daily practice is complex and filled with unique challenges. There is growing recognition that translating clinical AI into routine practice is not straightforward. Common obstacles, such as little to no effort spent replicating trials or reporting harm to patients from AI trials, persist across applications. Furthermore, AI built using machine learning often struggle with generalisation, potentially underperforming in various clinical environments. These hurdles highlight a critical issue in the effective deployment of clinical AI, and they could introduce new types of patient risks and obstruct the translation of research and investment into tangible clinical benefits [13]. The successful implementation of healthcare AI tools hinges on recognising and overcoming these challenges to ensure their reliability and efficacy in enhancing patient care. The journey towards mitigating these issues is as much about understanding and adjusting to the complexities of healthcare systems as it is about advancing AI technology. Ultimately, by cutting through the hype and unravelling the mysteries and challenges of AI in healthcare, we anticipate that this field of research will grow increasingly dynamic.

Funding: This research received no external funding.

Conflicts of Interest: The authors declare no conflicts of interest.

List of Contributions:

1. Roychowdhury, S. NUMSnet: Nested-U Multi-Class Segmentation Network for 3D Medical Image Stacks. *Information* **2023**, *14*, 333.
2. Taj, F.; Klein, M.C.A.; Van Halteren, A. Motivating Machines: The Potential of Modeling Motivation as MoA for Behavior Change Systems. *Information* **2022**, *13*, 258.
3. Qu, R.; Xiao, Z. An Attentive Multi-Modal CNN for Brain Tumor Radiogenomic Classification. *Information* **2022**, *13*, 124.
4. Bardhi, O.; Sierra-Sosa, D.; Garcia-Zapirain, B.; Bujanda, L. Deep Learning Models for Colorectal Polyps. *Information* **2021**, *12*, 245.
5. Uddin, M.J.; Ahamad, M.M.; Hoque, M.N.; Walid, M.A.A.; Aktar, S.; Alotaibi, N.; Alyami, S.A.; Kabir, M.A.; Moni, M.A. A Comparison of Machine Learning Techniques for the Detection of Type-2 Diabetes Mellitus: Experiences from Bangladesh. *Information* **2023**, *14*, 376.
6. Feng, Y.-Z.; Liu, S.; Cheng, Z.-Y.; Quiroz, J.C.; Rezazadegan, D.; Chen, P.-K.; Lin, Q.-T.; Qian, L.; Liu, X.-F.; Berkovsky, S.; et al. Severity Assessment and Progression Prediction of COVID-19 Patients Based on the LesionEncoder Framework and Chest CT. *Information* **2021**, *12*, 471.
7. Castillo-Olea, C.; Conte-Galván, R.; Zuñiga, C.; Siono, A.; Huerta, A.; Bardhi, O.; Ortiz, E. Early Stage Identification of COVID-19 Patients in Mexico Using Machine Learning: A Case Study for the Tijuana General Hospital. *Information* **2021**, *12*, 490.
8. Cingolani, A.; Kostopoulou, K.; Luraschi, A.; Pnevmatikakis, A.; Lamonica, S.; Kyriazakos, S.; Iacomini, C.; Segala, F.V.; Micheli, G.; Seguiti, C.; et al. HIV Patients' Tracer for Clinical Assistance and Research during the COVID-19 Epidemic (INTERFACE): A Paradigm for Chronic Conditions. *Information* **2022**, *13*, 76.
9. Zhou, H.; Luo, H.; Lau, K.K.-L.; Qian, X.; Ren, C.; Chau, P. Predicting Emergency Department Utilization among Older Hong Kong Population in Hot Season: A Machine Learning Approach. *Information* **2022**, *13*, 410.
10. Zhou, H.; Luo, H.; Lau, K.K.-L.; Qian, X.; Ren, C.; Chau, P. Public Health Implications for Effective Community Interventions Based on Hospital Patient Data Analysis Using Deep Learning Technology in Indonesia. *Information* **2024**, *15*, 41.
11. Pham, H.V.; Long, C.K.; Khanh, P.H.; Trung, H.Q. A Fuzzy Knowledge Graph Pairs-Based Application for Classification in Decision Making: Case Study of Preeclampsia Signs. *Information* **2023**, *14*, 104.
12. Ahmed, A.; Ramesh, J.; Ganguly, S.; Aburukba, R.; Sagahyroon, A.; Aloul, F. Investigating the Feasibility of Assessing Depression Severity and Valence-Arousal with Wearable Sensors Using Discrete Wavelet Transforms and Machine Learning. *Information* **2022**, *13*, 406.

References

1. Goodfellow, I.J.; Pouget-Abadie, J.; Mirza, M.; Xu, B.; Warde-Farley, D.; Ozair, S.; Courville, A.; Bengio, Y. Generative adversarial networks. *arXiv* **2014**, arXiv:1406.2661. [CrossRef]
2. Brown, T.B.; Mann, B.; Ryder, N.; Subbiah, M.; Kaplan, J.; Dhariwal, P.; Neelakantan, A.; Shyam, P.; Sastry, G.; Askell, A.; et al. Language models are few-short learners. *arXiv* **2020**, arXiv:2005.14165.
3. Bommasani, R.; Hudson, D.A.; Adeli, E.; Altman, R.; Arora, S.; von Arx, S.; Bernstein, M.S.; Bohg, J.; Bosselut, A.; Brunskill, E.; et al. On the opportunities and risks of foundation models. *arXiv* **2023**, arXiv:2108.07258.

4. Shneiderman, B. Human-centered AI: Ensuring human control while increasing automation. In Proceedings of the 5th Workshop on Human Factors in Hypertext, Barcelona, Spain, 28 June 2022; Article 1, pp. 1–2.
5. Degtiar, I.; Rose, S. A Review of Generalizability and Transportability. *Annu. Rev. Stat. Its Appl.* **2023**, *10*, 501–524. [CrossRef]
6. Blacklaws, C. Algorithms: Transparency and accountability. *Philos. Trans. R. Soc. A* **2018**, *376*, 20170352. [CrossRef] [PubMed]
7. Hutter, F.; Kotthoff, L.; Vanschoren, J. *Automated Machine Learning: Methods, Systems, Challenges*; The Springer Series on Challenges in Machine Learning; Springer International Publishing: Cham, Switzerland, 2019; ISBN 978-3-03005-317-8.
8. Singh, R.; Gill, S. Edge AI: A survey. *Internet Things Cyber-Phys. Syst.* **2023**, *3*, 71–92. [CrossRef]
9. Irvin, J.; Rajpurkar, P.; Ko, M.; Yu, Y.; Ciurea-Ilcus, S.; Chute, C.; Marklund, H.; Haghgoo, B.; Ball, R.; Shpanskaya, K.; et al. CheXpert: A large chest radiograph dataset with uncertainty labels and expert comparison. In Proceedings of the 33rd AAAI Conference on Artificial Intelligence and 31st Innovative Applications of Artificial Intelligence Conference and 9th AAAI Symposium on Educational Advances in Artificial Intelligence, Honolulu, HI, USA, 27 January–1 February 2019; p. 73.
10. Liu, S.; Graham, S.L.; Schulz, A.; Kalloniatis, M.; Zangerl, B.; Cai, W.; Gao, Y.; Chua, B.; Arvind, H.; Grigg, J.; et al. A deep learning-based algorithm identifies glaucomatous discs using monoscopic fundus photographs. *Ophthalmol. Glaucoma* **2018**, *1*, 15–22. [CrossRef] [PubMed]
11. Coiera, E. The fate of medicine in the time of AI. *Lancet* **2018**, *392*, 2331–2332. [CrossRef] [PubMed]
12. Tu, T.; Azizi, S.; Driess, D.; Schaekermann, M.; Amin, M.; Chang, P.-C.; Carroll, A.; Lau, C.; Tanno, R.; Ktena, I.; et al. Towards Generalist Biomedical AI. *arXiv* **2023**, arXiv:2307.14334.
13. Coiera, E.; Liu, S. Evidence synthesis, digital scribes, and translational challenges for artificial intelligence in healthcare. *Cell Rep. Med.* **2022**, *3*, 100860. [CrossRef] [PubMed]

Disclaimer/Publisher's Note: The statements, opinions and data contained in all publications are solely those of the individual author(s) and contributor(s) and not of MDPI and/or the editor(s). MDPI and/or the editor(s) disclaim responsibility for any injury to people or property resulting from any ideas, methods, instructions or products referred to in the content.

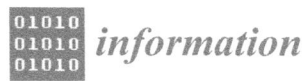

Article

Deep Learning Models for Colorectal Polyps

Ornela Bardhi [1,*], Daniel Sierra-Sosa [2], Begonya Garcia-Zapirain [1] and Luis Bujanda [3]

1. eVIDA Lab, Faculty of Engineering, University of Deusto, 48007 Bilbao, Spain; mbgarciazapi@deusto.es
2. Department of Computer Science & Information Technology, Hood College, Frederick, MD 21701, USA; sierra-sosa@hood.edu
3. Department of Gastroenterology, Instituto Biodonostia, Centro de Investigación Biomédica en Red de Enfermedades Hepáticas y Digestivas (CIBERehd), Universidad del País Vasco (UPV/EHU), 20014 San Sebastián, Spain; luis.bujandafernandezdepierola@osakidetza.eus
* Correspondence: ornela.bardhi@deusto.es

Abstract: Colorectal cancer is one of the main causes of cancer incident cases and cancer deaths worldwide. Undetected colon polyps, be them benign or malignant, lead to late diagnosis of colorectal cancer. Computer aided devices have helped to decrease the polyp miss rate. The application of deep learning algorithms and techniques has escalated during this last decade. Many scientific studies are published to detect, localize, and classify colon polyps. We present here a brief review of the latest published studies. We compare the accuracy of these studies with our results obtained from training and testing three independent datasets using a convolutional neural network and autoencoder model. A train, validate and test split was performed for each dataset, 75%, 15%, and 15%, respectively. An accuracy of 0.937 was achieved for CVC-ColonDB, 0.951 for CVC-ClinicDB, and 0.967 for ETIS-LaribPolypDB. Our results suggest slight improvements compared to the algorithms used to date.

Keywords: colon cancer; deep learning; detection; classification; localization; CNN; autoencoders

1. Introduction

Medical imaging has gained immense importance in healthcare throughout history. It has been used in diagnosing diseases, planning treatments, and assessing results. Furthermore, medical imaging is currently used in preventing illness, usually through screening programs. Aggregating it with demographic and other healthcare data can bring novel insights and help scientists discover breakthrough treatments [1].

A lot of research has been done in automating the delivery of medical imaging results. These results still rely on professional radiologists being present when finalizing them. However, automation can help radiologists be more efficient in their job and deliver results quicker.

A review of deep learning (DL) applications in medical imaging [2] shows that AI algorithms will have a significant impact in the healthcare field. The application areas span from digital pathology and microscopy to brain, eye, chest, breast, cardiac, abdomen, etc. These algorithms are for all types of imaging machines used nowadays: computed tomography (CT), ultrasound, MRI, X-ray, microscope, cervigram, photographs, endoscopy/colonoscopy, tomosynthesis (TS), mammography, etc. Most of these applications deal with classification, segmentation, or detection problems and convolutional neural networks (CNNs), auto-encoders (AE) or stacked auto-encoders (SAE), recurrent neural networks (RNNs), deep belief networks, and restricted Boltzmann machines (RBM) are the most used architectures for these settings. The architecture of some of the most used algorithms is depicted in Figure 1.

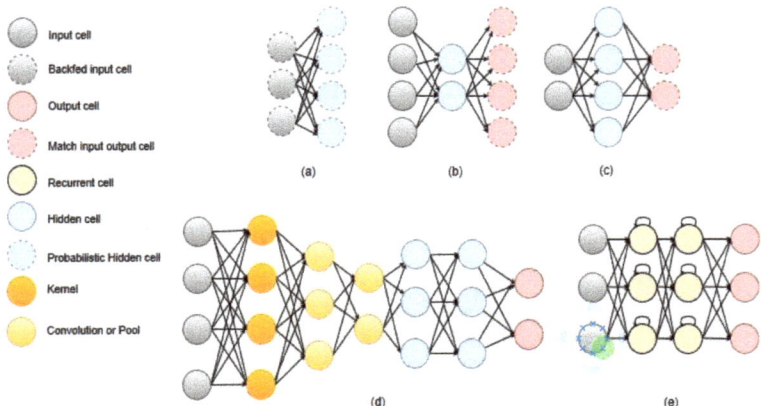

Figure 1. Graph representation of some of the commonly used architectures in medical imaging. (**a**) AE, (**b**) RBM, (**c**) RNN, (**d**) CNN, (**e**) MS-CNN.

In this paper, we focus on colorectal cancer (CRC) and how deep learning algorithms can help detect colon polyps. The World Health Organization, through the International Agency for Research on Cancer, has recognized colorectal cancer as responsible for around 881 thousand deaths, or 9.2% of the total cancer deaths [3]. The main concern is that the incidence rates have been rising, more than 1.85 million cases [3]. This increase could be prevented by conducting effective screening test [4]. However, a 2020 European study on colorectal cancer shows that total cancer mortality rates are predicted to decline, and these numbers for colorectal cancer are 4.2% in men and 8.3% in women [5]. These declines are expected in all age groups [6]. Another study done in the USA shows declining numbers in the USA as well [7]. The implementation of screening programs is an essential factor in the declining numbers various countries have seen. Colonoscopy is the preferred technique among the used screening tests to diagnose CRC. It is also used as a prevention procedure for CRC. CRC starts as growth in the lining of the colon or rectum. These growths are called polyps. Polyps are benign neoplasms; some types can transform into CRC over the years. Within the latter are adenomatous polyps and serrated polyps. Not all polyps develop into CRC. The adenomatous colon polyps (adenomas) and polyps larger than 1 cm have a higher risk of malignancy. Sometimes polyps are flat or hide between the folds of the colon, which makes their detection difficult.

One of the procedures to screen for colon polyps is the colonoscopy, which examines the large bowel and the distal part of the small bowel with a camera. The advantages of this procedure include visualization of the polyps and their removal before they grow bigger and, for biopsy purposes, if the medical personnel suspect a cancerous polyp. According to [7], colonoscopy is very well established as a procedure to prevent the development of CRC playing a significant role in rapid declines in incidence cases during the 2000s but not so much during the recent years. Another study on the impact of CRC screening mortality found that using colonoscopy indicates a more than 50% decline for CRC mortality [6]. Although colonoscopy has shown meaningful improvements, the colon polyp miss rate continues the same. A 2017 retrospective study done with 659 patients indicates that among these patients, the colon polyp miss rate was 17% (372 out of 2158 polyps), and 39% of patients (255 out of 659 patients) had at least one missed polyp [8]. As mentioned before, an undetected polyp, be it benign or malignant, may lead to a late CRC diagnosis, which is associated with a less than 10% survival rate for metastatic CRC. Many elements contribute to missed polyps during a colonoscopy. Two of them are the quality of bowel preparation and the experience of the colonoscopists [9]. While the first problem cannot be fixed by technology, the second one can, and computer-aided tools can assist colonoscopists in detecting polyps and reducing polyp miss rates.

The aims of this study are to give an overview of the recent deep learning algorithms used in colorectal images and videos and introduce a new model for colon polyp detection in images. The rest of the paper is organized as follows. Section 2 presents the recent techniques explicitly used in colon polyp detection, classification and localization in colonoscopy images and videos. Section 3 describes the databases we used to train, validate, and test our proposed model. Section 4 presents the results. We close the paper with Section 5, discussions and conclusions, where we also present the limitations and future work.

The key contributions of this paper are: (i) presenting the state-of-the-art in deep learning techniques to detect, classify, and localize colon polyps; and (ii) introducing the convolutional neural network with autoencoders (CNN-AE) algorithm for detection of polyps with no previous image pre-processing.

2. Background

Researchers have been applying deep learning techniques and algorithms in various healthcare applications. Considerable progress is seen in detecting colon polyps [10,11]. Having a public database of colon polyp images played a big role. Examples of such contributions include using a pre-trained deep convolutional neural network to detect colon polyps [10], dividing images into small patches or in sub-images to increase the database's size, and then classifying different regions of the same image [12]. Other works include exploring deep learning to automatically classify polyps using various configurations, such as training the CNN model from scratch or modifying different CNN architectures pre-trained in other databases and testing them in an 8-HD-endoscopic image database [13]. Authors in [14] take advantage of transfer learning, a technique where a model is trained on a task and later re-purposed and used for another task similar to the previous one. [14] uses CNN as a feature descriptor and to generate features for the classification of colon polyps. Another CNN was developed to detect hyperplastic and adenomatous polyps and classify them by modifying different low-level CNN layer features learned from non-medical datasets [15].

The authors in [16] use a deep CNN model as a transfer learning scheme. Besides image augmentation strategies for training deep networks, they propose two post-learning methods, automatic false-positive learning and offline learning. Shin & Balasingham (2017) [17] compare a handcraft feature method with a CNN method to classify colorectal images. For the handcraft feature approach, they use the shape and color features together with a support vector machine (SVM) for classification. On the other hand, the CNN approach uses three convolutional layers with pooling to do the same. They compare the strategies by testing them in three public polyp databases. Results show the CNN-based deep learning framework leads better classification performance by achieving an accuracy, sensitivity, specificity, and precision of over 90%. Authors in Korbar et al. [18] build an automatic image analysis method that classifies different types of colorectal polyps on whole-slide images with an accuracy of about 93%. Mahmood & Durr (2018) [19] use a deep CNN together with a conditional random field (CRF) called (CNN-CRF), a framework for estimating the depth of a monocular endoscopy. Estimated depth is used to reconstruct the topography of the surface of the colon from a single image. They train the framework on over 200,000 synthetic images of an anatomically realistic colon, which they generated by developing an endoscope camera model. The validation is done using endoscopy images from a porcine colon, transferred to a synthetic-like domain via adversarial training. The relative error of the CNN-CRF approach is 0.152 for synthetic endoscopy images and 0.242 for real endoscopy images. They show that the depth map can be used to reconstruct the mucosa topography.

Three 2020 studies focus more on polyp classification by approaching the problem in different ways. Carneiro et al. [20] studies the roles of confidence and classification uncertainty in deep learning models and proposes and tests a new Bayesian deep learning method to improve classification accuracy and model interpretability on a privately owned polyp image dataset. Gao et al. [21] use DL methods to establish colorectal lesion detection, positioning, and classification based on white light endoscopic images. The CNN model is used to detect whether the image contains lesions (CRC, colorectal adenoma, and other types of polyps), and the instance segmentation model is used to locate and classify the lesions on the images. They compare some of the most used CNN models to do so, such as ResNet50, AlexNet, VGG19, ResNet18, and GoogleNet. Song et al. [22] developed a computer-aided diagnostic system (CAD) for predicting colorectal polyp histology using deep-learning technology with near-focus narrow-band imaging (NBI) pictures of the privately-owned colorectal polyps image dataset. The performance of the CAD is validated with two test datasets. Polyps were classified into three histological groups. The CAD accuracy (81.3–82.4%) shows to be higher than that of trainee colonoscopists (63.8–71.8%) but comparable with that of expert colonoscopists (82.4–87.3%).

There are other works that are focused on colon polyp detection on colonoscopy videos besides images. Such work includes [23], where authors explore the idea of applying a deep CNN model to a large set of images taken from 20 videos approximately 5 h long (~500,000 frames). In [24], authors develop a three-dimensional (3D) CNN model and train it on 155 short videos. In [25] deep learning method called Y-Net is proposed that consists of two encoder networks with a decoder network that relies on efficient use of pre-trained and un-trained models with novel sum-skip-concatenation operations. The encoders are trained with a learning rate specific to encoders and the same for the decoder. Yu et al. (2017) [26] proposes an offline and online framework by leveraging the 3D fully convolutional network (3D-FCN). Their 3D-FCN framework is able to learn more representative spatial-temporal features from colonoscopy videos by showing more powerful discrimination capability. Their proposed online learning scheme deals with limited training data by harnessing the specific information of an input video in the learning process. They integrate offline learning to the online one to reduce the number of false positives, which brings detection performance improvements. Another work [27] includes using a deep CNN model based on inception network architecture trained in colonoscopy videos. They use only unaltered NBI video frames to train and validate the model. A test dataset of 125 videos of consecutively encountered diminutive polyps was used to test the model. However, the confidence mechanism of the model did not generate sufficient confidence to predict the detection of 19 polyps in the test set, which represented 15% of the polyps. In a more recent study, Poon et al. (2020) [11], the authors design an Artificial Intelligent Endoscopist (AI-doscopist) to localize polyps during colonoscopy with the purpose of evaluating the agreement between endoscopists and AI-doscopist for set localization. Another recent study that deals with colorectal videos is Wang et al. [28], which is the first double-blind, randomized controlled trial to assess the effectiveness of automatic polyp detection using the computer-aided detection (CADe) system during colonoscopy. To the best of our knowledge, this is also the only clinical trial that deals with the use of artificial intelligence (AI) in colorectal image/video detection, localization and/ or classification.

There are studies that train and test models in both images and videos. One of them is Yamada et al. [29], where they develop an AI system that detects early signs of colorectal cancer during colonoscopy by decomposing tensor metrics in the trained model. Their AI system consists of a Faster R-CNN and the VGG16 model. Table 1 summarizes the articles included in this minireview, together with some characteristics of these studies.

Table 1. Summary of the reviewed work.

Year	Authors	Nr of images	Format	Objective	Network	Metrics	Datasets	Novelties
2016	Yu et al. [26]	Train: 1.1 M non-med Test: 20	Video	Detection	3D-FCN	F1 = 78.6%, F2 = 73.9%	Asu-Mayo Clinic Polyp Database	An integrated framework with online and offline 3D representation learning
2017	Byrne et al. [27]	Train: 223 Test: 125	Video	Detection	DCNN based on inception network architecture	Accu = 94%, Sens = 98%, Spec = 83%, NPV = 97%, PPV = 90%	Private dataset	AI differentiating diminutive adenomas from hyperplastic polyps on unaltered videos of colon polyps. The model operates in quasi-real-time
2017	Shin & Balasingham [17]	Train: 1525 Test: 366	Image	Classification	HOG + SVM, Combined feature + SVM, CNN (gray), CNN(RGB)	Accu = 91.3%, Sens = 90.8%, Spec = 91.8%, Prec = 92.7%	CVC-Clinic, ETIS-Larib, Asu-Mayo	Compare handcraft feature based SVM method and CNN method for polyp image frame classification
2017	Korbar et al. [18]	Train: 2074 crop images Test: 239 full images	Image	Classification	AlexNet8, VGG19, GoogleNet22, ResNet50, ResNet101, ResNet152, ResNet152	Accu = 93.0%, Prec = 89.7%, Rec = 88.3%, F1 = 88.8%	Private dataset	Identify polyps and their types on whole-slide images by breaking them into smaller, overlapping patches
2018	Mahmood & Durr [19]	Synthetic colon: 100,000 Phantom colon: 100,000 Porcine colon: 1460	Image	Detection	CNN + CRF	RE = 0.242	synthetic data, real endoscopy images from a porcine colon	Synthetically generated endoscopy images
2018	Urban et al. [23]	Train: 8641 images Test: 20 videos	Image/Video	Detection	CNN	Accu = 96.4%, AUC ROC = 0.991	Private dataset	Localization model by optimizing the size and location, optimizing the Dice loss, and a variation of the "you only look once" algorithm ("internal ensemble")
2019	Yamada et al. [29]	Train: 4840 images Test: 77 videos	Image/Video	Detection	Faster R-CNN + VGG16	Sens = 97.3%, Spec = 99.0%, ROC = 0.975	Private dataset	Included 5000 images of more than 2000 lesions, and 3000 images of more than 500 non-polypoid superficial lesions It is nearly real-time processing

Table 1. *Cont.*

Year	Authors	Nr of images	Format	Objective	Network	Metrics	Datasets	Novelties
2020	Carneiro et al. [20]	940	Image	Classification	ResNet-101 & DenseNet-121	Accu = 51%, Avg Prec = 48% (Z = 0.7)	Private dataset (Australian & Japanese)	Deep learning classifier using classification uncertainty and calibrated confidence to reject the classification of test samples
2020	Gao et al. [21]	3413	Image	Detection + Classification	AlexNet, VGG19, ResNet18, GoogLeNet, ResNet50, Mask R-CNN	Accu = 93.0%, Sens = 94.3%, Spec = 90.6%	Private dataset	Detection and classification models based on white light endoscopic images
2020	Poon et al. [11]	Pre-trained: 1.2 M non-med images Fine-tuned: 291,090 polyp & non-med images Test: 144 videos	Video	Localizing	ResNet50 + YOLOv2 + a temporal tracking algorithm	Sens = 96.9%, Spec = 93.3%	CVC-ColonDB, CVC-ClinicDB, ETIS-LaribDB, AsuMayoDB, CU-ColonDB, ACP-ColonDB, Selected Google Images	Real-time AI algorithm for localizing polyps in colonoscopy videos, using different medical and non-medical datasets for training
2020	Song et al. [22]	Train: 12,480 image patches of 624 polyps Test: two DBs of 545 polyp images	Image	Classification	CAD based on NBI near-focus images + ResNet-50, DenseNet-201	Accu = 82.4%	Private dataset	A CAD system for predicting CR polyp histology using near-focus narrow-band imaging (NBI) pictures and deep-learning technology
2020	Wang et al. [28]	CADe group: 484 patients non-CADe group: 478 patients	Video	Detection	CAD + AI	ADR = 34%	Private dataset	The first double-blind, randomized controlled trial to assess the effectiveness of automatic polyp detection using a CADe system during colonoscopy.

Accu = accuracy, Prec = precision, Spec = Specificity, Sens = Sensitivity, Rec = recall, NPV = negative predictive value, PPV = positive predictive value, RE = relative error, ADR = adenoma detection rate, non-med = non-medical, CAD = computer-aided device, CADe = computer-aided detection.

Our model is a combination of CNN and autoencoders. This model was trained on three different colon polyp databases, CVC-ColonDB [30], CVC-ClinicDB [31], and ETIS-LaribPolypDB [32]. All these datasets are open source and can be used for research purposes to develop techniques to detect colon and rectal polyps making them in a way the standard datasets in the field.

3. Materials and Methods

3.1. Databases

In this study, we utilize 3 colorectal polyp image datasets, namely CVC-ColonDB, CVC-ClinicDB, and ETIS-LaribPolypDB. The first colorectal polyp image dataset to be made available for researchers is CVC-ColonDB, and it contains 380 images. All the images are part of 15 colonoscopy videos, and each sequence has various numbers of polyp pictures. The same group that published CVC-ColonDB later made available the CVC-ClinicDB dataset, which has 612 images taken from 29 sequences. The third dataset is ETIS-LaribPolypDB which has 196 images, Table 2. Each dataset consists of 2 main folders, the raw original images, and the masked images, the ground truths, of the corresponding one in the original image. Figure 2 shows images of polyps taken during several colonoscopies. As seen from the figure, polyps come in various shapes and sizes, and some of them are not significantly distinguishable from the mucosa of the colon.

Table 2. Databases used to train and test the CNN-AE model.

Datasets	Nr of Images
CVC-ColonDB [30]	380
CVC-ClinicDB [31]	612
ETIS-LaribPolypDB [32]	196

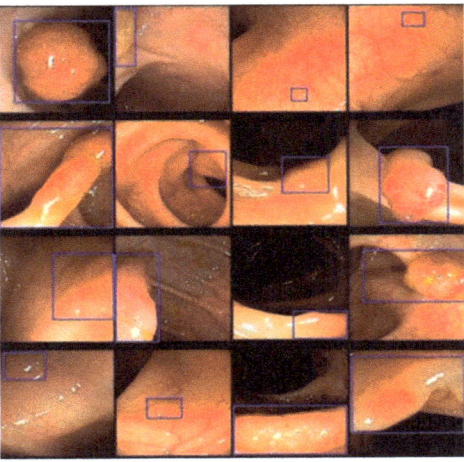

Figure 2. Different shapes and textures of colon polyps taken from colonoscopy videos.

3.2. The Proposed Model

There are some deep learning libraries that can be used to build a neural network model. One of them is TensorFlow [33], an open-source library created by Google and community contributors, currently on its 2.0 version. We used this library to train and test our convolutional encoder-decoder model. The model uses the same architecture as the SegNet architecture [34], an algorithm programmed using Caffe, another deep learning library created by Berkeley AI Research and community contributors. The training and testing were performed on a computer with NVIDIA Titan X GPU.

Figure 3 shows the architecture of the CNN-Autoencoder model. The model has two parts, the encoder and the decoder. The structure of the encoder is similar to some image classification neural networks such as the convolutional layer, which includes the batch normalization, the rectified linear unit (the ReLu) activation function, and the pooling layer. The decoder part has the inversed layers used in the encoder, such as deconvolution layers and de-max_pool layers.

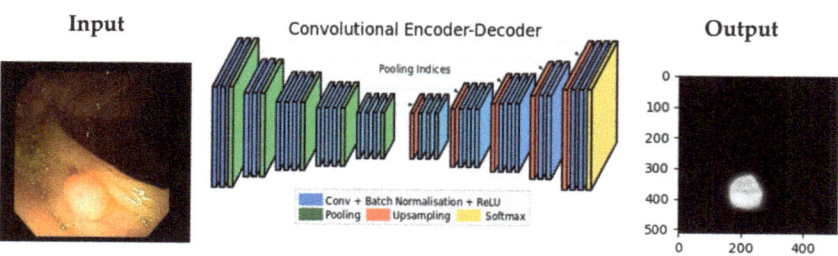

Figure 3. Convolutional encoder-decoder architecture.

The encoder part has 13 convolutional layers and 5 max_pooling layers, where the first 3 layers of the model have these characteristics: the first convolution layer is with stride 2, followed by the second convolution layer with stride 1, and a non-overlapping 2 × 2 window max_pooling layer with stride 2. As mentioned above, each decoder layer contains the corresponding layer of the encoder, which means the decoder network has 13 layers. The output of the last decoder is fed to the Softmax classifier, which produces for each pixel the probabilities if it is a polyp or a normal colon tissue. The network input-output dimensions are equal:

- use the same layer for the non-shrinking convolution layer.
- use transposed deconvolution for the shrinking convolution layer adjusted with the same parameters.
- use the nearest neighbor upsampling for the max_pooling layer.

Open source medical image datasets lack the number of images in them, often only a couple of hundred images. However, for deep learning algorithms to work, a large amount of data is needed. In the case of image databases, researchers have used image augmentation techniques to increase the number of training images. In our case, we used an image augmentation library in Python called Imgaug Library [35]. Figure 4 shows the results after applying some image augmentations that we used in our model, which include:

- Crop—parameter: px = (0, 16) which crops images from each side by 0 to 16 pixels chosen randomly.
- Fliplr—parameter: 0.5 which flips horizontally 50% of all images.
- Flipud—parameter: 0.5 which flips vertically 50% of all images.
- GaussianBlur—parameter: (0, 3.0), blurs each image with varying strength using gaussian blur (sigma between 0 and 3.0).
- Dropout—parameter: (0.02, 0.1), drop randomly 2 to 10% of all pixels (i.e., set them to black).
- AdditiveGaussianNoise—parameter: scale = 0.01*255, adds white noise pixel by pixel to images.
- Affine—parameter: translate_px = {"x": (-network.IMAGE_HEIGHT // 3, network.IMAGE_WIDTH // 3)}, applies translate/move of images (affine transformation).

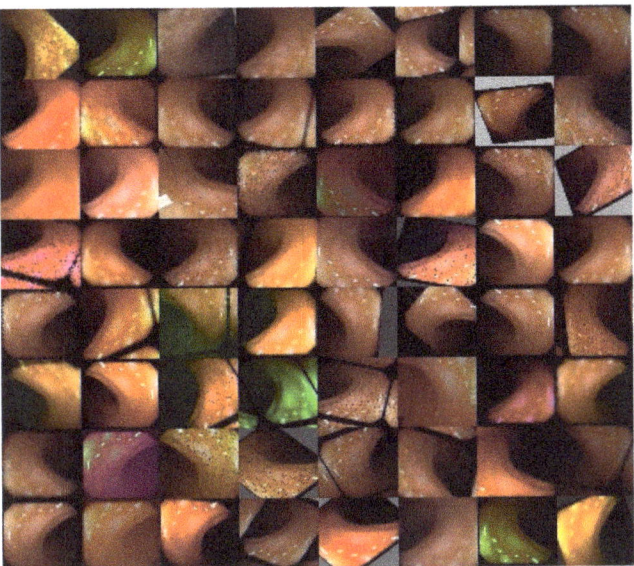

Figure 4. One image of colon polyp after applying different image augmentations.

By using image augmentation, we not only increased the number of images to train the model but also increased the robustness and reduced overfitting of our model. Another technique to deal with the overfitting problem was the Dropout technique with a rate of 0.2. Each dataset was divided into train set, validation set. Majority of the data in each dataset was used for training, 75%, 15% was used to validate and the other 15% to test the model.

4. Results

We trained the model on the selected databases using only the training sets and then we validated and tested with the validate and test sets. As each database has a different number of images, the time to train the model varied. The same batch size of 100 was used for all datasets. The accuracy and the total training time for each database are depicted in Table 3. The best accuracy was achieved on ETIS-LaribPolypDB's last batch with a score of 0.967.

Table 3. The accuracy and the total training time for each dataset.

Datasets	Best Accuracy	Batch	Total Time
ETIS-LaribPolypDB	0.967	1300	1120.48
CVC-ClinicDB	0.951	2200	2186.97
CVC-ColonDB	0.937	2000	3659.52

Apart from the accuracy results from each batch and the final test accuracy, we obtained the images that the algorithm predicted. The test input, test targets, and test predictions were set to gray scale before all the results were drawn. Figure 5 depicts one example from each dataset. The three columns represent the three datasets (left to right: ETIS-LaribPolypDB, CVC-ClinicDB, and CVC-ColonDB) and the three rows, from top to bottom, the test image, the test ground truth (target), and the result of the segment obtained from our model.

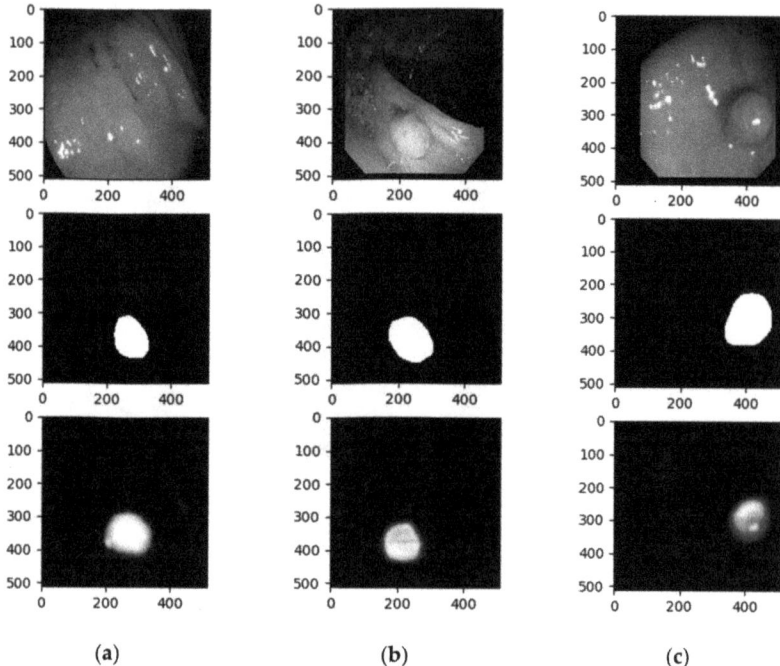

Figure 5. Images showing the results after training the convolutional encoder-decoder model on (**a**) ETIS-LaribPolypDB, (**b**) CVC-ClinicDB, and (**c**) CVC-ColonDB database.

As we presented in Figure 2, polyps have various shapes and characteristics, ranging from big and recognizable polyps to barely distinguishable circular shapes. In Figure 5, we can see that the polyp in the first column is not easily detectable by the human eye, while the polyp in the last is recognizable. This wide variation induces errors in polyp recognition.

5. Discussion and Conclusions

In the background section we presented many techniques and algorithms used these recent years. A quick glance at summary Tab 1 depicts how diverse these techniques are, but also how diverse the metrics to evaluate them are. Accuracy was one of the most used metrics followed by the other metrics such as precision, recall etc. Although the main topic is the same, colorectal polyps, comparing results is difficult. The first reason is the one we explained above, different metrics. The others are related to the objectives, for what purpose are these algorithms used (classification, segmentation, detection, or classification), and the databases these algorithms are trained.

Among the cited papers we find two other similar studies to ours, meaning they are focused on detection problem and use the same metric and database/s. By using the CNN-Autoencoder model, we obtained the highest accuracy of 96.7, which is slightly better than the current state-of-the-art models that calculated the accuracy, Table 4.

Table 4. Accuracy comparison for the proposed model and previously published studies on colon polyp detection.

Model	Accuracy (%)
CNN-Autoencoder (ours)	96.7
DLL [23]	96.4
AI-APD [24]	76.5

The main challenges with colonoscopy images seem to fall on the shape and texture of the polyps [18,22,26], and the quality of the images [21,22,26,27]. The quality of the images depends on the colonoscopy device itself [21,26] or on the expertise of the endoscopist [18,22,27]. Furthermore, in the case of polyp classification, class imbalance poses another problem [20]. Considering these challenges, we checked the image results and verified that indeed some of the segments the model predicted are not as expected. The unexpected bad masks are shown in Figure 6, and again this shows the implications that shape, and texture of the polyp has, but also the conditions the colonoscopy image was taken. The lighting used during the examination plays a negative role when it comes to colon polyp detection as the models misrecognize the normal tissue as a polyp. This phenomenon happens because the inner surface of the colon is smooth, and the light attached to the colonoscopy used by the endoscopists to exam the colon reflects, confusing the models to consider healthy colon tissues as polyps. We have to mention that the patient needs to prepare well and follow the doctor's instructions as per the normal colonoscopy session.

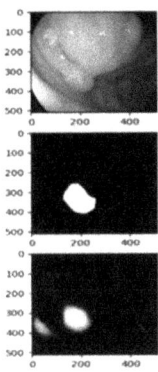

Figure 6. False detection of a polyp due to lighting conditions.

Technology has helped progress the medical field enormously, especially when it comes to medical imaging. Colorectal cancer has been one of the diseases which has gained attention, and many researchers have worked towards detecting and preventing such disease. CAD systems have shown that the polyp miss rate has gone down. However, research shows deep learning has shown even more progress aiding colonoscopists/endoscopists to perform better.

In this work, we presented the current state of the art of deep learning techniques in colon polyp detection, classification, segmentation and localization. We contributed by applying a novel algorithm CNN-AE for detection of polyps, which appears promising considering that no image preprocessing was performed prior to training the model. Our model shows better results than the current state of the art, although not very significant. We believe better results may be achieved if we increase the number of images in the dataset. Moreover, having a diverse range of polyp images may improve the algorithms performance. We tested the same model on other medical image databases, namely iris and pressure ulcer datasets, and the results obtained were better than with the colon polyp images. In future work we want to address these issues by making changes to the model and we will add other image augmentations currently not implemented in the Imgaug library. Besides the technical aspect, we want to address the lack of polyp image datasets. We are in the process of creating a bigger and more diverse dataset of colon polyp images. We will test the model as soon as we prepare the dataset which will be made available to researchers for academic purposes as well.

Author Contributions: Conceptualization, O.B., B.G.-Z. and L.B.; methodology, O.B., D.S.-S., B.G.-Z. and L.B.; software, O.B. and D.S.-S.; validation, D.S.-S. and O.B.; formal analysis, O.B. and D.S.-S.; investigation, O.B. and D.S.-S.; resources, B.G.-Z.; writing—original draft preparation, O.B.; writing—

review and editing, O.B., B.G.-Z., D.S.-S. and L.B.; visualization, O.B.; supervision, B.G.-Z.; project administration, B.G.-Z. and O.B.; funding acquisition, B.G.-Z. All authors have read and agreed to the published version of the manuscript.

Funding: O.B. received funding from the European Union's Horizon 2020 CATCH ITN project under the Marie Sklodowska-Curie grant agreement no. 722012.

Institutional Review Board Statement: Not applicable.

Informed Consent Statement: Not applicable.

Data Availability Statement: Not applicable.

Conflicts of Interest: The funders had no role in the design of the study; in the collection, analyses, or interpretation of data; in the writing of the manuscript, or in the decision to publish the results.

References

1. Esteva, A.; Robicquet, A.; Ramsundar, B.; Kuleshov, V.; DePristo, M.; Chou, K.; Cui, C. A guide to deep learning in healthcare. *Nat. Med.* **2019**, *25*, 24–29. [CrossRef]
2. Litjens, G.; Kooi, T.; Bejnordi, B.E.; Setio, A.A.A.; Ciompi, F.; Ghafoorian, M.; Van Der Laak, J.A.; Van Ginneken, B.; Sánchez, C.I. A survey on deep learning in medical image analysis. *Med. Image Anal.* **2017**, *42*, 60–88. [CrossRef]
3. World Health Organization and International Agency for Research on Cancer. Cancer Today. 2020. Available online: https://bit.ly/37jXYER (accessed on 17 November 2020).
4. Lieberman, D. Quality and colonoscopy: A new imperative. *Gastrointest. Endosc.* **2005**, *61*, 392–394. [CrossRef]
5. Carioli, G.; Bertuccio, P.; Boffetta, P.; Levi, F.; La Vecchia, C.; Negri, E.; Malvezzi, M. European cancer mortality predictions for the year 2020 with a focus on prostate cancer. *Ann. Oncol.* **2020**, *31*, 650–658. [CrossRef]
6. Zauber, A.G. The Impact of Screening on Colorectal Cancer Mortality and Incidence: Has It Really Made a Difference? *Dig. Dis. Sci.* **2015**, *60*, 681–691. [CrossRef]
7. Siegel, R.L.; Miller, K.D.; Jemal, A. Cancer statistics, 2020. *CA Cancer J. Clin.* **2020**, *70*, 7–30. [CrossRef]
8. Lee, J.; Park, S.W.; Kim, Y.S.; Lee, K.J.; Sung, H.; Song, P.H.; Yoon, W.J.; Moon, J.S. Risk factors of missed colorectal lesions after colonoscopy. *Medicine* **2017**, *96*, e7468. [CrossRef]
9. Bonnington, S.N.; Rutter, M.D. Surveillance of colonic polyps: Are we getting it right? *World J. Gastroenterol.* **2016**, *22*, 1925–1934. [CrossRef]
10. Tajbakhsh, N.; Shin, J.Y.; Gurudu, S.R.; Hurst, R.T.; Kendall, C.B.; Gotway, M.B.; Liang, J. Convolutional Neural Networks for Medical Image Analysis: Full Training or Fine Tuning? *IEEE Trans. Med. Imaging* **2016**, *35*, 1299–1312. [CrossRef] [PubMed]
11. Poon, C.C.; Jiang, Y.; Zhang, R.; Lo, W.W.; Cheung, M.S.; Yu, R.; Zheng, Y.; Wong, J.C.; Liu, Q.; Wong, S.H.; et al. AI-doscopist: A real-time deep-learning-based algorithm for localising polyps in colonoscopy videos with edge computing devices. *NPJ Digit. Med.* **2020**, *3*, 73.
12. Ribeiro, E.; Uhl, A.; Häfner, M. Colonic polyp classification with convolutional neural networks. In Proceedings of the IEEE 29th International Symposium on Computer-Based Medical Systems (CBMS), Dublin, Ireland, 20–24 June 2016.
13. Ribeiro, E.; Häfner, M.; Wimmer, G.; Tamaki, T.; Tischendorf, J.J.; Yoshida, S.; Tanaka, S.; Uhl, A. Exploring texture transfer learning for colonic polyp classification via convolutional neural networks. In Proceedings of the 2017 IEEE 14th International Symposium on Biomedical Imaging (ISBI 2017), Melbourne, Australia, 18–21 April 2017.
14. Ribeiro, E.; Uhl, A.; Wimmer, G.; Häfner, M. Exploring Deep Learning and Transfer Learning for Colonic Polyp Classification. *Comput. Math. Methods Med.* **2016**, *2016*, 6584725. [CrossRef]
15. Zhang, R.; Zheng, Y.; Mak, T.W.C.; Yu, R.; Wong, S.H.; Lau, J.Y.; Poon, C.C. Automatic Detection and Classification of Colorectal Polyps by Transferring Low-Level CNN Features from Nonmedical Domain. *IEEE J. Biomed. Health Inform.* **2017**, *21*, 41–47. [CrossRef]
16. Shin, Y.; Qadir, H.A.; Aabakken, L.; Bergsland, J.; Balasingham, I. Automatic Colon Polyp Detection Using Region Based Deep CNN and Post Learning Approaches. *IEEE Access* **2018**, *6*, 40950–40962. [CrossRef]
17. Shin, Y.; Balasingham, I. Comparison of hand-craft feature based SVM and CNN based deep learning framework for automatic polyp classification. In Proceedings of the 39th Annual International Conference of the IEEE Engineering in Medicine and Biology Society (EMBC), Jeju Island, Korea, 11–15 July 2017.
18. Korbar, B.; Olofson, A.M.; Miraflor, A.P.; Nicka, C.M.; Suriawinata, M.A.; Torresani, L.; Suriawinata, A.A.; Hassanpour, S. Deep Learning for Classification of Colorectal Polyps on Whole-slide Images. *J. Pathol. Inform.* **2017**, *8*, 30. [PubMed]
19. Mahmood, F.; Durr, N.J. Deep learning and conditional random fields-based depth estimation and topographical reconstruction from conventional endoscopy. *Med. Image Anal.* **2018**, *48*, 230–243. [CrossRef]
20. Carneiro, G.; Pu, L.Z.C.T.; Singh, R.; Burt, A. Deep learning uncertainty and confidence calibration for the five-class polyp classification from colonoscopy. *Med. Image Anal.* **2020**, *62*, 101653. [CrossRef]
21. Gao, J.; Guo, Y.; Sun, Y.; Qu, G. Application of Deep Learning for Early Screening of Colorectal Precancerous Lesions under White Light Endoscopy. *Comput. Math. Methods Med.* **2020**, *2020*, 8374317. [CrossRef]

22. Song, E.M.; Park, B.; Ha, C.A.; Hwang, S.W.; Park, S.H.; Yang, D.H.; Ye, B.D.; Myung, S.J.; Yang, S.K.; Kim, N.; et al. Endoscopic diagnosis and treatment planning for colorectal polyps using a deep-learning model. *Sci. Rep.* **2020**, *10*, 30. [CrossRef] [PubMed]
23. Urban, G.; Tripathi, P.; Alkayali, T.; Mittal, M.; Jalali, F.; Karnes, W.; Baldi, P. Deep Learning Localizes and Identifies Polyps in Real Time With 96% Accuracy in Screening Colonoscopy. *Gastroenterology* **2018**, *155*, 1069–1078.e8. [CrossRef] [PubMed]
24. Misawa, M.; Kudo, S.E.; Mori, Y.; Cho, T.; Kataoka, S.; Yamauchi, A.; Ogawa, Y.; Maeda, Y.; Takeda, K.; Ichimasa, K.; et al. Artificial Intelligence-Assisted Polyp Detection for Colonoscopy: Initial Experience. *Gastroenterology* **2018**, *154*, 2027–2029.e3. [CrossRef] [PubMed]
25. Mohammed, A.K.; Yildirim, S.; Farup, I.; Pederse, M.; Hovde, O. Y-Net: A deep Convolutional Neural Network for Polyp Detection. 2018. Available online: http://arxiv.org/abs/1806.01907 (accessed on 10 June 2020).
26. Yu, L.; Chen, H.; Dou, Q.; Qin, J.; Heng, P.A. Integrating Online and Offline Three-Dimensional Deep Learning for Automated Polyp Detection in Colonoscopy Videos. *IEEE J. Biomed. Health Inform.* **2017**, *21*, 65–75. [CrossRef]
27. Byrne, M.F.; Chapados, N.; Soudan, F.; Oertel, C.; Pérez, M.L.; Kelly, R.; Iqbal, N.; Chandelier, F.; Rex, D.K. Real-time differentiation of adenomatous and hyperplastic diminutive colorectal polyps during analysis of unaltered videos of standard colonoscopy using a deep learning model. *Gut* **2019**, *68*, 94. [CrossRef] [PubMed]
28. Wang, P.; Liu, X.; Berzin, T.M.; Brown, J.R.G.; Liu, P.; Zhou, C.; Lei, L.; Li, L.; Guo, Z.; Lei, S.; et al. Effect of a deep-learning computer-aided detection system on adenoma detection during colonoscopy (CADe-DB trial): A double-blind randomised study. *Lancet Gastroenterol. Hepatol.* **2020**, *5*, 343–351. [CrossRef]
29. Yamada, M.; Saito, Y.; Imaoka, H.; Saiko, M.; Yamada, S.; Kondo, H.; Takamaru, H.; Sakamoto, T.; Sese, J.; Kuchiba, A.; et al. Development of a real-time endoscopic image diagnosis support system using deep learning technology in colonoscopy. *Sci. Rep.* **2019**, *9*, 1–9. [CrossRef] [PubMed]
30. Bernal, J.; Sánchez, J.; Vilariño, F. Towards automatic polyp detection with a polyp appearance model. *Pattern Recognit.* **2012**, *45*, 3166–3182. [CrossRef]
31. Bernal, J.; Sánchez, F.J.; Fernández-Esparrach, G.; Gil, D.; Rodríguez, C.; Vilariño, F. WM-DOVA maps for accurate polyp highlighting in colonoscopy: Validation vs. saliency maps from physicians. *Comput. Med Imaging Graph.* **2015**, *43*, 99–111. [CrossRef] [PubMed]
32. Silva, J.; Histace, A.; Romain, O.; Dray, X.; Granado, B. Toward embedded detection of polyps in WCE images for early diagnosis of colorectal cancer. *Int. J. Comput. Assist. Radiol. Surg.* **2014**, *9*, 283–293. [CrossRef]
33. Abadi, M.; Barham, P.; Chen, J.; Chen, Z.; Davis, A.; Dean, J.; Devin, M.; Ghemawat, S.; Irving, G.; Isard, M.; et al. TensorFlow: A system for large-scale machine learning. In Proceedings of the 12th USENIX Conference on Operating Systems Design and Implementation, Savannah, GA, USA, 2–4 November 2016; pp. 265–283.
34. Badrinarayanan, V.; Kendall, A.; Cipolla, R. SegNet: A Deep Convolutional Encoder-Decoder Architecture for Image Segmentation. *IEEE Trans. Pattern Anal. Mach. Intell.* **2017**, *39*, 2481–2495. [CrossRef]
35. Jung, A. imgaug 0.2.5 [Internet]. 2017. Available online: http://imgaug.readthedocs.io/en/latest (accessed on 10 June 2020).

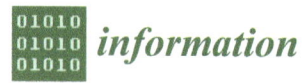 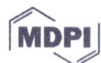

Article

Severity Assessment and Progression Prediction of COVID-19 Patients Based on the LesionEncoder Framework and Chest CT

You-Zhen Feng [1,†], Sidong Liu [2,†], Zhong-Yuan Cheng [1,†], Juan C. Quiroz [3], Dana Rezazadegan [4], Ping-Kang Chen [1], Qi-Ting Lin [1], Long Qian [5], Xiao-Fang Liu [6], Shlomo Berkovsky [2], Enrico Coiera [2], Lei Song [7,*], Xiao-Ming Qiu [8,*] and Xiang-Ran Cai [1,*]

[1] Medical Imaging Centre, The First Affiliated Hospital of Jinan University, Guangzhou 510630, China; fengyouzhen@jnu.edu.cn (Y.-Z.F.); chengzy@jnu.edu.cn (Z.-Y.C.); cpk1993@stu2019.jnu.edu.cn (P.-K.C.); linqiting@stu2018.jnu.edu.cn (Q.-T.L.)
[2] Centre for Health Informatics, Australian Institute of Health Innovation, Faculty of Medicine, Health and Human Sciences, Macquarie University, Sydney 2113, Australia; sidong.liu@mq.edu.au (S.L.); shlomo.berkovsky@mq.edu.au (S.B.); enrico.coiera@mq.edu.au (E.C.)
[3] Centre for Big Data Research in Health, University of New South Wales, Sydney 1466, Australia; juan.quiroz@unsw.edu.au
[4] Department of Computer Science and Software Engineering, Swinburne University of Technology, Melbourne 3000, Australia; drezazadegan@swin.edu.au
[5] Department of Biomedical Engineering, Peking University, Beijing 100871, China; longqianad@pku.edu.cn
[6] Tianjin Key Laboratory of Intelligent Robotics, Institute of Robotics and Automatic Information System, College of Artificial Intelligence, Nankai University, Tianjin 300350, China; liuxiaofang@nankai.edu.cn
[7] Department of Radiology, Xiangyang Central Hospital, Affiliated Hospital of Hubei University of Arts and Science, Xiangyang 441003, China
[8] Department of Radiology, Huangshi Central Hospital, Affiliated Hospital of Hubei Polytechnic University, Edong Healthcare Group, Huangshi 435002, China
* Correspondence: song580lei@gmail.com (L.S.); xiaomingqiu0714@gmail.com (X.-M.Q.); caixran@jnu.edu.cn (X.-R.C.)
† These authors contributed equally.

Abstract: Automatic severity assessment and progression prediction can facilitate admission, triage, and referral of COVID-19 patients. This study aims to explore the potential use of lung lesion features in the management of COVID-19, based on the assumption that lesion features may carry important diagnostic and prognostic information for quantifying infection severity and forecasting disease progression. A novel LesionEncoder framework is proposed to detect lesions in chest CT scans and to encode lesion features for automatic severity assessment and progression prediction. The LesionEncoder framework consists of a U-Net module for detecting lesions and extracting features from individual CT slices, and a recurrent neural network (RNN) module for learning the relationship between feature vectors and collectively classifying the sequence of feature vectors. Chest CT scans of two cohorts of COVID-19 patients from two hospitals in China were used for training and testing the proposed framework. When applied to assessing severity, this framework outperformed baseline methods achieving a sensitivity of 0.818, specificity of 0.952, accuracy of 0.940, and AUC of 0.903. It also outperformed the other tested methods in disease progression prediction with a sensitivity of 0.667, specificity of 0.838, accuracy of 0.829, and AUC of 0.736. The LesionEncoder framework demonstrates a strong potential for clinical application in current COVID-19 management, particularly in automatic severity assessment of COVID-19 patients. This framework also has a potential for other lesion-focused medical image analyses.

Keywords: chest CT; COVID-19; severity assessment; progression prediction; U-Net; RNN

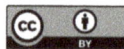

1. Introduction

The rapid escalation in the number of COVID-19 infections exceeded the capacity of healthcare systems to respond in many nations, and consequently reduced patient outcomes [1]. In such circumstances, it is of paramount importance to develop efficient diagnostic and prognostic models for COVID-19, so that the patients' care can be optimized.

Chest CT scans have been found to provide important diagnostic and prognostic information for COVID-19 [2–7]. Although there is still debate on the use of chest CT in screening and diagnosing COVID-19 cases [8], a surge of computational methods for chest CT have been developed to support medical decision making during the current pandemic [9–15]. Study population, model performance, and reporting quality vary substantially between studies. An in-depth comparison of these studies can be found in a recent systematic review [16].

In addition to diagnostic and screening models, several prediction models have been proposed based on an assessment of lung lesions. There are three typical classes of lesions that can be detected in COVID-19 chest CT scans: ground glass opacity (GGO), consolidation, and pleural effusion [3,4]. Imaging features of the lesions including shape, location, extent and distribution of involvement of each abnormality have been found to have good predictive power for mortality [17] or hospital stay [18]. These features, however, are mostly derived from the delineated lesions, and so depend heavily on lesion segmentation. Manual delineation of lesions often takes one to five hours, which substantially undermines clinical applicability of these methods.

Automatic lung lesion segmentation for COVID-19 has been actively investigated in recent studies [19,20]. A VB-Net model based on a neural network was proposed to segment the infection regions in CT scans [19]. This model, when trained using CT scans of 249 COVID-19 patients, achieved a Dice score of 0.92 between automatic and manual segmentations, and successfully reduced the delineation time to less than 4 min. In another recent study [20], a lesion segmentation model based on the 3D-Dense U-Net architecture was proposed and trained on CT scans of a combination of 160 COVID-19, 172 viral pneumonia, and 296 interstitial lung disease patients. Although the lesion masks were not compared voxel-to-voxel, the volumetric measures of lesions, such as percentage of opacity and consolidation, showed a high correlation (0.97–0.98) between automatic and manual segmentations.

Previous studies [19,20] have suggested that lesion features might be a useful biomarker for COVID-19 patient severity assessment, but the effectiveness of lesion features is yet to be verified. Lesion features may have additional applications in the management of COVID-19, which need to be investigated further. In this study, we aim to test the effectiveness of using lesion features in COVID-19 patients for disease severity assessment, and to explore the potential use of lesion features in predicting disease progression.

Automatic severity assessment and progression prediction will substantially facilitate admission, triage, and referral of patients. The first goal of this study is to develop a method for assessing severity of COVID-19 patients based on their baseline chest CT scans. Four severity types: mild, ordinary, severe, and critical, can be defined based on a core outcome set (COS) encapsulating clinical symptoms, physical and chemical detection, viral nuclei aid detection, disease process, etc. [21]. Supportive treatments, such as supplementary oxygen and mechanical ventilation, are usually required for severe and critical cases [22]. We represent the assessment severity task as a binary classification problem (i.e., to classify a patient as a mild/ordinary case (mild class) or a severe/critical case (severe class)).

The second goal of this study is to predict disease progression for the mild/ordinary cases based on their baseline CT scans. In other words, we aim to predict which of the mild/ordinary severity patients are likely to progress to the severe/critical category (converter class) in the short term (within seven days), and which patients would remain stable or recover (non-converter class), based on the assumption that lesion features may carry important prognostic information for forecasting disease progression. We again consider the task as a binary classification problem (i.e., to classify the non-converter cases and converter cases). Figure 1a presents an example of a COVID-19 case with mild symptoms. In less than seven days, the patient's symptoms rapidly worsened and progressed to severe. Figure 1b is an example of a non-converter case whose symptoms progressed slowly and remained mild seven days after the baseline CT scan.

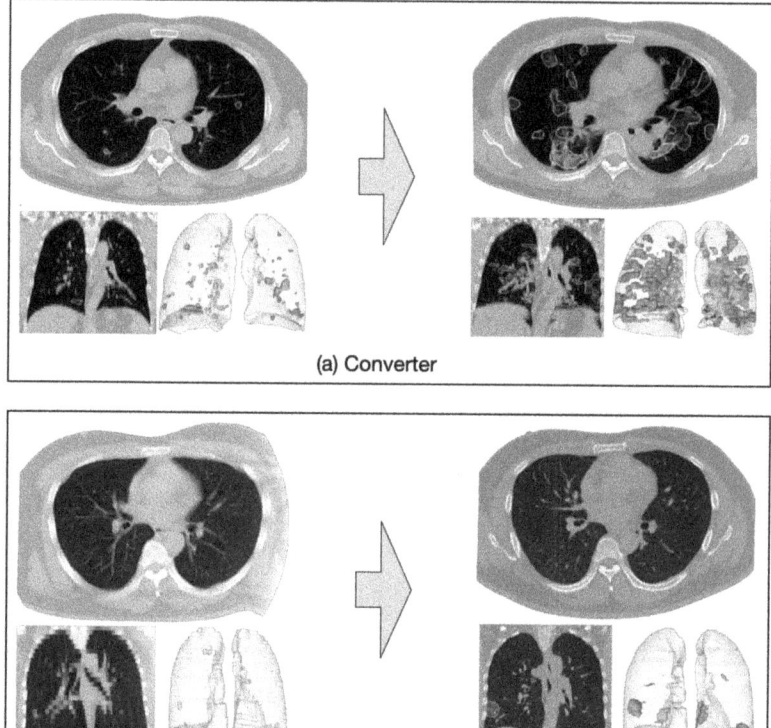

Figure 1. Examples of converter and non-converter cases. (**a**) A mild case progressed to severe within seven days; (**b**) a mild case did not progress to severe within seven days.

To achieve the above two goals, a novel LesionEncoder framework is proposed to detect lesions in CT scans and encode lesion features for automatic severity assessment and progression prediction. The LesionEncoder framework consists of two modules: (1) A U-Net module which detects lesions and extracts features from CT slices, and (2) a recurrent neural network (RNN) module for learning the relationship between feature vectors and classifying the sequence of feature vectors as a whole.

We applied the LesionEncoder framework for both severity assessment and progression prediction. With access to data of two COVID-19 confirmed patient cohorts from two hospitals, we trained our proposed model with CT scans of a cohort of patients from one hospital and tested it on an independent cohort from the other hospital. The models built on the LesionEncoder framework outperformed the baseline models that used lesion volumetric features and general imaging features, demonstrating a high potential for clinical applications in the current COVID-19 management, particularly in automatic severity assessment of COVID-19 patients. This framework may also have a strong potential in similar lesion-focused analyses, such as neuroimaging based diagnosis of brain tumors [23,24] and neurological disorders [25,26], CT-based lung nodule classification [27], and retinal imaging based ophthalmic disease detection [28].

2. Datasets

A total of 346 COVID patients confirmed by reverse transcription polymerase chain reaction (RT-PCR) were retrospectively selected from two local hospitals in the Hubei Province, China, namely Huang Shi Central Hospital (HSCH) and Xiang Yang Central Hospital (XYCH). Severity types of all patients at baseline and follow-up (in seven days) were assessed and confirmed by clinicians according to the COS for COVID-19 [21]. More details of the demographics and baseline characteristics of patients can be found in our previous study [29]. This analysis was approved by the Institutional Review Board of both hospitals, and written informed consent was obtained from all the participants.

Tables 1 and 2 illustrate, respectively, the demographics of patients for the development of a severity assessment model (Task 1—mild vs. severe) and a progression prediction model (Task 2—converter vs. non-converter). For both tasks, CT scans of the HSCH cohort were used for training the models, and CT scans of the XYCH cohort were used as an independent dataset to test the trained models. Patients may have either a lung-window scan, a mediastinal-window scan, or both in their baseline CT examination. All scans were included in the analysis. The total number of CT scans for Task 1 was 639, and that for Task 2 was 601. An internal validation set (20% of the training samples) was split from the training set and used to evaluate the model's performance during training.

Table 1. Demographics of the patients in Task 1 dataset.

Category	HSCH—Training Set	XYCH—Test Set	Total
Mild	7	1	8
Ordinary	212	104	316
Severe	7	6	13
Critical	4	5	9
Total patients	230	116	346
Total CT scans	433	206	639
Age (mean ± SD)	49.00 ± 14.4	47.5 ± 17.2	48.5 ± 15.4
Gender (female/male)	120/110	57/59	177/169

Table 2. Demographics of the patients in Task 2 dataset.

Category	HSCH—Training Set	XYCH—Test Set	Total
Non-converter	201	99	300
Converter	18	6	24
Total patients	219	105	324
Total CT scans	412	189	601
Age (mean ± SD)	48.4 ± 14.0	46.1 ± 16.6	47.7 ± 14.9
Gender (female/male)	113/106	55/50	168/156

Note that there is a highly imbalanced distribution of samples in the datasets (i.e., 324 (93.6%) patients in mild class for Task 1, and 300 (92.6%) patients in non-converter class for Task 2). A weighting strategy was used to address the imbalanced distribution in datasets, and the details are presented in Section 3.3.

3. Methods

Figure 2 gives an overview of the LesionEncoder framework, which consists of two modules: (1) A lesion encoder module for lesion detection and feature encoding, and (2) a RNN module for sequence classification. The lesion encoder module extracts features from individual CT slices; therefore, a CT scan with multiple CT slices can be represented as a sequence of feature vectors. The sequence classification module takes the sequence of feature vectors as input and then classifies the entire sequence collectively.

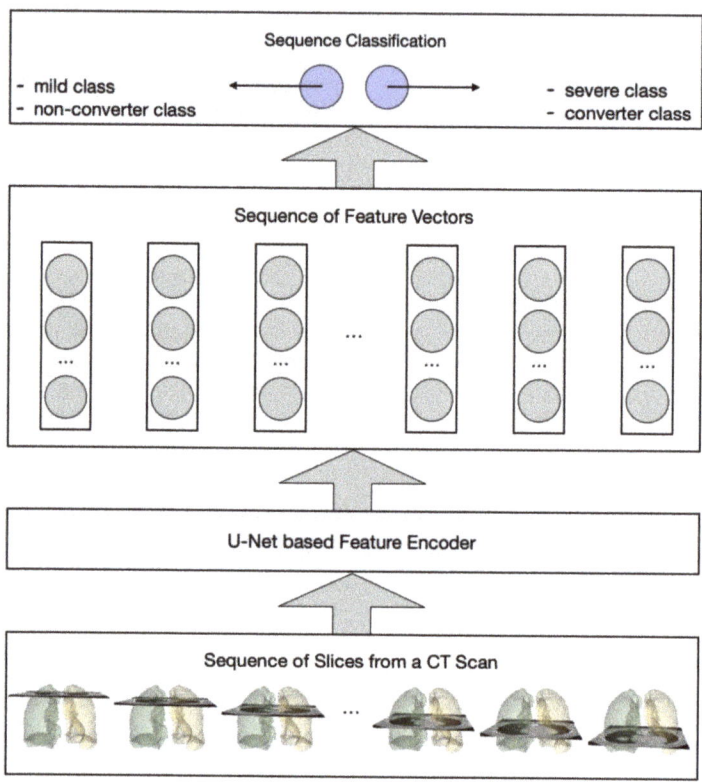

Figure 2. An overview of the proposed LesionEncoder framework.

3.1. Image Pre-Processing

All CT scans were pre-processed with intensity normalization, contrast limited adaptive histogram equalization, and gamma adjustment, using the same pre-processing pipeline as in our previous study [30]. We further performed lung segmentation on the CT slices using an established model—R231CovidWeb [31]. This model (The binary executable software for the lung segmentation model is available online (https://github.com/JoHof/lungmask (accessed on 11 February 2021))) was trained on a large and diverse dataset of non-COVID-19 CT scans and further fine-tuned with an additional COVID-19 dataset [32]. The CT slices with less than 3 mm^2 lung tissue were removed from our datasets, since they bear little or no information of the lung.

3.2. Lesion Encoder

The U-Net architecture [33] is adopted for the lesion encoder module. It consists of an encoder and a decoder, where the encoder captures the lesion features and the decoder maps lesion features back to the original image space. In other words, the encoder is responsible for extracting features from the input images (i.e., CT slices), whereas the decoder generates the segmentation maps (i.e., lesion masks). Figure 3 illustrates the encoder-decoder architecture of the lesion encoder module.

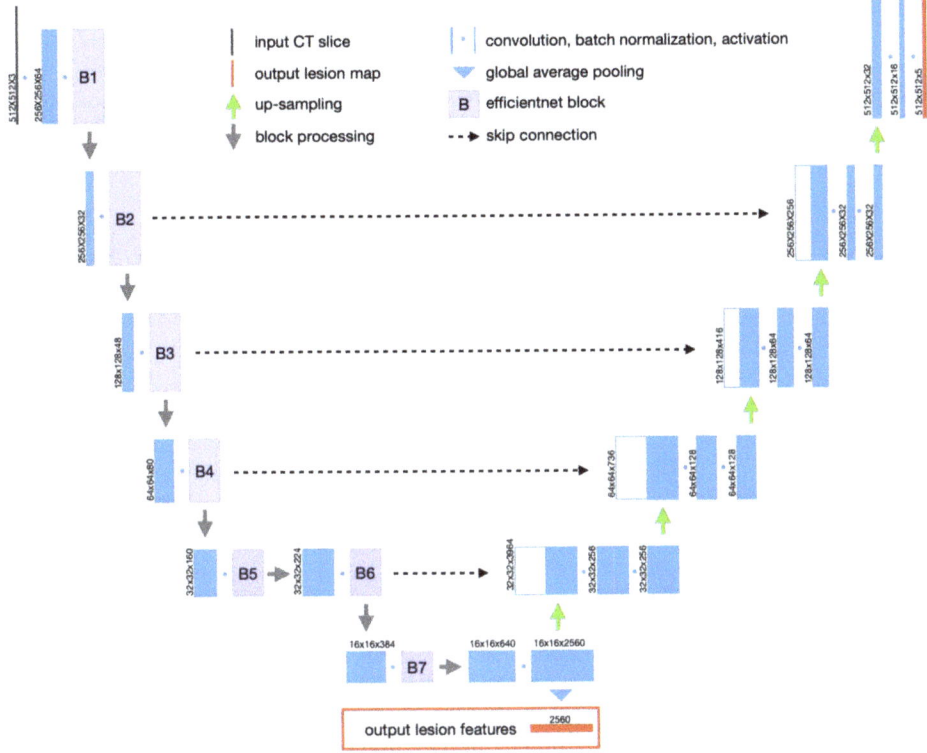

Figure 3. The U-Net architecture for lesion detection and feature encoding.

We used the EfficientNetB7 model [34] as the backbone to build the lesion encoder module, as it represents the state-of-the-art in object detection while being 8.4 times smaller and 6.1 times faster on inference than the best existing models in the ImageNet Challenge [35]. The ImageNet pre-trained weights were used to initialize the EfficientNetB7 model. There are 7 blocks in the EfficientNetB7 model, as shown in Figure 3. The skip connections were built between the expand activation layers in Blocks 2, 3, 4, and 6 and their corresponding up-sampling layers in our model. The output of the bottom layer is the final output feature vector representing the lesion features of the input slice.

A publicly available dataset was used to train the EfficientNetB7 U-Net, which consisted of 100 axial CT slices from 60 COVID-19 patients [32]. All the CT slices were annotated by an experienced radiologist with 3 different lesion classes, including GGO, consolidation, and pleural effusion. Since this dataset is very small, we applied different augmentations, including horizontal flip, affine transforms, perspective transforms, contrast manipulation, image blurring and sharpening, Gaussian noise, and random crops, to the dataset using the Albumentations library [36]. The model (The Tensorflow implementation of the EfficientNetB7 U-Net is available online (https://github.com/qubvel/segmentation_models (accessed on 11 February 2021))) was trained using Adam optimizer [37] with a learning rate of 0.0001 and 300 epochs.

The lesion encoder module was applied to process individual slices in a CT scan. For each CT slice, a high-dimensional feature vector (d = 2560) was derived. Independent component analysis (ICA) was performed on the training samples to reduce dimensionality (d = 64). The ICA model was then applied to the test samples, so that they have the same feature dimension as the training samples. The output of the lesion encoder is a sequence of feature vectors, which are then classified using a sequence classifier, as explained in the next section.

3.3. Sequence Classification

A RNN model was built for sequence classification. Its input is a sequence of feature vectors generated by the lesion encoder. The structure of the RNN model is illustrated in Table 3—two bidirectional long short-term memory (LSTM) layers, followed by a dense layer with a dropout rate of 0.5, and an output dense layer. For comparison purposes, another pooling model was created (Table 3)—using max pooling and average pooling to combine the slice-based feature vectors, as inspired by a previous study [9]. The difference between these two models is that the RNN model captures the relationship between feature vectors in a sequence, whereas the pooling model ignores such relationships.

Table 3. The architectures of the RNN model and the pooling model.

RNN Model	Pooling Model	
BiLSTM (64, return-sequences)	Global_Max_Pooling	Global_Average_Pooling
BiLSTM (32)	Concatenation	
Dense (64, ReLu, dropout = 0.5)	Dense (64, ReLu, dropout = 0.5)	
Dense (1, Sigmoid)	Dense (1, Sigmoid)	

Adam optimizer [37] with a learning rate of 0.001 was used for training the models in 100 epochs. A validation set (20%) was split from the training set for monitoring the training process. Every 20 epochs, the validation set was reselected from the training set, so that the model will be internally validated by all training samples during training. To address the imbalanced distribution in the datasets, we assigned different weights to the two classes (mild/non-converter class: 0.2, severe/converter class: 1.8) when training the models. In addition, if a patient has multiple CT scans, the scan with a higher probability of a positive prediction overrules the others when applying the models for inference.

3.4. Performance Evaluation

We tested the LesionEncoder framework with two configurations: (1) Using the pooling model as the classifier (LE_Pooling) and (2) using the RNN model as the classifier (LE_RNN). These methods were compared to 3 baseline methods. The first baseline method (BS_Volumetric) was inspired by a previous study [20], which was based on a Logistic Regression model using 4 lesion volumetric features as input: GGO percentage, consolidation percentage, pleural effusion percentage, and total lesion percentage. The second (BS_Pooling) and third (BS_RNN) baseline methods were based on the same classification models as in LE_Pooling and LE_RNN; however, the features were extracted from an EfficientNetB7 model without a lesion encoder module. The purpose of the second and third baseline models was to estimate the contribution of the lesion encoder. Following previous studies [38,39], sensitivity, specificity, accuracy, and area under curve (AUC) were used to evaluate the methods' performance. Receiver operating characteristic (ROC) curves were also compared between methods.

3.5. Development Environment

All the neural network models, including the EfficientNetB7 U-Net, the Pooling model and the RNN model, were implemented in Python (v3.6.9) and Tensorflow (v2.0.0). The models were trained using a Fujitsu server with Intel Xeon Gold 5218 GPU, 128 G memory, and NVidia V100 32 G GPU. The same server was used for image pre-processing, feature extraction, and classification.

4. Results

4.1. Lung and Lesion Segmentation

The lung masks generated using the R231CovidWeb model [31] and the lesion masks generated by the lesion encoder module were visually inspected by an experienced image analyst (S.L.). Overall, the lung segmentation results were visually reliable with few severe and critical cases having infection areas missed out in their lung masks. The lesion encoder achieved a Dice of 0.92 on the COVID-19 CT segmentation dataset [32]. Figure 4 presents four examples of the lung and lesion segmentation results (reconstructed using 3D Slicer (v4.6.2) [40]) of the COVID-19 patients, one for each severity class. It shows that higher severity of COVID-19 is reflected in CT scans as increasing number and volume of lesions.

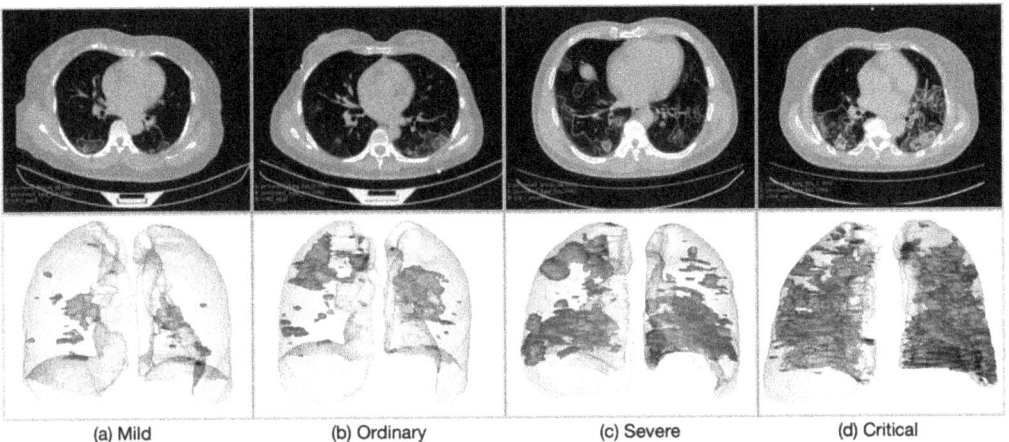

(a) Mild   (b) Ordinary   (c) Severe   (d) Critical

Figure 4. Examples of the patients in different severity groups: (**a**–**d**). The upper row presents the axial CT slices with the lung (red) and lesion (green: GGO; yellow: consolidation; brown: pleural effusion) boundaries overlaid on the CT slices. The lower row illustrates the 3D models of the lung and lesions.

4.2. Severity Assessment

Five different methods were compared in the automatic severity assessment of COVID-19 patients, including three baseline methods and two proposed methods, as described in Section 3.4. Table 4 illustrates the performance metrics of different methods on the severity assessment task, and Figure 5a shows the ROC curves of these methods. The three methods using lesion features (BS_Volumetric, LE_Pooling, and LE_RNN) consistently outperformed the models that did not use lesion features by a marked difference in sensitivity (>9.1%), specificity (>15.3%), accuracy (>14.7%), and AUC (>15.1%). In particular, BS_Volumetric achieved the highest AUC of 0.931, indicating that the lesion volumetric features were highly effective in distinguishing between severe and mild cases.

Table 4. Performance of different methods in baseline severity assessment. Bold font indicates best result in each performance metric achieved by the methods.

Method	Sensitivity	Specificity	Accuracy	AUC
BS_Volumetric	**0.818**	0.933	0.922	**0.931**
BS_Pooling	0.727	0.752	0.750	0.732
BS_RNN	0.727	0.771	0.767	0.749
LE_Pooling	**0.818**	0.924	0.914	0.900
LE_RNN	**0.818**	**0.952**	**0.940**	0.903

The proposed LE_RNN method achieved higher specificity (0.952) than the BS_Volumetric method (0.933), showing that the features captured by the lesion encoder might be useful in reducing the false positive rate compared with the volumetric features. When comparing the pooling models and RNN models, we found that the RNN models performed slightly better than the pooling models; and the impact of the sequence classifier on the classification performance was much lower than that of the lesion features.

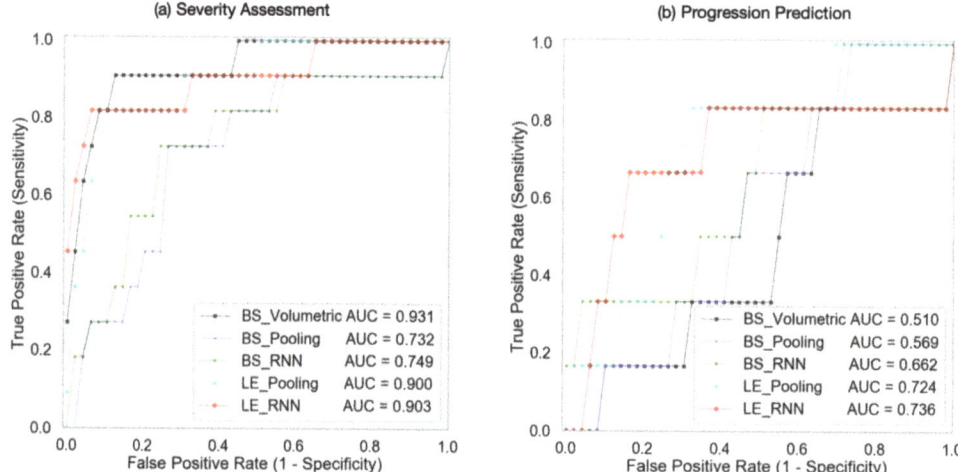

Figure 5. ROC curves of different models in (**a**,**b**).

4.3. Progression Prediction

The results of different methods in the prediction of disease progression task are presented in Table 5 and Figure 5b presents the ROC curves of these methods. The BS_Volumetric method performed poorly (sensitivity = 0.5, specificity = 0.465, accuracy = 0.467, AUC = 0.51), indicating that lesion volumetric features were not predictive of COVID-19 disease progression. This finding was not surprising, since the converter and non-converter cases both showed mild symptoms at baseline and presented a small quantity of lesions in the lungs. The BS_Pooling and BS_RNN methods achieved slightly better performance than BS_Volumetric, although they did not use any lesion features.

Table 5. Performance of different methods in prediction of disease progression. Bold font indicates best result in each performance metric achieved by the methods.

Method	Sensitivity	Specificity	Accuracy	AUC
BS_Volumetric	0.500	0.465	0.467	0.510
BS_Pooling	**0.667**	0.535	0.543	0.569
BS_RNN	**0.667**	0.535	0.543	0.662
LE_Pooling	**0.667**	0.737	0.733	0.724
LE_RNN	**0.667**	**0.838**	**0.829**	**0.736**

The LE_Pooling and LE_RNN methods outperformed the baseline methods with a substantial increase of 20–30% in specificity. LE_RNN was the best method in all the evaluation metrics (sensitivity = 0.667, specificity = 0.838, accuracy = 0.829, AUC = 0.736). The results indicate that the lesion features extracted by the lesion encoder may bear useful diagnostic information for predicting disease progression. However, it is still challenging to predict disease progression using the lesion features, and the low sensitivity (0.667) may restrict clinical applicability of the proposed methods.

5. Discussion

Clinical value in the management of COVID-19. The rapid spread of COVID-19 has put a strain on healthcare systems, necessitating efficient and automatic diagnosis and prognosis to facilitate the admission, triage, and referral of COVID-19 patients. Chest CT plays a key role in COVID-19 management by providing important diagnostic and prognostic information of patients. Several computational models have been developed to support automatic screening and diagnosis of COVID-19 [9–15]. There are also a few studies [19,20] using CT to quantify infection severity with a focus on development of lesion segmentation models. A few measures based on the lesion volumes have been proposed to quantify infection severity [19]; however, the intricate patterns of the lesion shape, texture, location, extent, and distribution were less investigated.

To capture the complex features in the lesions, we proposed a novel LesionEncoder framework. Two specific applications of this framework (i.e., assessment of severity and prediction of disease progression for COVID-19 patients) were explored in this study. To the best of our knowledge, this work represents the first attempt to predict COVID-19 patient disease progression using chest CT scans. Models built on this framework are able to take CT scans as input, detect, and extract features from the lesions, and quantify the severity or predict progression in a fully automated manner. The analysis of a high-resolution CT scan of $512 \times 12 \times 430$ voxels takes less than 1 min, which is substantially faster than radiologists' reading time. This can also save the burden of manual delineation of the lesions. The quantitative measures based on the features are of high clinical relevance, and can be used to support medical decision making or to track changes in patients.

We should note that this framework is not designed to analyze the COVID-19 suspects who are not confirmed by RT-PCR, or the covert/asymptomatic cases that are not documented [41–43]. The community-acquired pneumonia cases, such as viral pneumonia and interstitial lung disease patients, were also not considered in this study. As pointed out in a systematic review [44], normal controls and diseased controls will be needed for the development of screening or diagnostic models, thus the selection bias in the cohort may lead to a risk of overestimated performance. Since our model focuses on the confirmed and hospitalized COVID-19 cases; therefore, will not be exposed to such risk.

Models based on lesion features outperformed the baseline models without lesion features in both severity assessment and progression prediction. An interesting finding in severity assessment is that the lesion volumetric features are highly effective in distinguishing the severe cases from the mild cases. The features extracted by the lesion encoder did not improve the sensitivity of detecting the severe cases, but only reduced false positive predictions. This finding indicates that lesion volumetric features, such as GGO percentage and consolidation percentage, are prominent biomarkers in identifying the severe cases. The lesion encoder makes marginal contribution to severity assessment. In contrast, in progression prediction the models with the lesion encoder performed much better than those with volumetric features, indicating that the intricate pattern captured by the lesion encoder provide useful prognostic information for identifying the COVID-19 patients at higher risk of converting to the severe type. The LesionEncoder framework demonstrates a clinical applicability in COVID-19 management, particularly in the automatic severity assessment of COVID-19 patients (sensitivity = 0.818, specificity = 0.952, AUC = 0.931). However, it is still challenging to predict disease progression using lesion features, and the low sensitivity (0.667) may restrict clinical applicability of the proposed methods.

Technical contributions of the LesionEncoder framework. The technical contributions of this work are two-fold. Most importantly, this framework extends the use of lesion features beyond conventional lesion segmentation and volumetric analysis. There is a wealth of information in the lesions including shape, texture, location, extent, and distribution of involvement of the abnormality, that can be extracted by the lesion encoder. We demonstrated two novel applications of the lesion features in severity assessment and progression prediction. However, they also have a strong potential in a wide range of other clinical and research applications, such as supporting clinical decision making and providing insights of the pathological mechanism.

In addition, the proposed LesionEncoder framework attempts to address a common challenge in medical image analysis: how to reconcile local information and global information to improve medical image perception [45]. In this study, the slices from a CT scan were used as input for classification, but not every slice in the scan carries the same diagnostic/prognostic information. That is, the ground truth label of the entire scan cannot be propagated to label individual slices. For example, a CT slice with no lesion from a severe case might appear more 'normal' compared to a slice with some lesions from a mild case. Our proposed framework is a feasible approach to infer the holistic prediction with a focus on the analysis of region of interest. The RNN module in the framework is also a more sophisticated approach than the conventional feature fusion methods that use average pooling or max pooling to combine the local features. There are many analyses of the same nature, e.g., neuroradiologists may use features such as tumoral infiltration of surrounding tissues in MRI for tumor grading [46]; ophthalmologists may focus on lesions, such as hemorrhages and microaneurysms, hard exudates, and cotton-wool spots, when grading diabetic retinopathy [47]; and pathologists are more likely fixate on regions of highest diagnostic relevance when interpreting the biopsy whole slide images (WSI) [48]. The LesionEncoder framework may be generalizable to these lesion-focused medical image analyses.

Limitations. A limitation of this study is that we only had access to a retrospective cohort. Although it includes 639 CT scans of 346 patients, it is still a relatively small dataset compared to other datasets for development of deep learning models. It also refuted the idea of developing 3D deep learning models for scan-based classification. Since 3D models are usually more complicated than 2D models and have substantially more parameters, the small sample size will lead to undertrained models. In addition, there is a highly imbalanced distribution in the datasets. Among the 346 samples for the development of the severity assessment model, 324 (93.6%) patients were in the mild class. For the disease progression model, there are 300 (92.6%) patients in the non-converter class. Although this reflects the real distribution, it will be ideal to have more severe/converter class samples for training. To address this imbalance distribution problem, we used a class weighting strategy to give the positive class higher weight during training, and used a prediction weighting strategy during inference to enhance the prediction of the positive class if that patient has multiple scans. A larger sample size with more severe and converter cases in the datasets would help train more accurate and robust models as well as produce reliable performance estimates. Other techniques, such as synthetic minority oversampling [29], spherical coordinates transformation [49], and generative adversarial network [50], will be investigated in further study.

The lung masks generated using the R231CovidWeb model [31] and the lesion masks generated by the lesion encoder module were visually inspected by an experienced image analyst. The segmentation results were visually reliable, but the missed-out lung or lesion regions in the segmentation masks were noted in a few severe and critical cases. Since there were no lesion masks for our datasets, no quantitative analyses were performed to evaluate the automatic segmentation results. Further improvements can be made if the ground truth annotation of the lung and lesion can be provided to optimize the performance of the current lung segmentation model and lesion encoder module on our datasets.

Furthermore, it is still challenging for LesionEncoder alone to predict disease progression using lesion features. However, combining the proposed method with other biomarkers, such as short-time changes in neutrophil-to-lymphocyte ratio and urea-to-creatinine ratio [51] might further help stratify patients' severity.

There are a few recent studies that used explainable AI in chest CT segmentation and classification of COVID-19 patients, such as these based on class activation map [52], few-shot learning [53], and the shapely addictive explanations framework [29]. Another potential future extension of this work is to use explainable AI frameworks to explain the model's logics and decision-making processes, thereby unlocking the black box of deep learning and helping the end users to understand the models better.

6. Conclusions

In this study, a novel LesionEncoder framework was proposed to encode the enriched lesion features in chest CT scans for automatic severity assessment and progression prediction of COVID-19 patients. Models built on this framework outperformed the evaluated baseline models with a marked improvement. The lesion volumetric features were prominent biomarkers in identifying severe/critical cases, but intricate features captured by the lesion encoder were found effective in identifying the COVID-19 patients who have higher risks of converting to the severe or critical type. Overall, the LesionEncoder framework demonstrates a high clinical applicability in the current COVID-19 management, particularly in automatic severity assessment of COVID-19 patients.

An important future direction of this framework lies in the combination of clinical data and imaging data for better prediction performance, especially for the progression prediction, since clinical data may provide essential indicators of the clinical risks of the patients. Furthermore, the applications of the LesionEncoder framework to other types of lesion-focused analyses will be further investigated.

Author Contributions: The project was initially conceptualized and supervised by X.-R.C., X.-M.Q. and L.S. The patient data and imaging data were acquired by Y.-Z.F., Z.-Y.C. and D.R. The analysis methods were designed and implemented by S.L. and J.C.Q. The data were analyzed by S.L. and J.C.Q. The research findings were interpreted by P.-K.C., Q.-T.L., L.Q., X.-F.L., S.B. and E.C. All authors were involved in the design of the work. The manuscript was drafted by Y.-Z.F., S.L. and L.Q., and all authors have substantively revised it. All authors have read and agreed to the published version of the manuscript.

Funding: This project was funded by Natural Science Foundation of Guangdong Province (grant no. 2017A030313901), Guangzhou Science, Technology and Innovation Commission (grant no. 201804010239) and Foundation for Young Talents in Higher Education of Guangdong Province (grant no. 2019KQNCX005).

Institutional Review Board Statement: The study was conducted according to the guidelines of the Declaration of Helsinki, and approved by the Institutional Review Board of Xiang Yang Central Hospital and Huang Shi Central Hospital (approval number LL-2020-032-02, on 23 February 2020).

Informed Consent Statement: Informed consent was obtained from all subjects involved in the study.

Data Availability Statement: Not Applicable, the study does not report any data.

Acknowledgments: We acknowledge Fujitsu Australia Limited for providing the computational resources for this study. Special thanks to Eva Huang for proofreading this paper.

Conflicts of Interest: The authors have no conflict of interest nor any competing interest to declare.

Abbreviations

RNN—recurrent neural network; GGO—ground glass opacity; COS—core outcome set; LSTM—long short term memory; RT-PCR—reverse transcription polymerase chain reaction

References

1. Ji, Y.; Ma, Z.; Peppelenbosch, M.P.; Pan, Q. Potential association between COVID-19 mortality and health-care resource availability. *Lancet Glob. Health* **2020**, *8*, e480. [CrossRef]
2. Fang, Y.; Zhang, H.; Xie, J.; Lin, M.; Ying, L.; Pang, P.; Ji, W. Sensitivity of Chest CT for COVID-19: Comparison to RT-PCR. *Radiology* **2020**, *296*, E115–E117. [CrossRef]
3. Shi, H.; Han, X.; Jiang, N.; Cao, Y.; Alwalid, O.; Gu, J.; Fan, Y.; Zheng, C. Radiological findings from 81 patients with COVID-19 pneumonia in Wuhan, China: A descriptive study. *Lancet Infect. Dis.* **2020**, *20*, 425–434. [CrossRef]
4. Ng, M.-Y.; Lee, E.Y.; Yang, J.; Yang, F.; Li, X.; Wang, H.; Lui, M.M.-S.; Lo, C.S.-Y.; Leung, B.; Khong, P.-L.; et al. Imaging Profile of the COVID-19 Infection: Radiologic Findings and Literature Review. *Radiol. Cardiothorac. Imaging* **2020**, *2*, e200034. [CrossRef]
5. Ai, T.; Yang, Z.; Hou, H.; Zhan, C.; Chen, C.; Lv, W.; Tao, Q.; Sun, Z.; Xia, L. Correlation of chest CT and PT-PCR testing in coronavirus disease 2019 (COVID-19) in China: A report of 1014 cases. *Radiology* **2020**, *296*, E32E40. [CrossRef]
6. Huang, C.; Wang, Y.; Li, X.; Ren, L.; Zhao, J.; Hu, Y.; Zhang, L.; Fan, G.; Xu, J.; Gu, X.; et al. Clinical features of patients infected with 2019 novel coronavirus in Wuhan, China. *Lancet* **2020**, *395*, 497–506. [CrossRef]
7. Inui, S.; Fujikawa, A.; Jitsu, M.; Kunishima, N.; Watanabe, S.; Suzuki, Y.; Umeda, S.; Uwabe, Y. Chest CT Findings in Cases from the Cruise Ship "Diamond Princess" with Coronavirus Disease 2019 (COVID-19). *Radiol. Cardiothorac. Imaging* **2020**, *2*, e200110. [CrossRef]

8. The Royal Australian and New Zealand Colleague of Radiologists. Advice on Appropriate Use of CT Throughout the COVID-19 Pandemic. 2020. Available online: https://www.ranzcr.com/college/document-library/advice-on-appropriate-use-of-ct-throughout-the-covid-19-pandemic (accessed on 9 April 2020).
9. Li, L.; Qin, L.; Xu, Z.; Yin, Y.; Wang, X.; Kong, B.; Bai, J.; Lu, Y.; Fang, Z.; Song, Q.; et al. Artificial intelligence distinguishes COVID-19 from community acquired pneumonia on chest CT. *Radiology* **2020**, *296*, E65–E71. [CrossRef]
10. Song, Y.; Zheng, S.; Li, L.; Zhang, X.; Zhang, X.; Huang, Z.; Chen, J.; Wang, R.; Zhao, H.; Zha, Y.; et al. Deep learning Enables Accurate Diagnosis of Novel Coronavirus (COVID-19) with CT images. *medRxiv* **2020**, arXiv:2020.02.23.20026930. [CrossRef]
11. Gozes, O.; Frid-Adar, M.; Greenspan, H.; Browning, P.D.; Zhang, H.; Ji, W.; Bernheim, A.; Siegel, E. Rapid AI Development Cycle for the Coronavirus (COVID-19) Pandemic: Initial Results for Automated Detection & Patient Monitoring using Deep Learning CT Image Analysis. *arXiv* **2020**, arXiv:2003.05037.
12. Xu, X.; Jiang, X.; Ma, C.; Du, P.; Li, X.; Lv, S.; Yu, L.; Ni, Q.; Chen, Y.; Su, J.; et al. Deep Learning System to Screen Coronavirus Disease 2019 Pneumonia. *arXiv* **2020**, arXiv:2002.09334. [CrossRef]
13. Wang, S.; Kang, B.; Ma, J.; Zeng, X.; Xiao, M.; Guo, J.; Cai, M.; Yang, J.; Li, Y.; Meng, X.; et al. A deep learning algorithm using CT images to screen for Corona Virus Disease (COVID-19). *Eur. Radiol.* **2021**, *31*, 6096–6104. [CrossRef]
14. Chen, J.; Wu, L.; Zhang, J.; Zhang, L.; Gong, D.; Zhao, Y.; Chen, Q.; Huang, S.; Yang, M.; Yang, X.; et al. Deep learning-based model for detecting 2019 novel coronavirus pneumonia on high-resolution computed tomography: A prospective study. *medRxiv* **2020**, arXiv:2020.02.25.20021568.
15. Wang, L.; Wong, A. COVID-Net: A tailored deep convolutional neural network design for detection of COVID-19 cases from chest radiography images. *arXiv* **2020**, arXiv:2003.09871v1. [CrossRef] [PubMed]
16. Shi, F.; Wang, J.; Shi, J.; Wu, Z.; Wang, Q.; Tang, Z.; He, K.; Shi, Y.; Shen, D. Review of Artificial Intelligence Techniques in Imaging Data Acquisition, Segmentation, and Diagnosis for COVID-19. *IEEE Rev. Biomed. Eng.* **2021**, *14*, 4–15. [CrossRef]
17. Yuan, M.; Yin, W.; Tao, Z.; Tan, W.; Hu, Y. Association of radiologic findings with mortality of patients infected with 2019 novel coronavirus in Wuhan, China. *PLoS ONE* **2020**, *15*, e0230548. [CrossRef]
18. Qi, X.; Jiang, Z.; Yu, Q.; Shao, C.; Zhang, H.; Yue, H.; Ma, B.; Wang, Y.; Liu, C.; Meng, X.; et al. Machine learning-based CT radiomics model for predicting hospital stay in patients with pneumonia associated with SARS-CoV-2 infection: A multicenter study. *medRxiv* **2020**. [CrossRef]
19. Shan, F.; Gao, Y.; Wang, J.; Shi, W.; Shi, N.; Han, M.; Xue, Z.; Shen, D.; Shi, Y. Lung Infection Quantification of COVID-19 in CT Images with Deep Learning. *arXiv* **2020**, arXiv:2003.04655.
20. Chaganti, S.; Balachandran, A.; Chabin, G.; Cohen, S.; Flohr, T.; Georgescu, B.; Grenier, P.; Grbic, S.; Liu, S.; Mellot, F.; et al. Quantification of tomographic patterns associated with COVID-19 from chest CT. *arXiv* **2020**, arXiv:2004.01279.
21. Jin, X.; Pang, B.; Zhang, J.; Liu, Q.; Yang, Z.; Feng, J.; Liu, X.; Zhang, L.; Wang, B.; Huang, Y.; et al. Core outcome set for clinical trials on coronavirus disease 2019 (COS-COVID). *Engineering* **2020**, *6*, 1147–1152. [CrossRef]
22. Cascella, M.; Rajnik, M.; Cuomo, A.; Scott, C. *Features, Evaluation and Treatment Coronavirus (COVID-19)*; StatPearls: Treasure Island, FL, USA, 2020. Available online: https://www.ncbi.nlm.nih.gov/books/NBK554776/ (accessed on 2 September 2020).
23. Jian, A.; Jang, K.; Maurizio, M.; Liu, S.; Magnussen, J.; di Ieva, A. Machine learning for the prediction of molecular markers in glioma on magnetic resonance imaging: A systematic review and meta-analysis. *Neurosurgery* **2021**, *89*, 1. [CrossRef]
24. Gao, Y.; Xiao, X.; Han, B.; Li, G.; Ning, X.; Wang, D.; Cai, W.; Kikinis, R.; Berkovsky, S.; Di Ieva, A.; et al. Deep learning methodology for differentiating glioma recurrence from radiation necrosis using magnetic resonance imaging: Algorithm development and validation. *JMRI Med. Info.* **2020**, *8*, e19805. [CrossRef] [PubMed]
25. Zhang, C.; Song, Y.; Liu, S.; Lill, S.; Wang, C.; Tang, Z.; You, Y.; Gao, Y.; Klistorner, A.; Barnett, M.; et al. MS-GAN: GAN-based semantic segmentation of multiple sclerosis lesions in brain magnetic resonance imaging. In Proceedings of the 2018 Digital Image Computing: Techniques and Applications (DICTA), Canberra, ACT, Australia, 10–13 December 2018; pp. 1–8. [CrossRef]
26. Liu, S.; Cai, W.; Wen, L.; Feng, D.; Pujol, S.; Kikinis, R.; Fulham, M.; Eberl, S. Multi-channel neurodegenerative pattern analysis and its application in Alzheimer's disease characterization. *Comput. Med. Imaging Graph.* **2014**, *38*, 6–436. [CrossRef] [PubMed]
27. Zhang, F.; Song, Y.; Cai, W.; Liu, S.; Liu, S.; Pujol, S.; Kikinis, R.; Xia, Y.; Fulham, M.; Feng, D. Pairwise latent semantic association for similarity computation in medical imaging. *IEEE Trans. Biomed. Eng.* **2016**, *63*, 5. [CrossRef] [PubMed]
28. Liu, S.; Graham, S.L.; Schulz, A.; Kalloniatis, M.; Zangerl, B.; Cai, W.; Gao, Y.; Chua, B.; Arvind, H.; Grigg, J.; et al. A deep learning-based algorithm identifies glaucomatous discs using monoscopic fundus photographs. *Ophthal. Glaucoma* **2018**, *1*, 15–22. [CrossRef]
29. Quiroz, J.C.; Feng, Y.-Z.; Cheng, Z.-Y.; Rezazadegan, D.; Chen, P.-K.; Lin, Q.-T.; Qian, L.; Liu, X.-F.; Berkovsky, S.; Coiera, E.; et al. Development and Validation of a Machine Learning Approach for Automated Severity Assessment of COVID-19 Based on Clinical and Imaging Data: Retrospective Study. *JMIR Med. Inform.* **2021**, *9*, e24572. [CrossRef]
30. Liu, S.; Shah, Z.; Sav, A.; Russo, C.; Berkovsky, S.; Qian, Y.; Coiera, E.; Di Ieva, A. Isocitrate dehydrogenase (IDH) status prediction in histopathology images of gliomas using deep learning. *Sci. Rep.* **2020**, *10*, 7733. [CrossRef] [PubMed]
31. Hofmanninger, J.; Prayer, F.; Pan, J.; Rohrich, S.; Prosch, H.; Langs, G. Automatic lung segmentation in routine imaging is a data diversity problem, not a methodology problem. *arXiv* **2020**, arXiv:2001.11767v1. [CrossRef]
32. COVID-19 CT Segmentation Dataset. Available online: http://medicalsegmentation.com/covid19/ (accessed on 1 April 2020).
33. Ronneberger, O.; Fischer, P.; Brox, T. U-Net: Convolutional networks for biomedical image segmentation. *arXiv* **2015**, arXiv:1505.04597.

34. Tan, M.; Le, Q.V. Efficientnet: Rethinking model scaling for convolutional neural networks. *arXiv* **2019**, arXiv:1905.11946v3.
35. Deng, J.; Dong, W.; Socher, R.; Li, L.J.; Li, K.; Li, F.F. Imagenet: A large-scale hierarchical image database. In Proceedings of the 2009 IEEE Conference on Computer Vision and Pattern Recognition, Miami, FL, USA, 20–25 June 2009; pp. 248–255.
36. Buslaev, A.; Iglovikov, V.I.; Khvedchenya, E.; Parinov, A.; Druzhinin, M.; Kalinin, A.A. Albumentations: Fast and Flexible Image Augmentations. *Information* **2020**, *11*, 125. [CrossRef]
37. Kingma, D.P.; Ba, J. Adam: A method for stochastic optimization. *arXiv* **2014**, arXiv:1412.6980.
38. Do, D.T.; Le, N.Q.K. Using extreme gradient boosting to identify origin of replication in Saccharomyces cerevisiae via hybrid features. *Genomics* **2020**, *112*, 2445–2451. [CrossRef] [PubMed]
39. Le, N.Q.K.; Kha, Q.H.; Nguyen, V.H.; Chen, Y.-C.; Cheng, S.-J.; Chen, C.-Y. Machine Learning-Based Radiomics Signatures for EGFR and KRAS Mutations Prediction in Non-Small-Cell Lung Cancer. *Int. J. Mol. Sci.* **2021**, *22*, 9254. [CrossRef] [PubMed]
40. Fedorov, A.; Beichel, R.; Kalpathy-Cramer, J.; Finet, J.; Fillion-Robin, J.-C.; Pujol, S.; Bauer, C.; Jennings, D.; Fennessy, F.; Sonka, M.; et al. 3D Slicer as an image computing platform for the Quantitative Imaging Network. *Magn. Reson. Imaging* **2012**, *30*, 1323–1341. [CrossRef] [PubMed]
41. Nishiura, H.; Kobayashi, T.; Miyama, T.; Suzuki, A.; Jung, S.-M.; Hayashi, K.; Kinoshita, R.; Yang, Y.; Yuan, B.; Akhmetzhanov, A.R.; et al. Estimation of the asymptomatic ratio of novel coronavirus infections (COVID-19). *Int. J. Infect. Dis.* **2020**, *94*, 154–155. [CrossRef]
42. Li, R.; Pei, S.; Chen, B.; Song, Y.; Zhang, T.; Yang, W.; Shaman, J. Substantial undocumented infection facilitates the rapid dissemination of novel coronavirus (SARS-CoV2). *Science* **2020**, *368*, 489–493. [CrossRef] [PubMed]
43. Qiu, J. Covert coronavirus infections could be seeding new outbreaks. *Nature* **2020**. [CrossRef] [PubMed]
44. Wynants, L.; van Calster, B.; Collins, G.S.; Riley, R.D.; Heinze, G.; Schuit, E.; Bonten, M.M.J.; Dahly, D.L.; Damen, J.A.; Debray, T.P.A.; et al. Systematic review and critical appraisal of prediction models for diagnosis and prognosis of COVID-19 infection. *BMJ* **2020**, *369*, m1328. [CrossRef] [PubMed]
45. Krupinski, E.A. Medical image perception: Evaluating the role of experience. *Proc. SPIE* **2000**, *3959*, 281–289. [CrossRef]
46. Castillo, M. History and Evolution of Brain Tumor Imaging: Insights through Radiology. *Radiology* **2014**, *273*, S111–S125. [CrossRef]
47. Nayak, J.; Bhat, P.S.; Acharya, R.; Lim, C.M.; Kagathi, M. Automated Identification of Diabetic Retinopathy Stages Using Digital Fundus Images. *J. Med. Syst.* **2007**, *32*, 107–115. [CrossRef] [PubMed]
48. Brunye, T.; Carney, P.A.; Allison, K.H.; Shapiro, L.G.; Weaver, D.L.; Elmore, J.G. Eye Movements as an Index of Pathologist Visual Expertise: A Pilot Study. *PLoS ONE* **2014**, *9*, e103447. [CrossRef]
49. Russo, C.; Liu, S.; Di Ieva, A. Spherical coordinates transformation pre-processing in Deep Convolution Neural Networks for brain tumor segmentation in MRI. *arXiv* **2020**, arXiv:2008.07090. [CrossRef] [PubMed]
50. Jose, L.; Liu, S.; Russo, C.; Nadort, A.; Di Ieva, A. Generative adversarial networks in digital pathology and histopathological image processing: A review. *J. Pathol. Inform.* **2021**, *12*, 43. [CrossRef]
51. Solimando, A.G.; Susca, N.; Borrelli, P.; Prete, M.; Lauletta, G.; Pappagallo, F.; Buono, R.; Inglese, G.; Forina, B.M.; Bochicchio, D.; et al. Short-Term Variations in Neutrophil-to-Lymphocyte and Urea-to-Creatinine Ratios Anticipate Intensive Care Unit Admission of COVID-19 Patients in the Emergency Department. *Front. Med.* **2021**, *7*, 625176. [CrossRef]
52. Ye, Q.; Xia, J.; Yang, G. Explainable AI for COVID-19 CT Classifiers: An Initial Comparison Study. In Proceedings of the 2021 IEEE 34th International Symposium on Computer-Based Medical Systems (CBMS), Aveiro, Portugal, 7–9 June 2021; pp. 521–526. [CrossRef]
53. Voulodimos, A.; Protopapadakis, E.; Katsamenis, I.; Doulamis, A.; Doulamis, N. A Few-Shot U-Net Deep Learning Model for COVID-19 Infected Area Segmentation in CT Images. *Sensors* **2021**, *21*, 2215. [CrossRef]

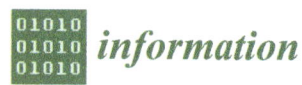 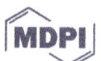

Article

Early Stage Identification of COVID-19 Patients in Mexico Using Machine Learning: A Case Study for the Tijuana General Hospital

Cristián Castillo-Olea [1,*], Roberto Conte-Galván [1], Clemente Zuñiga [2], Alexandra Siono [3], Angelica Huerta [4], Ornela Bardhi [5] and Eric Ortiz [6]

1. Ensenada Center for Scientifc Research and Higher Education, Ensenada 22860, Mexico; conte@cicese.mx
2. Tijuana General Hospital, Tijuana 22000, Mexico; drclementezuniga@gmail.com
3. Faculty of Engineering, CETYS University, Mexicali 21259, Mexico; alexandra.siono@cetys.edu.mx
4. Faculty of Medicine and Psychology, Autonomous University of Baja California, Mexicali 21100, Mexico; angelica.huerta.d@gmail.com
5. Independent Researcher, 1001 Tirana, Albania; alenroidhrab@gmail.com
6. comeMed Teleconsulting, Colonia Roma, Mexico City 6700, Mexico; dr.ericortiz.oncomed@gmail.com
* Correspondence: cristian.castillo2@gmail.com; Tel.: +52-5574302237

Citation: Castillo-Olea, C.; Conte-Galván, R.; Zuñiga, C.; Siono, A.; Huerta, A.; Bardhi, O.; Ortiz, E. Early Stage Identification of COVID-19 Patients in Mexico Using Machine Learning: A Case Study for the Tijuana General Hospital. *Information* 2021, 12, 490. https://doi.org/10.3390/info12120490

Academic Editors: Sidong Liu, Cristián Castillo Olea and Shlomo Berkovsky

Received: 13 October 2021
Accepted: 22 November 2021
Published: 24 November 2021

Publisher's Note: MDPI stays neutral with regard to jurisdictional claims in published maps and institutional affiliations.

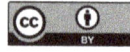

Copyright: © 2021 by the authors. Licensee MDPI, Basel, Switzerland. This article is an open access article distributed under the terms and conditions of the Creative Commons Attribution (CC BY) license (https:// creativecommons.org/licenses/by/ 4.0/).

Abstract: Background: The current pandemic caused by SARS-CoV-2 is an acute illness of global concern. SARS-CoV-2 is an infectious disease caused by a recently discovered coronavirus. Most people who get sick from COVID-19 experience either mild, moderate, or severe symptoms. In order to help make quick decisions regarding treatment and isolation needs, it is useful to determine which significant variables indicate infection cases in the population served by the Tijuana General Hospital (Hospital General de Tijuana). An Artificial Intelligence (Machine Learning) mathematical model was developed in order to identify early-stage significant variables in COVID-19 patients. Methods: The individual characteristics of the study subjects included age, gender, age group, symptoms, comorbidities, diagnosis, and outcomes. A mathematical model that uses supervised learning algorithms, allowing the identification of the significant variables that predict the diagnosis of COVID-19 with high precision, was developed. Results: Automatic algorithms were used to analyze the data: for Systolic Arterial Hypertension (SAH), the Logistic Regression algorithm showed results of 91.0% in area under ROC (AUC), 80% accuracy (CA), 80% F1 and 80% Recall, and 80.1% precision for the selected variables, while for Diabetes Mellitus (DM) with the Logistic Regression algorithm it obtained 91.2% AUC, 89.2% accuracy, 88.8% F1, 89.7% precision, and 89.2% recall for the selected variables. The neural network algorithm showed better results for patients with Obesity, obtaining 83.4% AUC, 91.4% accuracy, 89.9% F1, 90.6% precision, and 91.4% recall. Conclusions: Statistical analyses revealed that the significant predictive symptoms in patients with SAH, DM, and Obesity were more substantial in fatigue and myalgias/arthralgias. In contrast, the third dominant symptom in people with SAH and DM was odynophagia.

Keywords: machine learning; COVID-19; identification

1. Introduction

A novel coronavirus, known as Severe Acute Respiratory Syndrome (SARS-CoV-2), was identified in December 2019 as the cause of a respiratory illness called Coronavirus Disease 2019, or COVID-19 [1]. The origin of this virus is not yet confirmed, but an analysis of its genetic sequence suggests it is phylogenetically related to bat viruses similar to SARS (severe acute respiratory syndrome), making bats a possible key reservoir [2]. Symptoms of COVID-19 infection appear after an incubation period of approximately 5.2 days [3]. The period from the onset of COVID-19 symptoms to death ranges from 6 to 41 days with a median of 14 days [4]. This period depends largely on the age and the state of the patient's immune system [4].

The infection is transmitted through droplets generated by symptomatic patients when coughing or sneezing, but it can also occur through asymptomatic patients and even before the onset of symptoms [5].

The clinical features of COVID-19 are diverse, from an asymptomatic state to acute respiratory distress syndrome and multiorgan failure [5]. The most common early symptoms of COVID-19 illness are fever, cough, and fatigue, while other symptoms include headache, sputum production, hemoptysis, dyspnea, diarrhea, and lymphopenia [6]. Advanced age, cardiovascular disease, diabetes, chronic respiratory disease, hypertension, and cancer are said to increase the risk of death for people diagnosed with COVID-19.

Regarding COVID-19, as of 15 August 2021, there were 207,784,507 confirmed cases (410,464 new cases) and 4,370,424 deaths, while 4,462,336,040 vaccine doses have been reported worldwide [7,8]. Most estimates of fatality ratios have been based on cases detected through surveillance and calculated using crude methods, giving rise to widely variable estimates of CFR depending on the country—from less than 0.1% to over 25% [9].

Currently, in Mexico (August 2021), there are 3,310,989 estimated positives, with 261,384 estimated deaths, and 133,866 estimated actives. However, there are 3,108,438 confirmed cases, 5,527,343 negative, 477,811 suspected and 248,652 accumulated deaths. Of the confirmed cases, 53.56% have been women and 46.44% men. A total 5.6% of patients have been hospitalized, and 94.4% have been outpatients. Among the main comorbidities are hypertension (10.34%), Obesity (8.989%), diabetes (7.31%) and smoking (8.03%), with information updated on 16 August 2021. On the same date, the state of Baja California had 913 active cases, with 54,453 accumulated cases, and 8979 deaths. The state's capital, Mexicali, is the city with the highest number of cases in the state, with 21,778 accumulated cases, followed by Tijuana, our case study [10].

2. Background

Several authors have addressed the issue of SARS-CoV-2 from a technological point of view, with the development of artificial intelligence algorithms. There are models to predict the mortality rate [11]. Some studies present the detection of severely ill patients with COVID-19 from those with mild symptoms using clinical information and data from blood and urine tests [12]. Several artificial intelligence models have been used with Machine Learning and Deep Learning methods which have been used intensively for COVID-19. Although Machine Learning and Deep Learning methods show successful results in the COVID-19 cases tested, there are accounting challenges that can be considered to improve the quality of the research in that direction [13].

Table 1 summarizes the articles included in this minireview, together with some characteristics of these studies.

Table 1. Minireview of papers.

Authors.	Year	Objective	Learners	Metrics	Novelties
Li WT et al. [14].	2020	Classification	XGBoost	sensitivity of 92.5% and a specificity of 97.9%	Novel associations between clinical variables, including correlations between being male and having higher levels of serum lymphocytes and neutrophils. We found that COVID-19 patients could be clustered into subtypes based on serum levels of immune cells, gender, and reported symptoms.
Guan X et al. [15]	2020	Prediction	XGBoost	>90% precision and >85% sensitivity, as well as F1 scores >0.90	Proposed disease severity, age, serum levels of hs-CRP, LDH, ferritin, and IL-10 as significant predictors for death risk of COVID-19, which may help to identify the high-risk COVID-19 cases.

Table 1. *Cont.*

Authors.	Year	Objective	Learners	Metrics	Novelties
Delafiori J et al. [16]	2021	Diagnosis and risk assesment	gradient tree boosting (GDB) ADA tree boosting	96.0% of specificity and 83.1% of sensitivity 80.3% of specificity and 85.4% of sensitivity	Propose machine learning techniques to determine from databases the five main challenges in responding COVID-19 and how to overcome these challenges to save lives.
Allam M et al. [17]	2020	Diagnosis and prediction	Neural Networks	100% sensitivity and 99.9% specificity	The Abbott antibody test (SARS-CoV-2 IgG assay) has shown 100% sensitivity and 99.9% specificity thus far. The Abbott test finds whether the patient has IgG antibodies for COVID-19, which can stay for months to years after a person has recovered.
Assaf D et al. [18]	2020	Prediction	Classification and Regression Tree (CRT) model	Sensitivity, specificity, PPV, NPV and accuracy of 88.0%, 92.7%, 68.8%, 97.7% and 92.0%, respectively, with ROC AUC of 0.90.	The analysis of the database in this study found that most contributory variables to the models were APACHE II score, white blood cell count, time from symptoms to admission, oxygen saturation and blood lymphocytes count. Machine-learning models demonstrated high efficacy in predicting critical COVID-19 compared to the most efficacious tools available.
Naseem M et al. [19]	2020	Detection	Neural Networks	sensitivity of 90% and specificity of 96% respectively	Results were synthesized and reported under 4 themes. (a) The need of AI during this pandemic: AI can assist to increase the speed and accuracy of identification of cases and through data mining to deal with the health crisis efficiently, (b) Utility of AI in COVID-19 screening, contact tracing, and diagnosis: Efficacy for virus detection can a be increased by deploying the smart city data network using terminal tracking system along-with prediction of future outbreaks, (c) Use of AI in COVID-19 patient monitoring and drug development:
Arga KY [20]	2020	Prediction and diagnosis	Apache, Gleason and PASI	-	Machine learning is considered to help reduce diagnostic errors and unnecessary use of diagnostic tools through the development of rational algorithms. Indeed, the COVID-19 pandemic showed that digital health is invaluable, feasible, and not too far.
Majhi R et al. [21]	2020	Prediction	Nonlinear Regression (NLR), Decision Tree (DT) based regression, and random forest (RF) models	Evaluation metrics obtained using the Mean Absolute Percentage Error (MAPE). NLR = 0.24% DT = 0.18% RF = 0.02%	The algorithm predict the number of positive cases in India. In essence, the paper proposes a machine learning model that can predict the number of cases well in advance very effectively and also suggest some key inputs.

Table 1. Cont.

Authors.	Year	Objective	Learners	Metrics	Novelties
van der Schaar M et al. [22]	2020	Prediction	-	.	This paper summarizes the use of machine learning techniques in different studies to manage limited healthcare results, developing personalized treatment, informing policies and able effective collaboration and expediting clinical trials.
Das AK et al. [23]	2020	Prediction	Linear Regression	For liner regression (area under ROC curve = 0.830), calibration (Matthews Correlation Coefficient = 0.433; Brier Score = 0.036).	In this study, according to the random forest algorithm, age was the most important predictor followed by exposure, sex and province, whereas this order was sex, age, province and exposure as per logistic regression
Swapnarekha H et al. [24]	2020	Prognosis	Support Vector Machine (SVM), Rannom Forest RF, K-Means, XGBoost and linear regression	0.933 true positive rate, 0.74 true negative rate and 0.875 accuracy.	This article obtained good metrics for COVID-19 prediction. On the other hand, mentioned machined learning techniques used for classification and prediction to reduce the spread of coronavirus and understand the limitation of machine learning analysis, being: lack of information, accuracy of predictions, usage of advanced approaches, providing feasible solutions for developing countries and necessity of advance intelligent systems on symptom based identification of COVID-19.

3. Materials and Methods

This article is based on a study of COVID-19 patients at the Tijuana General Hospital, a public hospital that serves a very particular low-income population. Tijuana is a border city in northern Mexico next to San Diego, California, in the United States. Including neighboring Rosarito, the greater Tijuana region has a population of around 1,900,000 inhabitants, the majority Mexican nationals. However, there are also many migrants from other Central American, South American, and Caribbean countries living in unaccounted shantytowns, seeking to enter the United States in any way, either legal or illegally. While doing so, they temporarily live in Tijuana without a permanent job, a fixed salary, a steady place of work, or a regular postal address, and therefore, do not have access to social security or health services, and eventually fall ill, often due to a myriad of causes. The range of pathologies and diseases found in the city of Tijuana is much broader than those found in other cities with more homogeneous or steady populations, which further complicates medical and healthcare services for this specific segment of people. Tijuana General Hospital is one of the few public health institutions that serve this marginalized segment of the Tijuana population, hence the size and complexity of the challenges faced by its medical staff every day, as well as the diversity of pathologies met by the health professionals who treat them. In this article, we evaluate a group of COVID-19-diagnosed patients, who were treated at this Tijuana hospital during 2020.

3.1. Sample Size

The required sample size for this study was estimated considering the expected prevalence in studies carried out using bioimpedance analysis, 17% [25], assuming a margin of error of 5% and a confidence interval of 95%. According to these criteria, a total of 185 patients were needed in order to obtain the desired results. The average age of the studied population was 55 years, while the average hospital length of stay duration was six days.

Patients arrived mainly from the Tijuana and Rosarito urban and suburban areas. This research included patient medical history, pharmacology, PCR testing and biochemical data.

3.2. Database

Information on 185 patients with 99 variables was collected for each of them to create the database, the description of the variables can be found in Appendix A. Table 1 shows the gender criteria for evaluating patients at the Tijuana General Hospital, which serves a low-income population in the Tijuana and Rosarito areas of Baja California, with a higher percentage of men than women as seen from the Table 2.

Table 2. Evaluation Criteria.

Gender	%	Kg-m^2	SpO
Women	39.46%	<6.1 kg/m^2	>95%
Men	60.54%	<8.5 kg/m^2	>95%

3.3. Bedford's Law

Benford's Law validation method was used in order to make sure the data was consistent, in order to develop an efficient study. Benford's Law, or the Law of First Digits, is a tool used in different fields of science, with a method to suggest a mathematical pattern in the distribution of the first digits in a dataset that does not display a uniform distribution, but rather are arranged in such a way that the digit "1" is the most frequent, followed by "2", then "3", and so on, down to "9". This model suggests that, within a random set of data, the first digit of approximately 30.10% of the numbers will be "1". Several studies have used this technique to validate and evaluate veracity in databases with information about COVID-19 [26,27].

By using Benford's Law as a validation method, it was demonstrated that there is consistency in the data collected from the Tijuana General Hospital, as the curve of our current information is close to the curve generated by the percentages established by Benford's Law. For this comparison, "length of stay" data were used, as within the database that was used, most information is described by binary numbers (0 and 1), while the variable "length of stay" is a defined variable. For this, in addition to the graph function, two Excel functions were used:

Left: This function allowed the first digit to be taken to the left of the number within the "length of stay" column.

Countif: This function allows to count the frequency of each of the digit numbers without considering 0.

Figure 1 shows the comparison results between Bedford's Law and "length of stay" which suggest that the data is consistent.

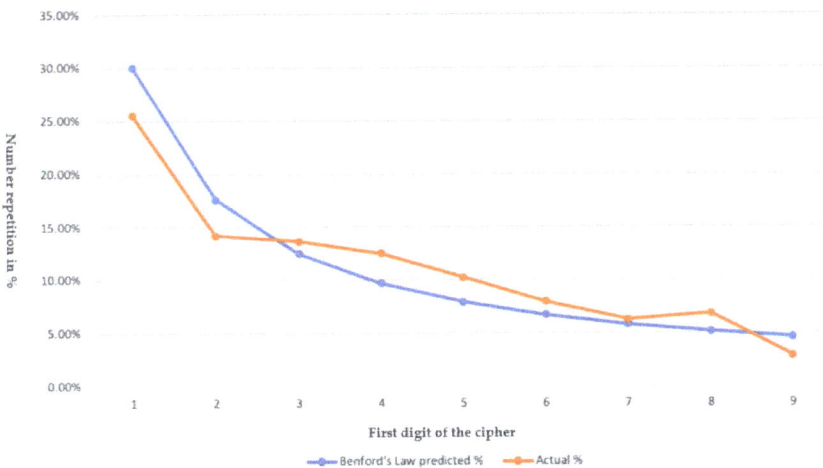

Figure 1. Benford's Law curve comparison with the curve generated by the actual data from "length of stay".

The distribution by first digit numbers in the data can be seen in Table 3. Invalidating the data, the comparison suggests that according to Benford's law, the results obtained from this analysis for the Tijuana Hospital database are accurate.

Table 3. Data compared with Bedford's Law.

Benford's Law	Actual	R.E. *
	Tijuana cases [1]	
30.10%	25.57%	−15.01%
17.61%	14.20%	−19.30%
12.49%	14.00%	9.12%
9.69%	12.50%	22.89%
7.92%	10.23%	29.16%
6.69%	7.95%	18.83%
5.80%	6.25%	7.75%
5.12%	6.82%	33.20%
4.58%	2.84%	1.73%

[1] Considering "length of stay" for validation. * Relative Error.

3.4. Machine Learning Analysis

For the evaluation of each dataset, the following classifiers were used: Decision Tree (DT), Support Vector Machine (SVM), Random Forest (RF), Multi-Layer Perceptron Neural Network (MLPNN), Naive Bayes (NB), Logistic Regression (LR) and AdaBoost (AB). The configuration for each algorithm were suggested by Orange. These configurations are shown in Table 4. The algorithms were evaluated by stratified k-fold cross-validation, where the data was iteratively examined by ten folds, using nine folds for training and 1-fold for testing; with this method, the data can be divided into equal parts, which gives better results, avoiding generalization which means possible errors when new data is used for predictions with the trained models.

Table 4. Configurations used for each learner in the analysis.

Learner	Configuration for Learners
RF	A number of trees: 10, minimum subsets split: 5, maximum tree depth: unlimited.
kNN	Number of neighbors: 3, metric: Euclidean, weight: uniform
SVM	Type: SVM Regression, C = 1, ε = 0.1, Kernel= Radial Basis Function (RBF), exp $(-auto\,|x-y|^2)$, numerical tolerance: 0.001
MLPNN	Hidden layers: 100, activation: ReLu, solver: Adam, alpha: 0.0001, maximum iterations: 200, replicable training: True.
NB	
AB	Base estimator: tree, number of estimators: 50, algorithm (classification): Samme. r, loss (regression): Linear
DT	Type: binary tree, internal nodes < 5, maximum depth: 100, splitting: 95%.

The datasets for each analysis were created by feature selection; for this, HAS, DM, and Obesity were selected as targets due to their importance in the development of COVID-19. After selecting the targets, the complete database was analyzed iteratively with each of the chosen targets. The process of selecting the most relevant features was done by using the DT and comparing the results with the rank, using the following scoring methods: gain ratio, Gini, X^2, ReliefF and Fast Correlation Based Filter (FCBF). The algorithm followed for the scoring techniques is shown in Table 5.

Table 5. Rank Scoring Algorithms.

Method	Algorithm
Gain Ratio	$IG(Ex,a) = H(Ex) - \sum_{v \in values\,(a)} \left(\frac{|\{x \in Ex | value(x,a) = v\}|}{|Ex|} * H(\{x \in Ex | value(x,a) = v\}) \right)$
Gini	$G = \frac{\sum_{i=1}^{n} * \sum_{j=1}^{n} * |x_i - x_j|}{2\sum_{i=1}^{n} * \sum_{j=1}^{n} * x_j}$
X^2	$X = \frac{m - Np}{\sqrt{Npq}}$
ReliefF	$W_i = W_i - (x_i - nearHit_i)^2 + (x_i - nearMiss_i)^2$
FCBF	$H(X) = -\sum_i P(x_i) log_2(P(x_i))$

4. Results

Given that the comorbidities prevalent in patients of the analyzed database are SAH with 49% of patients, DM with 34% of patients, and Obesity with 11% of patients, it was decided to take these three diseases independently as a target to find the variables that were most related to these diseases present in patients with COVID-19, determining the factors involved where the information had to be pre-processed. The Decision Tree and ranking methods were used to determine the variables with the most significant impact. Tables 6–8 show the resulting datasets after the analysis. Dataset 1 in each table was determined by using all of the existing variables in the database; then, for dataset 2, the selection of features was determined by choosing the ones closer to the root within the first ten levels; finally, to assess dataset 3, ranking results were considered, regardless of the variables "Tos" (cough), "Fiebre" (fever), "Disnea" (dyspnea), and "Dolor de cabeza/Cefalea (headache)" as these were established by the World Health Organization as official COVID-19 symptoms, and by using them for analysis they performed better obtaining an increase in the dataset scores, therefore by dismissing them the research found other significant variables.

Table 6. Datasets for HAS as a target (variable names in Spanish).

Dataset	Target HAS
Dataset 1	Edad, género, grupo etario, DM, ECV, Hepáticas, SNC, Neumopatía, Cáncer, Inmunosupresión, Obesidad, Otros (1), Comorbilidades, Fiebre, Mialgias/artralgias, Fatiga, Odinogafia/ardor faringeo, Tos, Disnea, Dolor Toracico, Congestión Nasal, Rinorrea, Expectoración Diarrea, Náusea, Anorexia, Vómito, Cefalea, Mareo, Hispomia/Anosmia, Ageusia, Conjuntivitis, Saturación >90, Saturación 80–90%, Saturación < 80%, Leucopenia, Leucocitosis, Neutropenia, Neutrofilia, Linfopenia, Linfocitosis, Eosinopenia, Trombocitopenia, Trombocitosis, TP normal, TP alargado, INR normal, INR Alto, TTPa normal, TTPa alargado, Creatinina normal, Creatinina alta, Ferritina normal, Ferritina alta, Dímero D normal, Dímero D Alto, Fibrinógeno normal, Fibrinógeno Alto, PCR normal, PCR alta, Procalcitonina normal, Procalcitonina alta, Troponina normal, Troponina alta, CPK normal, CPK alta, CK-MB normal, CK-MB alta, Albúmina baja, Albúmina normal, Bilirrubina total normal, Bilirrubina total alta, ALT/TGP normal, ALT/TGP alta, AST/TGO normal, AST/TGO alta, DHL normal, DHL alta, DHL > 1000, Fosfatasa alcalina normal, Fosfatasa alcalina alta, Muestra, POSITIVA, Mayor 50%, Moderado, Grave, Oseltamivir, Ceftriaxona, Claritromicina, Azitromicina, Levofloxacino, Otros (2), Hidroxicloroquina/Cloroquina, Tocilizumab, Esteroides, Pronación, Respondedor, Respondedor parcial, No respondedor, Alta por mejoría, Defunción, Días de estancia hospitalaria.
Dataset 2	Comorbilidades, Edad, Tos, CK-MB Normal, INR Alto, DM, Cefalea, Neutrofilia, Dímero, Leucocitos, Neumopatía, Obesidad, Días de estancia, CPK alta, Saturación 90, Eosinopenia, TP Alargado y Odinofagia
Dataset 3	Comorbilidades, Edad, CK-MB Normal, CK-MB Alto, DM, Neutrofilia, Dímero D Alto, Leucocitosis, Neumopatía, Obesidad, Dias de estancia, Otros (1)

Table 7. Datasets for DM as a target (variable names in Spanish).

Dataset	Target DM
Dataset 1	Edad, género, grupo etario, HAS, ECV, Hepáticas, SNC, Neumopatía, Cáncer, Inmunosupresión, Obesidad, Otros (1), Comorbilidades, Fiebre, Mialgias/artralgias, Fatiga, Odinogafia/ardor faringeo, Tos, Disnea, Dolor Toracico, Congestión Nasal, Rinorrea, Expectoración Diarrea, Náusea, Anorexia, Vómito, Cefalea, Mareo, Hispomia/Anosmia, Ageusia, Conjuntivitis, Saturación > 90, Saturación 80–90%, Saturación < 80%, Leucopenia, Leucocitosis, Neutropenia, Neutrofilia, Linfopenia, Linfocitosis, Eosinopenia, Trombocitopenia, Trombocitosis, TP normal, TP alargado, INR normal, INR Alto, TTPa normal, TTPa alargado, Creatinina normal, Creatinina alta, Ferritina normal, Ferritina alta, Dímero D normal, Dímero D Alto, Fibrinógeno normal, Fibrinógeno Alto, PCR normal, PCR alta, Procalcitonina normal, Procalcitonina alta, Troponina normal, Troponina alta, CPK normal, CPK alta, CK-MB normal, CK-MB alta, Albúmina baja, Albúmina normal, Bilirrubina total normal, Bilirrubina total alta, ALT/TGP normal, ALT/TGP alta, AST/TGO normal, AST/TGO alta, DHL normal, DHL alta, DHL > 1000, Fosfatasa alcalina normal, Fosfatasa alcalina alta, Muestra, POSITIVA, Mayor 50%, Moderado, Grave, Oseltamivir, Ceftriaxona, Claritromicina, Azitromicina, Levofloxacino, Otros (2), Hidroxicloroquina/Cloroquina, Tocilizumab, Esteroides, Pronación, Respondedor, Respondedor parcial, No respondedor, Alta por mejoría, Defunción, Días de estancia hospitalaria.

Table 7. Cont.

Dataset	Target DM
Dataset 2	Edad, Neutropenia, Comorbilidades, Cáncer, Claritromicina, HAS, linfocitosis, Ferritina normal, Hepáticas, SNC, Leucopenia, Inmunosupresión, eosinofilia, ferritina alta, Troponina normal, vómito, INR alto, CM-KB alta, Disnea, TTP alargado, Levofloxacino, Fatiga, AST/TGO alta, bilirrubina total alta, fiebre, creatinina alta, INR normal, Diarrea, Augesia.
Dataset 3	Edad, Género, HAS, Obesidad, Otros (1), Comorbilidades, Leucocitosis, Creatinina normal, Creatinina alta, Procalcitonina alta, Levofloxacino, Hidroxicloroquina

Table 8. Datasets for Obesity as a target (variable names in Spanish).

Dataset	Target Obesity
Dataset 1	Edad, género, grupo etario, HAS, DM, ECV, Hepáticas, SNC, Neumopatía, Cáncer, Inmunosupresión, Otros (1), Comorbilidades, Fiebre, Mialgias/artralgias, Fatiga, Odinogafia/ardor faringeo, Tos, Disnea, Dolor Toracico, Congestión Nasal, Rinorrea, Expectoración Diarrea, Náusea, Anorexia, Vómito, Cefalea, Mareo, Hispomia/Anosmia, Ageusia, Conjuntivitis, Saturación > 90, Saturación 80–90%, Saturación < 80%, Leucopenia, Leucocitosis, Neutropenia, Neutrofilia, Linfopenia, Linfocitosis, Eosinopenia, Trombocitopenia, Trombocitosis, TP normal, TP alargado, INR normal, INR Alto, TTPa normal, TTPa alargado, Creatinina normal, Creatinina alta, Ferritina normal, Ferritina alta, Dimero D normal, Dimero D Alto, Fibrinogeno normal, Fibrinogeno Alto, PCR normal, PCR alta, Procalcitonina normal, Procalcitonina alta, Troponina normal, Troponina alta, CPK normal, CPK alta, CK-MB normal, CK-MB alta, Albumina baja, Albumina normal, Bilirrubina total normal, Bilirrubina total alta, ALT/TGP normal, ALT/TGP alta, AST/TGO normal, AST/TGO alta, DHL normal, DHL alta, DHL > 1000, Fosfatasa alcalina normal, Fosfatasa alcalina alta, Muestra, POSITIVA, Mayor 50%, Moderado, Grave, Oseltamivir, Ceftriaxona, Claritromicina, Azitromicina, Levofloxacino, Otros (2), Hidroxicloroquina/Cloroquina, Tocilizumab, Esteroides, Pronación, Respondedor, Respondedor parcial, No respondedor, Alta por mejoría, Defunción, Días de estancia hospitalaria
Dataset 2	Saturación 80–90, Edad, Cefalea, Género, Levoflaxina, GRAVE, Hisponia/asmonia, Linfopeni, a Neumopatía, Fosfatasa alcalina normal, Creatinina normal, días de estancia, PCR alta
Dataset 3	Saturación 80–90, Edad, Género, Levoflaxina, GRAVE, Hisponia/asmonia, Linfopenia Neumopatía, Fosfatasa alcalina normal

After the analysis of each dataset, the obtained results are shown in Tables 9–11; where the best scores are shown in bold font for each method.

Table 9. Highest scores from a dataset with HAS as a target.

Model	AUC	CA	F1	Precision	Recall
Tree Decision	0.814	0.784	0.784	0.784	0.784
SVM	0.867	0.762	0.762	0.762	0.762
Random Forest	0.866	0.784	0.784	0.784	0.784
Neural Network	0.876	0.773	0.773	0.773	0.773
Naive Bayes	0.832	0.757	0.755	0.761	0.757
Logistic Regression	**0.910**	**0.800**	**0.800**	**0.801**	**0.800**
AdaBoost	0.860	0.811	0.811	0.811	0.811

Table 10. Highest scores from a dataset with DM as a target.

Model	AUC	CA	F1	Precision	Recall
Tree	0.867	0.881	0.878	0.882	0.881
SVM	0.934	0.886	0.885	0.886	0.886
Random Forest	0.877	0.849	0.847	0.847	0.849
Neural Network	0.871	0.816	0.812	0.813	0.816
Naive Bayes	0.849	0.838	0.838	0.838	0.838
Logistic Regression	0.912	0.892	0.888	0.897	0.892
AdaBoost	0.827	0.843	0.844	0.844	0.843

Best model: Logistic Regression with 0.934 of AUC, 0.886 of CA, 0.885 of F1, 0.886 of Precision, and 0.886 of Recall.

Table 11. Highest scores from a dataset with Obesity as a target.

Model	AUC	CA	F1	Precision	Recall
Tree	0.700	0.876	0.869	0.864	0.876
SVM	0.643	0.838	0.831	0.824	0.838
Random Forest	0.807	0.903	0.872	0.912	0.903
Neural Network	**0.834**	**0.914**	**0.899**	**0.906**	**0.914**
Naive Bayes	0.793	0.865	0.845	0.833	0.865
Logistic Regression	0.778	0.881	0.856	0.851	0.881
AdaBoost	0.697	0.881	0.879	0.876	0.881

Best model: Neural Network with 0.834 of AUC, 0.914 of CA, 0.899 of F1, 0.906 of Precision and 0.914 of Recall.

As shown in Table 8, the highest score using as target HAS was obtained with the Logistic Regression algorithm, using the default parameters with a cost strength of 1.00 (C-1) and Ridge-type regularization (L2), which shows 91.0% Area under ROC (AUC), 80% Classification Accuracy (CA), 80% F1, and 80.1%, Precision and Recall for selected variables in Dataset 3 in Table 6 as possible variables essential to consider for a more accurate determination of vulnerability in people with HAS.

On the other hand, when targeting DM patients, the best-functioning model using the default parameters already mentioned above was found to be Logistic Regression, obtaining 91.2% AUC, 89.2% CA, 88.8% F1, 89.7% precision, and recall 89.2% for selected variables from dataset 3 in Table 7.

While the Neural Network algorithm showed better results for patients with Obesity, obtaining 83.4% AUC, 91.4% CA, 89.9% F1, 90.6% Accuracy, and 91.4% Recall (See Table 11).

The prevalent symptoms present in people with different comorbidities, and statistical analysis was performed without considering cough, fever, dyspnea, and headache as part of the symptoms for the same reason mentioned above. In people with HAS, DM, and Obesity, the presence of fatigue and myalgias/arthralgias was greater; while the third dominant symptom in people with HAS and DM was odynophagia, instead of people with Obesity, this symptom was positioned with the eighth, occupied the third position with chest pain (See Figures 2–4).

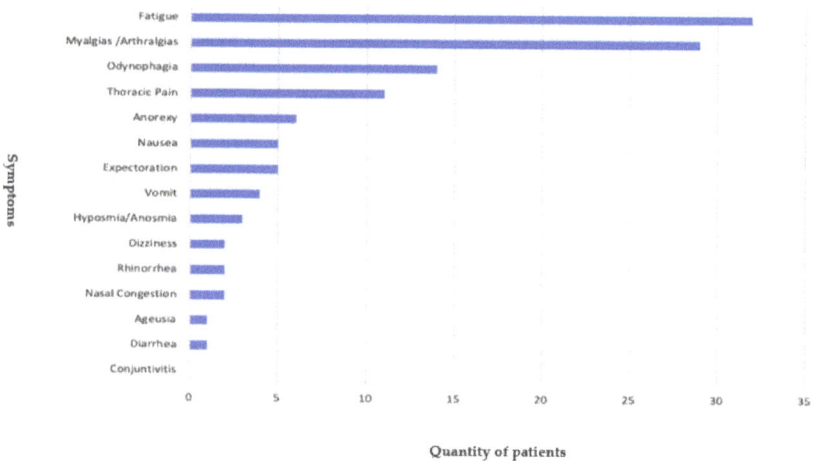

Figure 2. Frequency of symptoms in patients with DM.

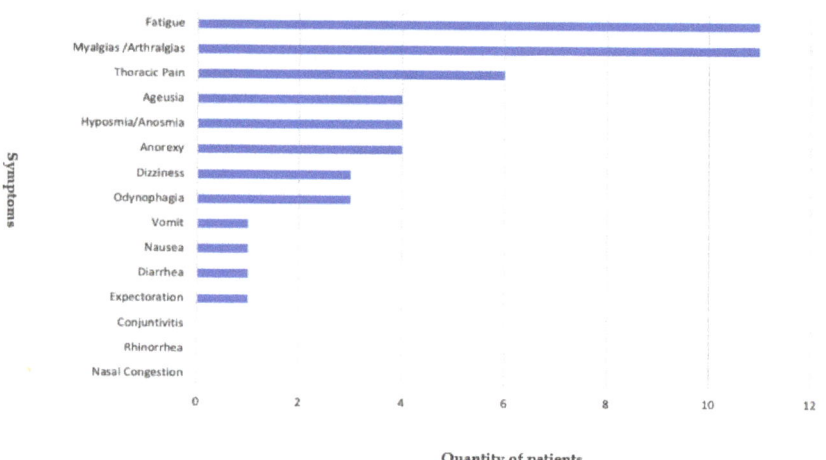

Figure 3. Frequency of symptoms in patients with HAS.

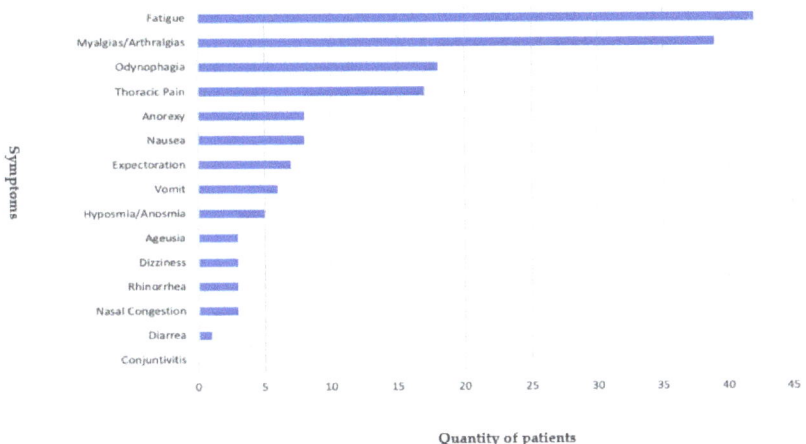

Figure 4. Frequency of symptoms in patients with Obesity.

5. Discussion

Obesity, diabetes, and hypertension are high-prevalence comorbidities in the Mexican population. In 2018, approximately 1/4 of the Mexican people had high blood pressure, while 71.2% of people over the age of 20 had a prevalence of obesity and overweight. These two conditions are considered to be significant risk factors for developing other diseases such as diabetes since 90% of people with diabetes in Mexico are overweight and obese [28].

In processing the information in this study, the prevalence of these three diseases considered as risk factors for COVID-19 infection could be noted. For this reason, it was decided to carry out an analysis using Artificial Intelligence (Machine Learning) techniques, aiming for each of these diseases, looking for any relationship between the symptoms and conditions of people suffering from these comorbidities.

After reviewing the medical literature, it was found that COVID-19 causes chronic inflammation in patients with obesity, along with other diseases considered as risk factors, such as lack of vitamin D and intestinal dysbiosis, which result in deficiencies in the functioning of the immune system in the face of infections. On the other hand, Obesity has a negative impact on respiratory mechanics as it is affected due to the resistance generated by lack of elasticity in the chest box [29,30]. Both diabetes and high blood pressure are diseases more present in the elderly, one of the reasons why these diseases are thought to be closely related to COVID-19, due to the fact that people with advanced age are highly vulnerable to COVID-19. The reason diabetes could have a high impact on the condition of patients with COVID-19 may be due to a disruption generated in the endocrine system where the COVID-19 virus affects angiotensin-converting Enzyme 2 (ECA2), which is responsible for anti-inflammatory regulation, vasodilators, and the process of releasing sodium into the urine. Another function of ECA2 is to offer protection to different organs, including those that are part of the pulmonary and cardiovascular systems, which is why the absence of this enzyme is related to the involvement of the lungs and the development of hypertension [31,32].

Different authors mentioned in a report of the analysis carried out with a database of 3894 patients in Italy [33], obtaining values for a death risk target with an accuracy rating of 83.4%, F1 value of 90.4%, specificity of 30.8%, and Recall of 95.2% when using Random Forest over a dataset with variables such as Glomerular Filtration Rate (eGFR), C- Reactive Protein (CRP), Age, Diabetes, Sex, Hypertension, Smoking, Lung Disease, Myocardial Infection, Obesity, Heart Failure, and Cancer, demonstrating this as vulnerable to those who exhibit the above-mentioned comorbidities. To achieve a comparison between the variables established with the results of this analysis, the scores of the three targets used

(HAS, Diabetes, and Obesity) were taken into account and the average was calculated, obtaining values of 84.50% for CA, 83.43% of F1, 84.76% Precision, and 84.53% of Recall.

On the other hand, a study of Brazilian patients shows their scores at 86% for CA, 92% for AUC, 28% of Precision, 86% of Recall, and 42% of F1 for the Logistic Regression model, where the results show that there is a high relationship between patients over 60 years of age with breathing difficulties, fever, cough, rhinorrhea, odynophagia, diarrhea, headache, heart disease, pneumopathies, kidney disease, diabetes, smoking, Obesity, and hospitalization with those who come down with COVID-19 [34].

This analysis provides a complete and accurate perspective of the current situation in Tijuana since having information from a single source allows us to know the current situation of those served at the Tijuana General Hospital, who are mostly part of low-income or economically disadvantaged family groups. Since 41.9% of the Mexican population is economically disadvantaged [35], it is important to understand the comorbidities and symptoms present in this group, which results in more vulnerable people and increases expenditures in public sector hospitals regarding space and medical equipment, which often is extremely limited. Since the study was done considering typical human patients, regardless of their geographical and ethnic origin, a similar genomic situation can be assumed with migrant patients from both parts of Mexico and regions such as Central America, South America, and the Caribbean.

6. Conclusions

The values of the prevalent comorbidity found in this study were as follows: 49% in patients with HAS; 34% in patients with DM; and 11% in patients with Obesity, corresponding to the population segment that was served at the General Hospital of Tijuana during the aforementioned dates.

The deaths reported during the evaluated period of the total number of patients evaluated in this study were 42 subjects, from a population universe of 185 patients evaluated, with a fatality rate of 22%, a non-representative sample but within the data that places Mexico with a fatality rate (Case fatality) of 8.8% compared to other fatality rates in Latin America, such as Peru (3.5%), Colombia (2.6%), Chile (2.5%), Brazil (2.4%), and 2–3% globally [36].

A total of 52 different medicines were prescribed, where Steroids (16.1%), azithromycin (10.9%), enoxaparin (8.2%), levofloxacin (7.3%), hydroxyquinone (6.6%), omeprazole (6.2%), and acetaminophen (6.2%) were most commonly used. The rest, presenting themselves with a <6.0% per drug, correspond as a whole to 38.5% and are classified as "other".

The values obtained for each dataset evaluating Obesity, DM, and HAS in this study using Artificial Intelligence, specifically with various Machine Learning techniques, have been compared with values presented in other similar academic/medical publications, particularly those for HAS were obtained with the Logistic Regression algorithm obtaining 91.0% AUC, CA, F1 and Recall 80%, and accuracy 80.1%. For Diabetes, the Logistic Regression algorithm obtained 91.2% AUC, 89.2% CA, 88.8% F1, 89.7% accuracy, and recall 89.2%, obtaining similar results for Hypertension and Diabetes, while improved results were obtained in the case of Obesity using the Neural Network algorithm, obtaining 83.4% AUC, 91.4% CA, 89.9% F1, 90.6% Accuracy and 91.4% Recall.

The results presented here confirm the convenience of using Logistic Regression algorithms in the dataset presented when evaluating HAS as a target; Similarly, Logistic Regression's algorithms were the most successful in evaluating DM as a target; while finally, Neural Network algorithms showed the best results for the case of Obesity as a target, in the specific sample case of 185 patients with limited or non-existing financial resources, who suffered these medical conditions, and who were served at the Tijuana General Hospital during the year 2020.

With these results, we can conclude that the use of Artificial Intelligence using Machine Learning techniques has been effectively used to identify the early stages of COVID-19 in patients in Baja California.

Author Contributions: Conceptualization, C.C.-O., C.Z., R.C.-G., E.O.; Data curation, C.C.-O., A.S.; Methodology, C.C.-O., A.S., R.C.-G., A.H.; Project administration, C.C.-O., R.C.-G., E.O., C.Z.; Supervision, R.C.-G., E.O., O.B., C.Z.; Validation, C.C.-O., O.B., E.O., C.Z. and R.C.-G.; Writing—original draft, C.C.-O., A.S., R.C.-G., O.B.; Writing—review & editing, C.C.-O., O.B., C.Z. and E.O. All authors have read and agreed to the published version of the manuscript.

Funding: This research was funded by a postdoctoral fellowship from the Consejo Nacional de Ciencia y Tecnología (National Council of Science and Technology).

Institutional Review Board Statement: The study was conducted according to the guidelines of the Declaration of Helsinki, and approved by the Ethics Committee of Hospital General de Tijuana protocol code 171101-20 on 12 April 2020.

Informed Consent Statement: Informed consent was obtained from all subjects involved in the study.

Data Availability Statement: Not applicable.

Acknowledgments: The authors would especially like to express their gratitude to the Mexican National Council of Science and Technology (CONACYT) for the Postdoctoral scholarship 334844.

Conflicts of Interest: The authors declare no conflict of interest.

Appendix A

Table A1. Description of variables.

Variable	Description
Edad	Age
Género	Gender (Female/Male)
Grupo etario	Grupo etario
HAS	Defined by two levels according to the 2017 American College of Cardiology/American Heart Association (ACC/AHA) guidelines: (1) Elevated blood pressure, with a systolic pressure (SBP) between 120—129 mm Hg and diastolic pressure (DBP) less than 80 mm Hg, and (2) stage 1 hypertension, with a SBP of 130 to 139 mm Hg or a DBP of 80 to 89 mm Hg
DM	Diagnosis by meeting any of the criteria: Fasting glucose ≥ 126 mg/dL (7.0 mmol/L). Fasting is defined as the absence of caloric intake for at least 8 h OR 2 h postprandial glucose ≥ 200 mg/dL (11.1 mmol/L). The test should be performed as described by the WHO, using a glucose load containing the equivalent of 75 g of anhydrous glucose dissolved in water. OR Glycated hemoglobin $\geq 6.5\%$ (48 mmol/mol). The test must be performed in a laboratory using a method that is certified by NGSP and standardized for the DCCT assay. OR In a patient with classic symptoms of hyperglycemia or hyperglycemic crisis, a random plasma glucose ≥ 200 mg/dL (11.1 mmol/L).
ECV	Neurological alteration is characterized by its sudden onset, generally without warning, with symptoms lasting 24 h or more, causing sequelae and death.
Hepaticas	Primary or secondary diseases that affect liver tissue.
SNC	Central Nervous System.

Table A1. Cont.

Variable	Description
Neumopatía	Lung disease is a generic term to describe diseases that affect the lungs. It should not be confused with the term pneumonia, which specifically refers to infection of the lung by a virus or bacteria.
Cancer	Any of a large number of diseases characterized by the development of abnormal cells that divide uncontrollably and have the ability to infiltrate and destroy normal body tissue.
Inmunosupresión	Suppression or reduction of immune reactions. It may be due to the deliberate administration of immunosuppressive drugs used in the treatment of autoimmune diseases or in recipients of transplanted organs to avoid rejection. It can also be secondary to pathological processes such as immunodeficiencies, tumors, or malnutrition.
Obesidad	A condition characterized by the excessive accumulation and storage of fat in the body and which in an adult is typically indicated by a body mass index of 30 or more.
Otros	Other types are of diseases not classifiable in the previous variables.
Comorbilidades	A concomitant but unrelated disease process or disease; is commonly used in epidemiology to indicate the coexistence of two or more disease processes.
Otros Especificar	Other types are of diseases not classifiable in the previous variables, where the type is specified.
Fiber	Temperature above the normal range due to an increase in the body temperature set point. There is no agreed upper limit for normal temperature with sources using values between 37.2 and 38.3 °C (99.0 and 100.9 °F) in humans.
Mialgias/arthralgias	Muscle or joint pain.
Fatigue	Difficulty starting or maintaining physical or mental activity voluntarily.
Odinofagia/ardor faringeo	Feeling of pain when swallowing.
Tos	Sudden and acute expulsion of air from the lungs that acts as a protective mechanism to clear the airways or as a symptom of a pulmonary disorder.
Disnea	Difficulty breathing.
Dolor toracico	Localized chest pain, regardless of its etiology.
Congestión nasal	A feeling of blockage or obstruction in the nasal cavity and/or sinuses due to inflammation of the mucous lining of the nose.
Rinorrea	Flow or abundant emission of fluid from the nose.
Expectoración	Expulsion through coughing or sputum or other secretions formed in the respiratory tract.
Diarrhea	It consists of the expulsion of three or more liquid stools, with or without blood, in 24 h, which adopt the shape of the container that contains them.
Nausea	Feeling sick or sick in the stomach that may appear with an urgent need to vomit.
Anorexia	It is used to denote lack of appetite or lack of appetite that can occur in very different circumstances.
Vómito	Violent expulsion through the mouth of what is contained in the stomach.

Table A1. Cont.

Variable	Description
Cefalea	They are painful and disabling primary disorders such as migraine, tension headache, and cluster headache.
Mareo	Feeling of vertigo and instability in the head and discomfort in the stomach that can lead to the urge to vomit and loss of balance.
Hyposmia/Anosmia	Decreased or absent sense of smell.
Ageusia	Decreased or absent sense of taste.
Conjunctivitis	Inflammation or irritation of the conjunctiva.
Saturación >90	Oxygen saturation in ambient air >90%.
Saturación 80–90%	Oxygen saturation in ambient air of 80–90%.
Saturación <80%	Oxygen saturation in ambient air <80%.
Leucopenia	Reduction in circulating white blood cell count <4000/mcL.
Leukocytosis	A white blood cell count greater than 11,000/mm^3,
Neutropenia	When the neutrophil numbers are below 1500–1800 per mm3.
Neutrophilia	Neutrophil blood values equal to or less than 7700/microL.
Linfopenia	Total lymphocyte count <1000/mcL.
Linfocitosis	When the lymphocyte count is greater than 4000 per microliter.
Eosinopenia	Reduction in circulating eosinophils <0.01 $\times$ 10^9/L.
Eosinophilia	A count of more than 500 eosinophils per microliter of blood.
Thrombocytopenia	Decrease in the absolute number of platelets in the peripheral blood below 150,000 per µL.
Trombocitosis	Platelet count greater than 600,000 per µL.
TP normal	TP in blood with a range of 11 to 13.5 s.
TP alargado	TP in blood >13.5 s.
INR normal	INR with a value between 0.9 to 1.3.
INR Alto	INR with a value >1.3.
TTP normal	APTT in blood in a range of 25 to 35 s.
TTP alrgado	APTT in blood >35 s.
Creatinine normal	The normal range for creatinine is 0.7 to 1.3 mg/dL (61.9 to 114.9 µmol/L) for men and 0.6 to 1.1 mg/dL (53 to 97.2 µmol/L) for women.
Creatinine alta	Values >1.3 mg/dL for men and >1.1 mg/dL for women.
Ferritin normal	The range of normal values for ferritin are: Men: 12 to 300 nanograms per milliliter (ng/mL) Women: 12 to 150 ng/mL.
ferritin alta	Ferritin values in Men of >300 nanograms per milliliter (ng/mL), in women >150 ng/mL.
Dimero D normal	The normal range for D-dimer is less than 0.5 micrograms per milliliter.
Dimero D Alto	D-dimer >0.5 micrograms per milliliter.
Fibrinogen normal	The normal range for fibrinogen is 200 to 400 mg/dL (2.0 to 4.0 g/L).
Fibrinogeno Alto	Fibrinogen value >400 mg/dL.
PCR normal	0 y 5 mg/dl
PCR alta	above 5 mg/dl
Procalcitonina normal	Normal blood procalcitonin values are less than 0.5 ng/mL

Table A1. Cont.

Variable	Description
Procalcitonina alta	Procalcitonin values in blood >0.5 ng/mL
Troponina normal	Troponin in blood, within the reference limit up to 0.04 ng/mL.
Tropoonina alta	Troponin in blood >0.04 ng/mL.
CPK normal	Normal values for creatine phosphokinase (CPK) are between 32 and 294 U/L for men and 33 to 211 U/L for women.
CPK alta	CPK values greater than 294 U/L for men and greater than 211 U/L for women
CK-MB normal	CK-MB blood values within a range of 5 to 25 IU/L.
CK-MB alta	CK-MB blood values >25 IU/L.
Albumina baja	Albumin in blood <3.4 g/dL.
Albumina normal	Albumin in blood with a range of 3.4 to 5.4 g/dL.
Bilirrubina total normal	Total blood bilirubin values of 3–1.9 mg/dL
Bilirrubina total alta	Total blood bilirubin values >1.9 mg/dL
ALT/TGP normal	ALT blood values in a range of 10–40 IU/L.
ALT/TGP alta	ALT blood values >40 IU/L.
AST/TGO normal	AST blood values in a range of 10–34 IU/L.
AST/TGO alta	AST blood values >34 IU/L.
DHL normal	DHL blood value in a range of 105–333 IU/L
DHL alta	DHL blood value >333 IU/L.
DHL > 1000	DHL > 1000
Fostasa alcalina normal	Alkaline phosphatase blood value in a range of 44–147 IU/L
Fosfatasa alcalina alta	Alkaline phosphatase blood value >147 IU/L.
POSITIVA	PCR sample for COVID-19 positive.
MODERADO	Clinical or radiographic evidence of lower respiratory tract disease, with an oxygen saturation greater than or equal to 94%.
GRAVE	Oxygen saturation <94%, respiratory rate > or equal to 30 breaths/minute, pulmonary infiltrates >50%.
Oseltamivir	A drug that selectively inhibits the neuraminidase enzyme found in influenza A and B viruses, preventing infected cells from releasing viral particles. Its action is greater against influenza A viruses.
Ceftriaxone	Antibiotic of the third generation cephalosporin class, which has broad-spectrum actions against Gram-negative and Gram-positive bacteria.
Claritromicina	Macrolide antibiotic active against gram positives, gram negatives, it is also active against spirochetes, Chlamydophila and several intracellular pathogens.
Azitromicina	Broad-spectrum antibiotic from the group of Macrolides that act against various gram-positive and gram-negative bacteria.
Levofloxacin	Antibacterial fluoroquinolone, used to treat infections caused by sensitive germs.
Otros	Other medications
Especificar	Specify

Table A1. *Cont.*

Variable	Description
Hidroxicloroquina/ Cloroquina	Commonly prescribed aminoquinoline for the treatment of uncomplicated malaria, rheumatoid arthritis, chronic discoid lupus erythematosus, and systemic lupus erythematosus.
Tocilizumab	Humanized monoclonal antibody that inhibits interleukin 6 receptors.
Esteroides	A group of chemicals classified by a specific carbon structure. Steroids include drugs used to relieve inflammation, such as prednisone and cortisone.
Pronación	Anatomical position of the human body characterized by: Body position lying face down and head on its side.
Responder	That responds to a stimulus.
Responder parcial	That responds little to a stimulus.
No respondedor	Non responder
Alta por mejoría	Discharge for improvement
Defunción	Death
Días de estancia hospitalaria	Days of hospital stay.

References

1. Helmy, Y.A.; Fawzy, M.; Elaswad, A.; Sobieh, A.; Kenney, S.P.; Shehata, A.A. The COVID-19 pandemic: A comprehensive review of taxonomy, genetics, epidemiology, diagnosis, treatment, and control. *J. Clin. Med.* **2020**, *9*, 1225. [CrossRef]
2. Shereen, M.A.; Khan, S.; Kazmi, A.; Bashir, N.; Siddique, R. COVID-19 infection: Origin, transmission, and characteristics of human coronaviruses. *J. Adv. Res.* **2020**, *24*, 91–98. [CrossRef]
3. Guan, W.J.; Ni, Z.Y.; Hu, Y.; Liang, W.H.; Ou, C.Q.; He, J.X.; Liu, L.; Shan, H.; Lei, C.L.; Hui, D.S.; et al. Early Transmission Dynamics in Wuhan, China, of Novel Coronavirus–Infected Pneumonia. *N. Engl. J. Med.* **2020**, *382*, 1199–1207.
4. Wang, W.; Tang, J.; Wei, F. Updated understanding of the outbreak of 2019 novel coronavirus (2019-nCoV) in Wuhan, China. *J. Med. Virol.* **2020**, *92*, 441–447. [CrossRef] [PubMed]
5. Singhal, T. A Review of Coronavirus Disease-2019 (COVID-19). *Indian J. Pediatrics* **2020**, *87*, 281–286. [CrossRef]
6. Rothan, H.A.; Byrareddy, S.N. The epidemiology and pathogenesis of coronavirus disease (COVID-19) outbreak. *J. Autoimmun.* **2020**, *109*, 102433. [CrossRef]
7. Wu, Z.; Mcgoogan, J.M. Characteristics of and Important Lessons from the Coronavirus Disease 2019 (COVID-19) Outbreak in China. *JAMA* **2020**, *323*, 1239. [CrossRef] [PubMed]
8. World Health Organization. WHO Coronavirus (COVID-19) Dashboard. 2021. Available online: https://covid19.who.int/ (accessed on 15 August 2021).
9. World Health Organization. Estimating Mortality from COVID-19. Scientific Brief. 2020. Available online: https://apps.who.int/iris/bitstream/handle/10665/333642/WHO-2019-nCoV-Sci_Brief-Mortality-2020.1-eng.pdf?sequence=1&isAllowed=y (accessed on 10 May 2020).
10. Secretaría de Salud. COVID-19 Tablero México. COVID-19 Tablero México. 2020. Available online: https://coronavirus.gob.mx/datos/ (accessed on 16 August 2021).
11. Yadaw, A.S.; Li, Y.C.; Bose, S.; Iyengar, R.; Bunyavanich, S.; Pandey, G. Clinical predictors of COVID-19 mortality. *medRxiv* **2020**. Available online: https://pubmed.ncbi.nlm.nih.gov/32511520/ (accessed on 11 July 2021).
12. Yao, H.; Zhang, N.; Zhang, R.; Duan, M.; Xie, T.; Pan, J.; Peng, E.; Huang, J.; Zhang, Y.; Xu, X.; et al. Severity Detection for the Coronavirus Disease 2019 (COVID-19) Patients Using a Machine Learning Model Based on the Blood and Urine Tests. *Front. Cell Dev. Biol.* **2020**, *8*, 683. Available online: https://www.ncbi.nlm.nih.gov/pmc/articles/PMC7411005/ (accessed on 11 June 2021). [CrossRef] [PubMed]
13. Alyasseri, Z.A.A.; Al-Betar, M.A.; Doush, I.A.; Awadallah, M.A.; Abasi, A.K.; Makhadmeh, S.N.; Alomari, O.A.; Abdulkareem, K.H.; Adam, A.; Damasevicius, R.; et al. *Review on COVID-19 Diagnosis Models Based on Machine Learning and Deep Learning Approaches. Expert Systems*; John Wiley and Sons Inc.: Hoboken, NJ, USA, 2021. Available online: https://www.ncbi.nlm.nih.gov/pmc/articles/PMC8420483/ (accessed on 11 June 2021).
14. Li, W.T.; Ma, J.; Shende, N.; Castaneda, G.; Chakladar, J.; Tsai, J.C.; Apostol, L.; Honda, C.O.; Xu, J.; Wong, L.M.; et al. Using machine learning of clinical data to diagnose COVID-19: A systematic review and meta-analysis. *BMC Med. Inform. Decis. Making* **2020**, *20*, 247. [CrossRef]

15. Guan, X.; Zhang, B.; Fu, M.; Li, M.; Yuan, X.; Zhu, Y.; Peng, J.; Guo, H.; Lu, Y. Clinical and inflammatory features based machine learning model for fatal risk prediction of hospitalized COVID-19 patients: Results from a retrospective cohort study. *Ann. Med.* **2021**, *53*, 257–266. [CrossRef] [PubMed]
16. Delafiori, J.; Navarro, L.C.; Siciliano, R.F.; de Melo, G.C.; Busanello, E.N.B.; Nicolau, J.C.; Sales, G.M.; de Oliveira, A.N.; Val, F.F.A.; de Oliveira, D.N.; et al. COVID-19 Automated Diagnosis and Risk Assessment through Metabolomics and Machine Learning. Analytical Chemistry. *Am. Chem. Soc.* **2021**, *93*, 2471–2479. [CrossRef]
17. Allam, M.; Cai, S.; Ganesh, S.; Venkatesan, M.; Doodhwala, S.; Song, Z.; Hu, T.; Kumar, A.; Heit, J.; COVID-19 Study Group. COVID-19 Diagnostics, Tools, and Prevention. *Diagnostics* **2020**, *10*, 409. [CrossRef]
18. Assaf, D.; Gutman, Y.; Neuman, Y.; Segal, G.; Amit, S.; Gefen-Halevi, S.; Shilo, N.; Epstein, A.; Mor-Cohen, R.; Biber, A.; et al. Utilization of machine-learning models to accurately predict the risk for critical COVID-19. *Intern. Emergency Med.* **2020**, *15*, 1435–1443. [CrossRef] [PubMed]
19. Naseem, M.; Akhund, R.; Arshad, H.; Ibrahim, M.T. Exploring the Potential of Artificial Intelligence and Machine Learning to Combat COVID-19 and Existing Opportunities for LMIC: A Scoping Review. *J. Primary Care & Community Health* **2020**, *11*, 215013272096363. [CrossRef]
20. Arga, K.Y. COVID-19 and the Futures of Machine Learning. *OMICS A J. Integr. Biol.* **2020**, *24*, 512–514. [CrossRef]
21. Majhi, R.; Thangeda, R.; Sugasi, R.P.; Kumar, N. Analysis and prediction of COVID-19 trajectory: A machine learning approach. *J. Public Aff.* **2020**, e2537. [CrossRef]
22. Van Der Schaar, M.; Alaa, A.M.; Floto, A.; Gimson, A.; Scholtes, S.; Wood, A.; McKinney, E.; Jarrett, D.; Lio, P.; Ercole, A. How artificial intelligence and machine learning can help healthcare systems respond to COVID-19. *Mach. Learn.* **2020**, *10*, 1–14. [CrossRef]
23. Das, A.K.; Mishra, S.; Saraswathy Gopalan, S. Predicting COVID-19 community mortality risk using machine learning and development of an online prognostic tool. *PeerJ* **2020**, *8*, e10083. [CrossRef]
24. Swapnarekha, H.; Behera, H.S.; Nayak, J.; Naik, B. Role of intelligent computing in COVID-19 prognosis: A state-of-the-art review. *Chaos Solitons Fractals* **2020**, *138*, 109947. [CrossRef]
25. Silva, L.; Figueiredo Filho, D. Using Benford's law to assess the quality of COVID-19 register data in Brazil. *J. Public Health* **2020**, *43*, 107–110. [CrossRef]
26. Lee, K.; Han, S.; Jeong, Y. COVID-19, flattening the curve, and Benford's law. *Phys. A Stat. Mech. Appl.* **2020**, *559*, 125090. [CrossRef] [PubMed]
27. Panorama Epidemiologico. Enfermedades No Transmisibles. Secretaría de Salud. 2018. Available online: https://epidemiologia.salud.gob.mx/gobmx/salud/documentos/pano-OMENT/Panorama_OMENT_2018.pdf (accessed on 17 November 2021).
28. Petrova, D.; Salamanca-Fernández, E.; Rodríguez Barranco, M.; Navarro Pérez, P.; Jiménez Moleón, J.; Sánchez, M. La obesidad como factor de riesgo en personas con COVID-19: Posibles mecanismos e implicaciones. *Atención Primaria* **2020**, *52*, 496–500. [CrossRef]
29. Monteagudo, D.E. La obesidad: Posibles mecanismos que explican su papel como factor de riesgo de la COVID-19. *Revista Cubana de Alimentación y Nutrición* **2020**, *30*, 12.
30. Pérez-Martínez, P.; Carrasco Sánchez, F.J.; Carretero Gómez, J.; Gómez-Huelgas, R. Resolviendo una de las piezas del puzle: COVID-19 y diabetes tipo 2. *Rev. Clin. Esp.* **2020**, *220*, 507–510. [CrossRef]
31. Giralt-Herrera, A.; Rojas-Velázquez, J.; Leiva-Enríquez, J.; Giralt-Herrera, A.; Rojas-Velázquez, J.; Leiva-Enríquez, J. Relación entre COVID-19 e Hipertensión Arterial. Scielo.sld.cu. Available online: http://scielo.sld.cu/scielo.php?pid=S1729-519X2020000200004&script=sci_arttext&tlng=en (accessed on 18 November 2020).
32. Di Castelnuovo, A.; Bonaccio, M.; Costanzo, S.; Gialluisi, A.; Antinori, A.; Berselli, N.; Blandi, V.; Bruno, R.; Guaraldi, G. Common cardiovascular risk factors and in-hospital mortality in 3,894 patients with COVID-19: Survival analysis and machine learning-based findings from the multicentre Italian CORIST Study. *Nutr. Metab. Cardiovasc. Dis.* **2020**, *30*, 1899–1913. [CrossRef]
33. De Souza, F.S.H.; Hojo-Souza, N.S.; Dos Santos, E.B.; Da Silva, C.M.; Guidoni, D.L. Predicting the disease outcome in COVID-19 positive patients through Machine Learning: A retrospective cohort study with Brazilian data. *Front. Artif. Intell.* **2021**, *4*, 579931. Available online: https://www.medrxiv.org/content/10.1101/2020.06.26.20140764v1 (accessed on 22 February 2021). [CrossRef] [PubMed]
34. Comunicado de Prensa No. 10. Coneval.org.mx. 2019. Available online: https://www.coneval.org.mx/SalaPrensa/Comunicadosprensa/Documents/2019/COMUNICADO_10_MEDICION_POBREZA_2008_2018.pdf (accessed on 22 February 2021).
35. Hopkins, J. Mortality Analyses-Johns Hopkins Coronavirus Resource Center. Johns Hopkins Coronavirus Resource Center. 2021. Available online: https://coronavirus.jhu.edu/data/mortality (accessed on 21 February 2021).
36. Cao, Y.; Hiyoshi, A.; Montgomery, S. COVID-19 case-fatality rate and demographic and socioeconomic influencers: Worldwide spatial regression analysis based on country-level data. *BMJ Open* **2020**, *10*, e043560. [CrossRef] [PubMed]

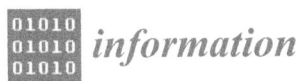

Article

HIV Patients' Tracer for Clinical Assistance and Research during the COVID-19 Epidemic (INTERFACE): A Paradigm for Chronic Conditions

Antonella Cingolani [1,2], Konstantina Kostopoulou [3], Alice Luraschi [1,4], Aristodemos Pnevmatikakis [3,*], Silvia Lamonica [1], Sofoklis Kyriazakos [3,5], Chiara Iacomini [1,4], Francesco Vladimiro Segala [2], Giulia Micheli [2], Cristina Seguiti [2], Stathis Kanavos [3], Alfredo Cesario [1,3], Enrica Tamburrini [1,2], Stefano Patarnello [2], Vincenzo Valentini [1,2,4] and Roberto Cauda [1,4]

[1] Fondazione Policlinico A. Gemelli IRCCS, 00168 Rome, Italy; antonella.cingolani@unicatt.it (A.C.); alice.luraschi@policlinicogemelli.it (A.L.); silvia.lamonica@policlinicogemelli.it (S.L.); chiara.iacomini@policlinicogemelli.it (C.I.); acesario@innovationsprint.eu (A.C.); enrica.tamburrini@unicatt.it (E.T.); vincenzo.valentini@policlinicogemelli.it (V.V.); roberto.cauda@policlinicogemelli.it (R.C.)
[2] Infectious Diseases Department, Università Cattolica del Sacro Cuore, 00168 Rome, Italy; fvsegala@gmail.com (F.V.S.); micheli93giulia@gmail.com (G.M.); cseguiti@gmail.com (C.S.); stefano.patarnello@gemelligenerator.it (S.P.)
[3] Innovation Sprint, 1200 Brussels, Belgium; kkostopoulou@innovationsprint.eu (K.K.); skyriazakos@innovationsprint.eu (S.K.); skanavos@innovationsprint.eu (S.K.)
[4] Gemelli Generator, Fondazione Policlinico A. Gemelli IRCCS, 00168 Rome, Italy
[5] BTECH, Department of Business Development and Technology, Aarhus University, 7400 Herning, Denmark
* Correspondence: apnevmatikakis@innovationsprint.eu

Citation: Cingolani, A.; Kostopoulou, K.; Luraschi, A.; Pnevmatikakis, A.; Lamonica, S.; Kyriazakos, S.; Iacomini, C.; Segala, F.V.; Micheli, G.; Seguiti, C.; et al. HIV Patients' Tracer for Clinical Assistance and Research during the COVID-19 Epidemic (INTERFACE): A Paradigm for Chronic Conditions. *Information* 2022, 13, 76. https://doi.org/10.3390/info13020076

Academic Editors: Sidong Liu, Cristián Castillo Olea and Shlomo Berkovsky

Received: 2 January 2022
Accepted: 28 January 2022
Published: 5 February 2022

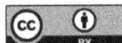

Copyright: © 2022 by the authors. Licensee MDPI, Basel, Switzerland. This article is an open access article distributed under the terms and conditions of the Creative Commons Attribution (CC BY) license (https://creativecommons.org/licenses/by/4.0/).

Abstract: The health emergency linked to the SARS-CoV-2 pandemic has highlighted problems in the health management of chronic patients due to their risk of infection, suggesting the need of new methods to monitor patients. People living with HIV/AIDS (PLWHA) represent a paradigm of chronic patients where an e-health-based remote monitoring could have a significant impact in maintaining an adequate standard of care. The key objective of the study is to provide both an efficient operating model to "follow" the patient, capture the evolution of their disease, and establish proximity and relief through a remote collaborative model. These dimensions are collected through a dedicated mobile application that triggers questionnaires on the basis of decision-making algorithms, tagging patients and sending alerts to staff in order to tailor interventions. All outcomes and alerts are monitored and processed through an innovative e-Clinical platform. The processing of the collected data aims into learning and evaluating predictive models for the possible upcoming alerts on the basis of past data, using machine learning algorithms. The models will be clinically validated as the study collects more data, and, if successful, the resulting multidimensional vector of past attributes will act as a digital composite biomarker capable of predicting HIV-related alerts. Design: All PLWH > 18 sears old and stable disease followed at the outpatient services of a university hospital (n = 1500) will be enrolled in the interventional study. The study is ongoing, and patients are currently being recruited. Preliminary results are yielding monthly data to facilitate learning of predictive models for the alerts of interest. Such models are learnt for one or two months of history of the questionnaire data. In this manuscript, the protocol—including the rationale, detailed technical aspects underlying the study, and some preliminary results—are described. Conclusions: The management of HIV-infected patients in the pandemic era represents a challenge for future patient management beyond the pandemic period. The application of artificial intelligence and machine learning systems as described in this study could enable remote patient management that takes into account the real needs of the patient and the monitoring of the most relevant aspects of PLWH management today.

Keywords: HIV; COVID-19; e-Clinical assistance; outcome prediction

1. Background

People living with HIV infection (PLWH), particularly those with immunodeficiency and immune dysregulation, may be at increased risk of morbidity and mortality during SARS-CoV-2 infection [1]. Although the literature data do not appear to be in complete agreement, several papers have documented an increased risk of severe disease and death associated with HIV cofactor during COVID-19 infection [2–5].

In Italy, the impact of the COVID-19 pandemic on National Health Service facilities has primarily involved infectious disease facilities, with potential consequences on HIV diagnosis, treatment, and prevention. The model for the management and control of HIV infection in Italy has been based, since the development of Law No. 135/90, on the central role of the infectious diseases' structures, through an articulation of care services in acute inpatient wards, day hospital structures, dedicated outpatient clinics for the taking charge and treatment, and integrated home care structures.

The results obtained by the entire care system dedicated to the treatment of PLWH risk being compromised by the impact of COVID-19 on the National Health Service, and in particular on the infectious diseases structures, which are central to the strategy of intervention and control of the new pandemic. The negative impact may involve both the provision of care in acute wards, in particular for people with newly diagnosed HIV and late presentation (AIDS presenters), as well as outpatient facilities for the care and management of chronic patients with stable HIV infection, with possible losses in follow-up and reduced continuum of care.

This scenario could persist in the continuation of the COVID-19 pandemic, resulting in serious harm to people living with HIV, as reported by global health agencies (WHO, UNAIDS) [6,7], the European Parliament, and the European Commission, which already pointed out a step back from the WHO 90-90-90 target and fear a strong risk of failure to meet the 2030 SDG targets, reminding governments of the importance of ensuring HIV care and prevention services even in these times of COVID-19 emergencies.

The "Istituto Superiore di Sanità" has drawn up a plan that foresees and encourages the use of telemedicine to allow hospital structures to use tele-consultation and remote management of chronic patients [8]. Tele-consultation and telemedicine in general are applications that allow, in these moments when travel is by definition limited, to monitor patients suffering from chronic pathologies, who need regular and constant care and control. This concept has been stressed also by international guidelines on the management of PLWH [9–12].

People living with HIV/AIDS (PLWHA) represent a typology of patients for whom telemedicine could, particularly in pandemic times, represent an extremely useful tool of support and clinical management [13–16]. People living with HIV today are people who have a life expectancy very similar to that of the general population, due to the extraordinary effect that antiretroviral therapies have produced on survival and on the reduction of HIV-related morbidity [17]. Nowadays, PLWHA patients face a chronic condition with all the consequences that this situation entails (symptoms, side effects of the drugs, management of adherence and quality of life, periodic supply of drugs, blood samples to check the tolerability of the drugs, any new clinical events that may occur, needing advice from other specialists, etc.).

Since the end of February 2020, the Fondazione Policlinico Gemelli continues to represent a reference center for the care of patients affected by COVID-19. For this reason, during these months the outpatients' clinics of the FPG that take care of patients with chronic pathologies have been able to provide services and visits only if mandatory, with inevitable repercussions on the management of chronicity in all its aspects.

With the persisting of pandemic restrictions, it is essential to find ways of managing these patients remotely to allow continuity of care that will inevitably not reflect what happened in pre-epidemic periods. Moreover, it seems to be crucial in this period, to quickly identify potential sources for spreading of SARS-CoV-2 diffusion and transmission among potentially high-risk population such as PLWHA. In addition, the pandemic experience has provided insight into how the pressure on the healthcare system from carefully selected patients affected by chronic diseases can be mitigated through the use of remote care systems without losing a proper doctor-patient interaction.

For these reasons, we designed a pilot study for PLWH with stable chronic disease, with the objective of creating an "integrated clinical assistance" through an efficient operating model to "follow" the patient, capture the evolution of his/her disease, provide assistance and care, and interact also to establish proximity and relief through a remote collaborative model. Here, we describe the entire protocol including rationale and design of the study, with particular regard to the technical description of the innovative aspects of integrated care inherent in the study itself. Moreover, some very preliminary results on the learning of models to predict alerts of interest are shown.

2. Methods
2.1. Study Design, Duration, and Setting

This is an interventional monocentric study. The first phase of the study has been based on the set up of a mobile application for both Android and iOS that can be downloaded on the patient smartphone. This app is set up with functionalities to support and achieve objectives such as health and quality of life monitoring, antiretroviral treatment adherence, and assessment of SARS-CoV-2 infection risk.

In a future phase, it is foreseen to connect data self-reported by using the application and the clinical data from the electronic reporting system of the hospital to provide the clinicians with an overview as complete as possible.

The different monitoring aspects of the system are shown in Figure 1 and include:

(1) Self-reported prescreening on symptoms and signs compatible with SARS-CoV-2 infection, possible access to healthcare facilities, possible results of swabs/serologies, and evaluation of hospitalization risk due to COVID-19, on the basis of selected self-reported stress tests.
(2) Specific self-reported aspects to monitor patients' life (quality of life, anxiety, depression, HIV-related symptoms, adherence to treatments) through triggered standardized questionnaires, to be filled in by patients at specific timepoints. Additional questionnaires will be then triggered according to patients' answers to the first generic questionnaire (EQ 5D-3L) identifying specific unmet needs, with a sequential approach based on a predefined algorithm. All reported outcomes, triggered or self-reported, will be always accessible on the app in a dedicated area, the "health diary", for patients and on a dedicated dashboard for physicians. Patients' self-reported data also generate tailored alerts on the basis of their actual needs and predefined scores in order to provide physicians with useful information for patient management.
(3) Important parameters for drug management (BMI, MDRD). These data will be calculated periodically on the basis of individual lab results and they will be used to adjust dose of drugs.
(4) Drug adherence is monitored through linkage of self-reported information on adherence with hospital pharmacy's refill data and laboratory results (plasma HIV/RNA).
(5) Periodic blood sample control through an alerting system of laboratory results that, in the case of abnormal values, will warn physicians via tailored alerts.
(6) Any new onset of symptoms/side effects: patients can report any symptoms/side effects on a specific area of the app, and this report will appear as an alert to the physician.
(7) Support tools for patients such as FAQs, User Guide, and disease-specific information.
(8) Notifications containing different kind of information and/or recommendations are automatically sent to patients on the basis of their answers to questionnaires, lab results, or drugs refill.
(9) An automated feedback system to the treating physician to highlight those situations that need attention. This includes self-reported symptoms (i.e., bothersome symptoms), any self-reported mental health issues, any changes in periodic laboratory tests,

any problems with adherence to antiretroviral therapy, and any symptoms or signs consistent with a risk of SARS-CoV-2 infection.

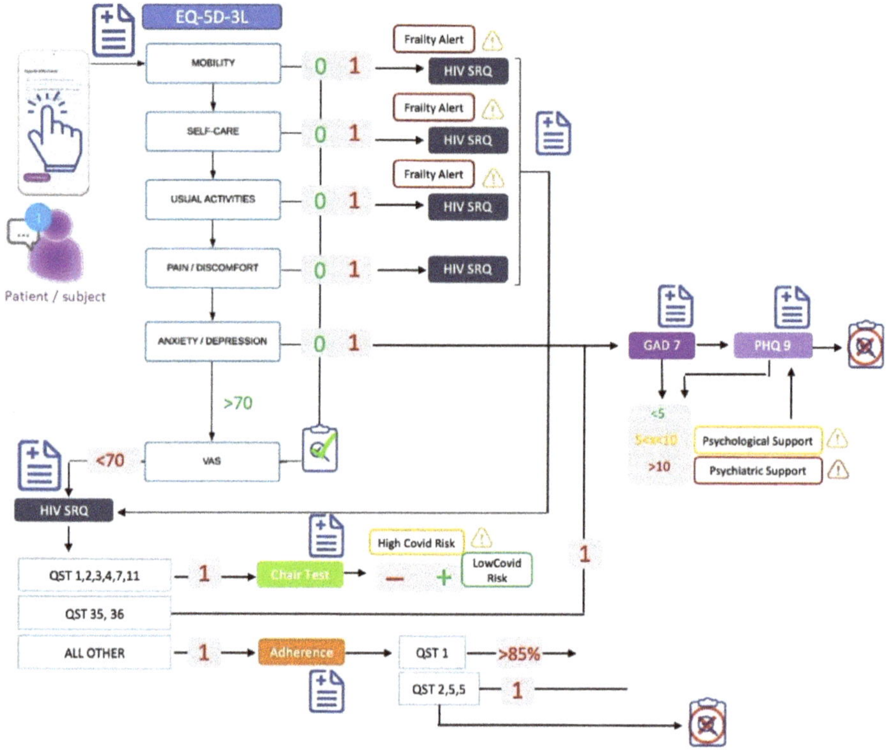

Figure 1. Questionnaires triggering system. The patient is sent a monthly notification to answer the EQ-5D-3L [18] questionnaire. If an alteration in any of the domains of the questionnaire is reported, the patient is automatically notified of a more specific questionnaire to which the altered domain refers: HIVSRQ [19], GAD-7 [20], PHQ9 [21]. If the EQ5D VAS is <70%, then all the above questionnaires are notified, including the treatment adherence questionnaire [22]. With regard to HIVSRQ, if symptoms compatible with SARS-CoV-2 infection are reported, the patient is asked for an in-depth investigation of COVID and risk of hospitalization (chair stress test, CST). In case of alteration to each questionnaire, a report of need for intervention is sent to the attending physician (psychological support, psychiatric support, intervention on symptoms, intervention on low adherence to ART, intervention on COVID-19 risk).

2.2. Study Population

All PLWHA, on antiretroviral therapy treated in Fondazione Policlinico Universitario "A. Gemelli" IRCCS (FPUAG IRCCS) of Rome, Italy, who will be considered eligible, will be enrolled and asked to install the app on their smartphone.

2.2.1. Inclusion Criteria

- Patients' age >18 years.
- Patients able to use apps and smartphone devices without any caregivers or, in the case of patient unable to use them, patients with caregiver able to use apps and smartphone devices.
- Patients able to provide informed consent.

2.2.2. Exclusion Criteria

- Patients not able to use smartphone devices and applications without the presence of caregivers.
- Recent diagnosis of HIV infection (<3 months).
- Any unstable clinical condition requiring hospitalization.

2.3. Data Collection

The study is based on standardized data collection procedures able to efficiently process large amounts of data and provide the physicians with a panel of useful information to evaluate patients' health conditions, quality of life, mental health, how HIV impacts their QoL, and to monitor eventual worsening.

Five different data sources were used for data collection: 4 internal to the electronic data reporting system of the hospital and 1 external (Healthentia app).

From the electronic data reporting system of the hospital, we defined eight structured variables (laboratory exams, drugs refill from pharmacy, weight, height, gender, study degree, civil status).

A standard ETL procedure was developed for the extraction of such data using SAS Institute software analytics tool and SAS® Vyia® (Cary, NC 27513, USA), which refreshes on daily basis in order to continuously include both new enrolled patients and new data from patients already registered to the app (new laboratory exams, drugs refill for pharmacy, etc.).

Hospital data are integrated with real-world data coming from the Healthentia app (Innovation Sprint Sprl, Brussels, Belgium), through which will be collected symptoms potentially related to SARS-CoV-2 infection, symptoms related to HIV, adherence to treatments, quality of life, anxiety, and depression. The collected data are already outlined in Figure 1. They are collected via questionnaires (validated and custom ones) and during a functional test.

We employ validated questionnaires for HIV-related symptoms through the questionnaire "HIV Symptom Rating Questionnaire (HIVSRQ)", health-related quality of life through the questionnaires "EQ-5D-3L" (comprising the following five dimensions: mobility, self-care, usual activities, pain/discomfort, and anxiety/depression), anxiety through "General Anxiety Disorder-7 (GAD-7)", and depression through "Patient Health Questionnaire-9 (PHQ-9)".

We employ custom (non-validated) questionnaires to collect adherence to antiretroviral therapy, SARS-CoV-2 infection assessment (tracking of symptoms related to SARS-CoV2 infection for its early detection), the result of a swab test, and the SARS-CoV-2 vaccine.

Finally, we employ the chair stand test (functional test), during which the oxygen saturation (one of the most important parameters to assess the risk of hospitalization for patients with SARS-CoV-2) is monitored.

Each questionnaire mentioned above has many questions, i.e., results to many attributes of the data. The question of which of the attributes is of high importance in predicting the outcomes of interest is addressed by analyzing the decisions of the learnt models in Section 4.3.

Data will be collected for a duration of 2 years starting from 1 January 2021. About 1500 patients currently followed up at the Infectious Diseases Clinic met the inclusion criteria. These patients represent the share of patients without urgent clinical needs or whose periodic medical examination can be carried out every 4–6 months.

On the basis of previous experiences on such a kind of studies, we found that up to 30% of the patients could be interested in being enrolled in such a study and using Healthentia. As such, with expected recruited population of 450 patients, we aimed at analyzing at least 220 patients who actively used the app in order to accurately describe our recruited population with a confidence interval of 95% and margin of error of 5%.

Unfortunately, the pandemic has only allowed us to recruit 61 patients at this point, since the beginning of the study in January 2021. Recruitment is still active though, with the latest patients being enrolled in November 2021 in an ongoing process. The enrolment process across time and some demographic information about the study population is given in Figure 2.

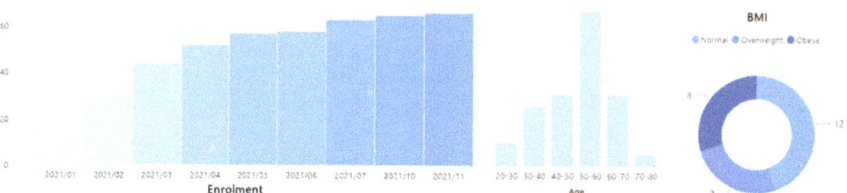

Figure 2. Enrolment of patients in the first year of the study and their age and body mass index distribution.

2.4. Workflow Structure

INTERFACE is an interventional study with a purpose of collecting, as previously described, real-world data (RWD) regarding patient outcomes and parameters. In order to be enrolled to the study, patients have to sign an informed consent form declaring their awareness about data sharing for research purpose or use the eConsent process available on the app. Patients are enrolled on the study by downloading the application for free from the AppStore or Google Play, installing it on their own smartphone and registering. Patients can retire themselves from the study by uninstalling the application without any formal communication, and they can obtain the definitive elimination of collected data at any moment.

Data flow from the Healthentia app to a protected Microsoft Azure Server cloud environment where Healthentia SaaS Solution is hosted by Innovation Sprint, and there is a point-to-point cryptographic encryption of the data that makes it impossible for third parties to read the information in transit in clear text. FPUAG IRCCS, as the data controller with the right of access, use, and management of data for research purposes, has access to Innovation Sprint's servers.

The study is conducted in the framework of Gemelli Generator Real-World Data facility (G2 RWD), the innovative research center of FPUAG IRCSS. Within the Gemelli Generator Real-World Data (G2 RWD) architecture, INTERFACE data collected using Healthentia will be integrated with clinical data and stored in a dedicated research Data Mart (i.e., organized subsets of data on a specific area of knowledge) in FPUAG IRCCS servers. In coherence with G2 RWD roles, if necessary, selected supervisors will be authorized to access the pseudo-anonymized data and identify patients for eventual clinical needs according to the collected data.

2.5. Efficacy Indicators

In order to evaluate the effectiveness of this project, after 2 years, we will consider the following indicators:

1. Proportion, characteristics, and cofactors of self-reported outcomes and changes in them according to the epidemic situation and during the time of the study.
2. Proportion of clinical intervention provided following alert messages received.
3. Proportion of unmet needs as generated by patients' reported outcomes.
4. Proportion of intervention on drug regimen modification according to parameters recorded.
5. Number of PLWHA with self-reported symptoms/signs of COVID-19 who can be correctly and timely allocated to different in-hospital access.
6. Prevalence of PLWHA regularly followed as outpatients with confirmed COVID-19.

3. Healthentia e-Clinical Environment

For the purposes of INTERFACE, a very comprehensive and adaptive e-Clinical environment, provided by the partner company Innovation Sprint, has been customized to meet the needs of INTERFACE protocol. The e-Clinical environment is based on Healthentia solution, which facilitates clinical trial optimization, accelerates trial processes, reduces failure rates, and validates drug/intervention efficacy and effectiveness with RWD insights. Healthentia is a Class I Medical Device with CE mark, a medical decision support software intended for monitoring of non-vital parameters to support decision making during clinical trials, according to RWD gathered from patients taking part in the clinical investigation.

Healthentia extends the use of traditional electronic patient-reported outcomes (ePRO)/electronic clinical outcomes assessment (eCOA) applications by adding lifestyle, behavioral, and health-related data collected from smartphones and internet of things (IoT) devices. Applying artificial intelligence (AI) and machine learning techniques on these data, one can discover behavioral biomarkers and cluster patients into behavioral phenotypes, which allows the activation of smart services for the prediction of clinical outcomes, the generation of prevention alarms, and the linking of phenotypes with intervention efficacy. Furthermore, on the basis of reported outcomes, the AI module is able to generate automatic alerts in the case of adverse events. These automatic and prevention alarms support decision making by the investigator during clinical trial for the benefit of the individual patient's health. The main components that are utilized for the purposes of the INTERFACE study are:

ePRO/eCOA—The ePRO/eCOA component is responsible for the communication with the mobile application that runs in iOS and Android devices. The component has all functionalities and services that are consumed by the smartphone app via Healthentia API. The Healthentia app interacts with the ePRO/eCOA component to allow the patient from the comfort of their home to:

- fill in health-related and quality of life questionnaires from their device;
- log events for symptoms, school/work absence, treatment, or hospitalization, etc.;
- receive ad hoc messages from the system or the investigator of a study;
- receive automatic messages from the system or the investigator of a study;
- receive notification for filling in questionnaires or medication reminders;
- find protocol/treatment or device-related information;
- contact the investigator;
- use the chatbot functionality for questions and virtual coaching.

The ePRO/eCOA component also includes the questionnaire editor and scheduler. The questionnaire editor allows the investigator to create or edit questionnaires that will be delivered to the patients. The editor provides the functionality to create complicated questionnaires with advanced routing between questions, and even between questionnaires as well as multiple types of questions and user interfaces, e.g., single, multiple, image selection, location-based, etc. The questionnaire scheduler is the functionality that is used by the investigators to create rules for the automatic submission of questionnaires to specific recipients. These rules may include the registration date, or even the answers from the subject and the auto-tagging of a subject into a certain category.

Smart services—Further to the currently supported features of Healthentia, i.e., collecting data from patients, the wealth of information collected is used in real time by the Healthentia machine learning (ML) services to provide useful insights for clinical endpoints. On the basis of the patients' data, models are learned both for predictive and generative purposes. Predictive models can estimate future clinical outcomes from current and past data. Once such predictors of outcomes are validated, they are considered biomarkers for the particular outcomes at hand. Unlike traditional biomarkers, these models form composite digital biomarkers by non-linearly combining various information attributes to predict the wanted outcome. Such predictive models are shown in Section 4.3, but the results there are considered preliminary, and the models are not yet validated into biomarkers. Generative models are built by modelling patient clusters and can be used to generate synthetic data. Different clustering algorithms can be used to derive the clusters, which can then be validated by verifying that all patients in a cluster exhibit some common outcome. When this is verified, the cluster models are validated into phenotypes. In Figure 3, the lifecycle of RWD in Healthentia is described.

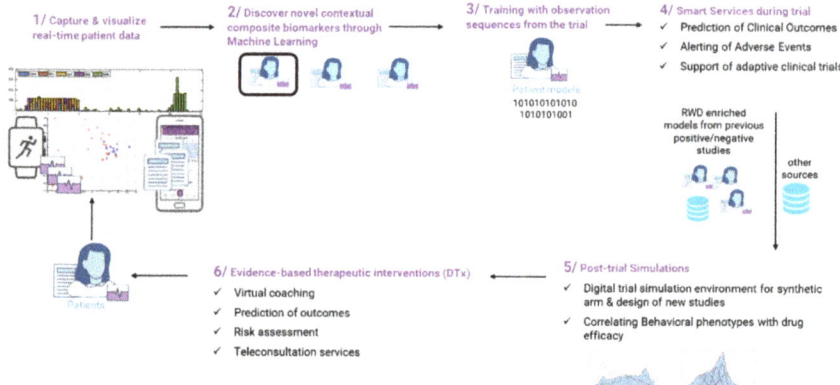

Figure 3. The lifecycle of RWD in Healthentia.

The lifecycle of RWD in Healthentia can be described in six steps. In step 1, data are captured and visualized at real-time basis. In step 2, digital composite biomarkers are discovered, and patients are clustered using ML algorithms. For this purpose, physiological, psychological, and sociological data are used. In step 3, training of the selected patient model is performed by means of observational sequences from the trial in order to allow smart services to be applied, such as prediction of clinical outcomes and alarms (see step 4). At the end of a study, the investigator can further use the derived patients' models to run in silico trials (see step 5), while the enriched models can be utilized for digital therapeutic (DTx) services, such as the orchestration of virtual coaching messages.

In the case of the INTERFACE study, patients will be grouped in phenotypes on the basis of ML processing of the RWD, and a digital composite biomarker will be derived, consisting of several dimensions, for each of the data points captured, e.g., questionnaire scores and scales. This digital composite biomarker will then be optimized by identifying which of the dimensions will have significant impact to the endpoints, and when an AI training process is followed, it will be used to predict future outcomes. The digital composite biomarker can then be used for future in silico studies and/or driving DTx decisions for HIV patients.

4. Data Analysis

The sample will be described using a descriptive analysis with the aim of analyzing how health conditions, mental health, and quality of life changes during the use of Healthentia.

Qualitative variables will be summarized with percentage frequency tables by analyzing questionnaires filled in by patients.

Quantitative variables will be described using the minimum, maximum, mean, median, standard deviation, and interquartile range; then, through histogram and box plot, we will see the shape of the data distribution. Normality of continuous variables will be checked using the Kolmogorov–Smirnov test.

Inferential techniques, defined after a data exploration phase, will be then used with the aim of implementing a Guardian Bot, a software able to automatically detect earlier predictors of a worsening trend of the main disease or of SARS-CoV-2 infection occurrence. In this manuscript, we only present preliminary results regarding the construction of a machine learning model for predicting the alerts shown in Figure 1.

4.1. Interface Integration with Generator Real World Data

INTERFACE will leverage on the overall architecture and capabilities of Gemelli GENERATOR Real-World Data facility (G2 RWD), the innovative research center of FPUAG IRCCS, with the principal aim to transform data and information into actionable knowledge while fully respecting the privacy, data integrity, and intellectual property for the benefit of all.

Indeed, if the main purpose of INTERFACE is totally in line with G2 RWD objectives: the exploitation of G2 RWD framework represents a quality guarantee for INTERFACE both in terms of data collection, quality, and analysis and of data privacy and protection. Actually, G2 RWD architecture has been approved by the Local Ethical Committee and widely used in FPUAG IRCCS with good results [23].

The architecture and methods that G2 RWD will contribute for INTERFACE are based on:

- the creation and update of a dedicated Data Mart (organized subsets of data on a specific area of knowledge) in which all data collected both for the app and from the electronic data reporting system of the hospital are correctly stored and organized, in order to be easily accessible and understandable for physicians;
- Mathematical and statistical tools available, ranging from the traditional qualitative-quantitative analysis techniques to the more advanced artificial intelligence algorithms, to provide new modeling hypotheses to be tested and validated with clinicians for research purposes;
- The data architecture, defined to provide the highest degree of protection, in accordance with all GDPR and security requirements.

4.2. Data Privacy and Data Protection

All privacy matters are analyzed with the Policlinico Gemelli Data Protection Officer (DPO) so that every G2 RWD study will be compliant with GDPR Italian and European directives and regulation (EU Directive 2016/679 and under Italian Laws: Decreto Legislativo 196/2003, Decreto Legislativo 101 2018, Autorizzazione Generale Garante 9/2016). The data architecture that supports RWD studies has been designed to provide the highest degree of protection, in accordance with all GDPR and security requirements. In this respect, RWD provides "protection by design" in each step of the process.

4.3. Learning Models to Predict Alerts

The questionnaire pipeline of Figure 1 is triggered once per month, and depending on the answers of the patients, the maximum number of questions answered is 255. When there is no need to answer some questions, they are assigned to the default "no problem" state. As a result of the answers given, four types of alerts might be issued:

- Frailty alert, binary (OK, alert);
- HIV symptoms alert, binary (OK, alert);
- Adherence alert, binary (OK, alert); and,
- Psychological/psychiatric support alert, tristate (OK, psychological, psychiatric).

Given the current state of the patient, i.e., the answers to the questionnaires of the current month, the alerts are fully determined. The machine learning (ML) goal of INTERFACE is to predict the alarms given the patient history. The history is determined as the questionnaire answers of part months, and it can span one month (predict the alarms in the current month given the questionnaire answers of the previous month) or more. The input vectors comprise the individual answers in a history window of n months, i.e., of $255 \cdot n$ attributes, $n = 1, 2, \ldots$, while the output vectors comprise of the four attributes for the four alerts.

The patients answer the questionnaires on a monthly basis. Thus, a patient being n months in the INTERFACE study provides $N - n$ pairs of input and output vectors. Since there are not a lot of patients in the study, especially for long durations, large values of the history window drastically reduce the number of available vectors, albeit they increase the actual information each vector caries. The lack of adequate vectors to learn ML models is a typical situation where vectors are contributed on a monthly or even weekly basis.

Although the alerts are not really rare, raising them is not the common state. Hence, the state of the output attributes is far from balanced, with the majority of the vectors indicating "no problem" and only few of them resulting to alerts. Thus, the ML problem at hand is a heavily imbalanced one, and therefore the accuracy is not a good performance metric for the predictors. We employ balanced accuracy [24] instead.

The lack of data and the imbalance nature of the model learning task make it a particularly hard to tackle. The situation is depicted in Table 1. The number of available vectors (198 for $n = 1$ or 149 for $n = 2$) forbids the use of neural network [25] predictors of any usable depth. Training of random forests [26] though a few estimators is possible, and this is the selected ML algorithm training our INTERFACE predictive models.

Table 1. Volume of data per history depth and outcome state.

Attribute	History (Months)	Counts per State		
		#1	#2	#3
Frailty	1	186	13	N/A
	2	143	6	N/A
HIV symptoms	1	139	60	N/A
	2	100	49	N/A
Adherence	1	190	9	N/A
	2	141	8	N/A
Psychological, psychiatric	1	163	25	11
	2	124	18	7

N/A: not applicable.

For the same reason, the split of the available vectors in training, validation, and testing sets is not practical. Instead, we train and validate the models using k-fold cross-validation [27]. We split the data in k folds of size 5 each (39 for $n = 1$ or 29 for $n = 2$) and use $k - 1$ of them for training and 1 for validation. We repeat the training 30 times for each fold selection and select the highest balanced accuracy of the 10 as the balanced accuracy of the fold. We average the balanced accuracies of the $k - 1$ folds to obtain the balanced accuracy for one configuration of the random forest. We vary the number of estimators as different configurations and select the best of them all.

The number of estimators (trees) of the random forest are varied in the training. The tree creation parameters are as follows: bootstrap samples are used instead of the complete dataset when building trees, randomly selected at consecutive training sessions. The quality of tree node splits is measured using Gini impurity and best split is sought for considering the square root of the total number of features. Tree nodes are expanded until they contain a single sample, with the number of leaf nodes being unlimited. Even though the different class population is not balanced, no attempt has been made to assign different weights to the different classes.

The average training balanced accuracy for one month is 92%, while for two months it is the perfect 100%. Such a training gives us no generalization confidence however, and therefore we proceed with the k-fold cross-validation scheme discussed above. The resulting average balance accuracy across all four outcomes as a function of the number of random forest estimators is shown in Figure 4. Note that the maximum performance for two months of history generally increased for a larger number of estimators, while for one month, the algorithm found an optimum point at a small number of estimators. The reason that the cross-validation did not result in better results for two months of history is because of the fewer vectors available, with the problem at hand having double the features.

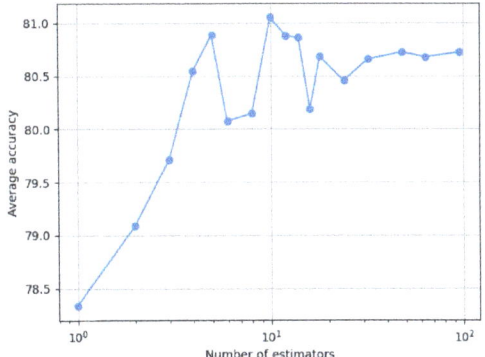 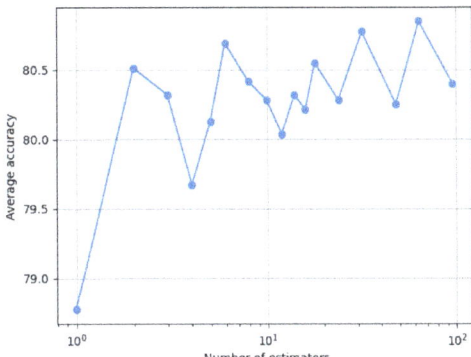

Figure 4. Balanced accuracy for the RF classifiers averaged over all four outcomes as a function of the number of estimators for one (**left**) and two months (**right**) memory.

The decisions of the classifier are analyzed using Shapley Additive explanations (SHAP) analysis [28]. SHAP analysis is applied on every decision, yielding the effect of each attribute in the feature vector towards a positive or negative prediction. These attributes are questions in the different questionnaires, and thus the SHAP analysis actually yields the on average most important questions to ask for each outcome. This is shown in Figure 5.

Two notes are in order. Firstly, the ranking of the questions shown in Figure 5 is averaged across all the population. It is interesting to discover how this ranking varies when considering the different individuals. Unfortunately, there are too few different patients with many decisions (many months in the study) to conduct this analysis just yet. This brings us to the second note: Since the data we currently have at hand are limited, we cannot actually claim that the most important factors from a clinical viewpoint are found. Instead, at this point the analysis is more of a machine learning rather than of clinical importance. That being said, we observe that the overall health question of the ED-5D questionnaire is always high in importance. The frailty and adherence alerts seem to have a very large dependency on their most important attribute, the rest being quite lower, while the rest of the alarms have a more even dependency on the different attributes. Most of the important factors for the psychological/psychiatric alarm fall in the anxiety/pessimism categories.

Finally, the most important factors for the decisions based on one month history are compared to those based on two months in Figure 6. The attributes whose names finished with a "-1" were those of the oldest month. Note that many of the most important attributes were from the oldest month, with the current one not ranking high, such as the PHQ sleep, preference to die or lack of interest, or the GAD ability to control worries or to sit up. On the other hand, in some cases, the attributes of the two months of history appeared in pairs, such as the most important pair of EQ_5D health of the previous and this month or the EQ_5D pain.

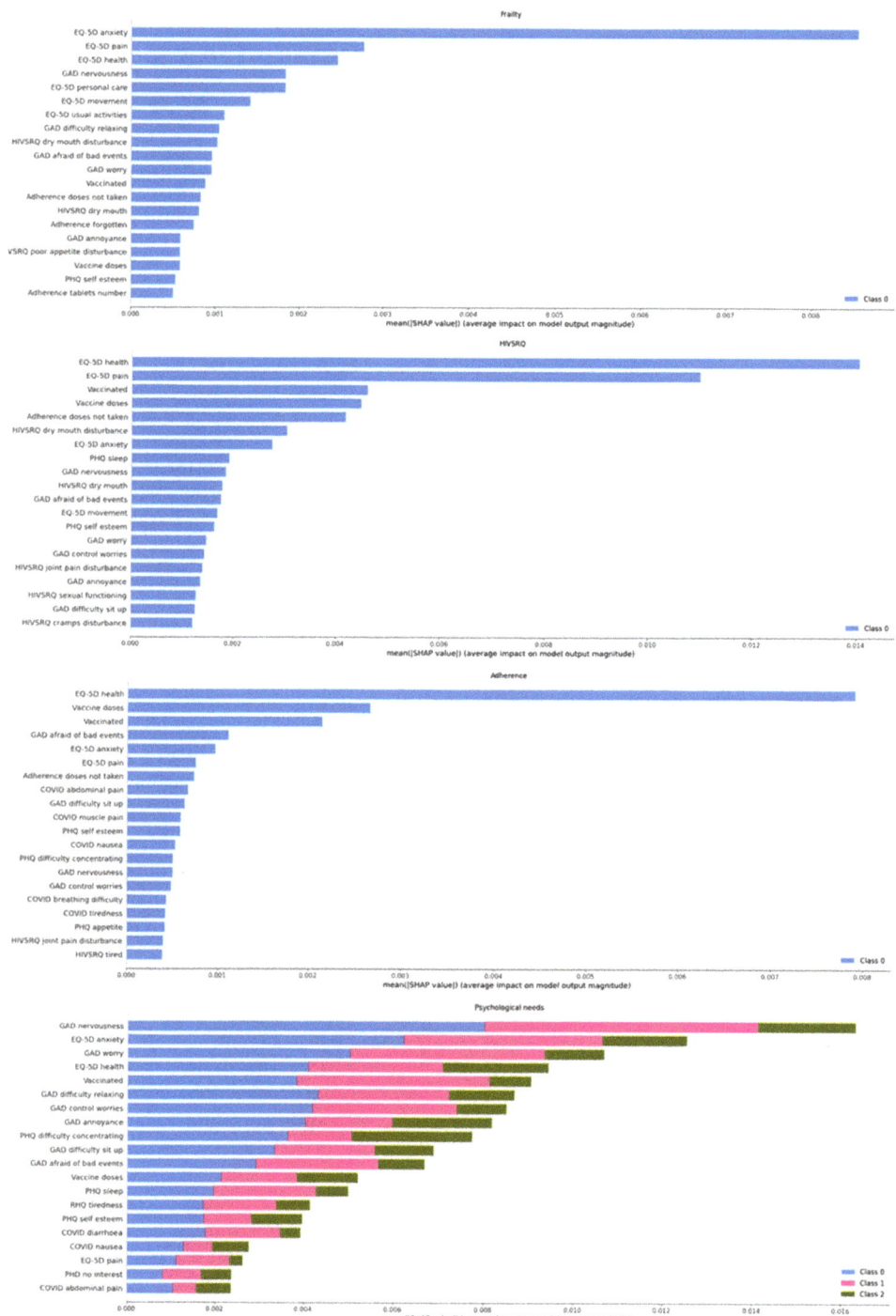

Figure 5. SHAP analysis of the classifier decisions to obtain the most important attributes affecting the decisions of either positive or negative outcomes.

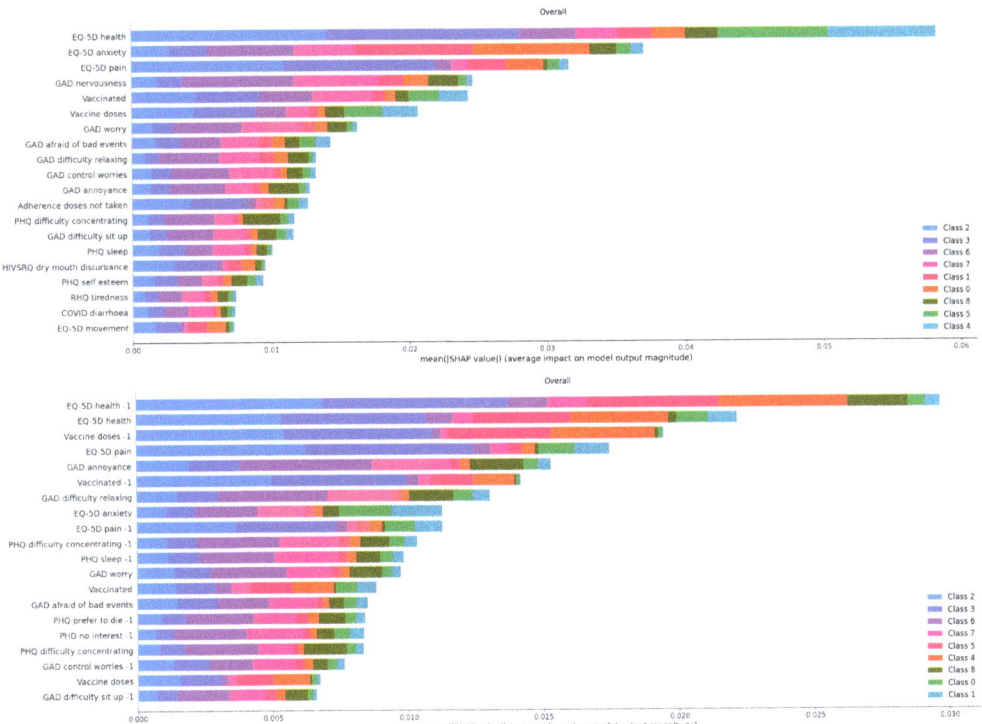

Figure 6. Comparison of the most important factors of the prediction (across all outcomes) for one month history (**top**) and two months history (**bottom**).

5. Ethical Aspects

The protocol has been approved by Local Ethical Committee (Protocol n 3436).

6. Discussion

During the COVID-19 pandemic, medical care for PLWHA is at risk of being compromised, calling into question the excellent results achieved in this field. The main scientific societies have produced guidelines suggesting how to ensure an adequate standard of care during this phase, promoting different models of care involving tools such as telemedicine [29,30].

Moreover, during the COVID-19 pandemic, machine learning and artificial intelligence systems are being used increasingly more accurately to optimize the care of people, identify predictive factors for the diagnosis and prognosis of the disease itself, and for the monitoring of mental health [31–34].

In the protocol described here, we propose a study based on the integration of telemedicine and telemonitoring with a standardized approach translating the huge amount of data collected on the day-to-day experience, integrating with historical health data, into useful insight and medical practices based on patients' experience and lessons learned by the artificial intelligence approach. In more detail, the system is expected to improve clinical decision making by providing physicians with additional data about patient needs and behaviors. For example, it may help clinicians to detect mood disturbances that do not impair patient daily activities, such as persistent depressive disorder. The system is indeed presenting to every recruited patient validated questionnaires for depression screening. In turn, in our system, these questionnaires are designed to trigger specific alerts that are then displayed directly to the attention of the clinician, enabling them, eventually, to refer the target patient to mental health services. We thus believe that our system will help clinicians to assess mental health issues in people living with HIV during the COVID-19 pandemic. Alternatively, when clinical data from the electronic reporting system of the hospital will be integrated, the system is designed to draw to the physician attention altered lab results directly on his/her smartphone, empowering the clinician, even in the outpatient setting, to act promptly in case of major disturbances. A final example of how we expect our system to improve clinical care is adherence to ARV therapy, which is, in our view, a substantial challenge during the present pandemic. This will be possible by selected questionnaires (able to trigger specific "low adherence" alerts to the doctor's attention), along with drawing to the clinician's attention the latest results of patient's viral load. Moreover, what has been demonstrated, even if only preliminarily, in the predictive model on future alert detection, suggests that such a model may be of fundamental importance in optimizing the clinical management of PLWH. The possibility of detecting problems related to mental health or adherence to treatment, for example, may allow the prediction of a tailored management of the patient with consequent optimization of resources. For instance, we have already observed that several mental health issues have been identified among the enrolled patients and we believe that this evidence could be a useful tool to draw attention to the need to provide patients with a more effective support at this regard.

It has been reported that telemedicine is variably accepted by patients, precisely because of the risk of "depersonalization" that such a tool may carry [35]. Moreover, in recent years, the attention of research and the HIV patient community is increasingly focused on what is called the "fourth 90", i.e., everything that concerns the global health status of patients, their quality of life, and their feeling [35]. For these reasons, developing an e-health tool that complements but does not replace care, and that focuses on what is defined as "patients reported outcomes", could address multiple unmet needs that remote care of HIV patients has not yet solved.

It has been reported that the adoption of remote healthcare has exposed critical gaps in access, such as socioeconomic disparities that may prevent many vulnerable persons from benefiting from telehealth innovations, namely, defined as "digital divide" [36]. In order to mitigate this problem, the present study will make use of strategies both inherent in the product (easy access modes, user guide, explanatory videos, etc.) and strategies to involve the community of patients for the support of people with different social or educational frailties.

The difficulties potentially encountered by PLWHA during the pandemic are also shared with patients suffering from other chronic diseases. In our opinion, this study could represent a model of integrated management also for other chronic pathologies such as oncological pathologies for two fundamental reasons: Firstly, because oncology has long paid relevant attention to the aspects reported directly by patients in terms of quality of life, symptoms, experience with the care system, etc., leading to consider PROs as potential hard outcomes in the design of clinical trials [37]. Secondly, because the oncological patient presents many aspects of linkage to the care center that are very similar to what is reported for PLWHA in terms of continuity of care and "personalization" of care. Finally, the study is beginning to yield enough monthly data to facilitate learning of predictive models for the alerts of interest. Such models are learnt for one or two months of history of the questionnaire data. No attempt has yet been carried out to integrate with the hospital data.

7. Conclusions

The development of such an e-health system may respond to clinical care needs for a specific type of chronicity such as HIV infection. In particular, in this COVID-19 pandemic period, such a system can be an important tool for managing the quality of life of the HIV patient. The COVID-19 pandemic is having a deleterious impact on the physical and, above all, mental health of the chronic population and also on the HIV-infected population [38], and the identification of tools capable of identifying physical and mental health problems and producing interventions tailored to the specific needs of the patient represents a significant improvement in the standard of care for people with HIV, even in the absence of physical access to the reference healthcare facilities. Moreover, it can represent a simple and widely useful system to perform a prescreening for chronic patients during the COVID-19 epidemic in order to prevent potential transmission clusters within the hospital as much as possible.

Early evidence that the prediction of the alerts of interest can be made is given. As on the one side, the study yields more data points, facilitating more training and the inclusion of more months of history, and on the other side, the hospital data augment the data attributes at hand, we expect the prediction to become more accurate. Upon reaching this point, the SHAP analysis of the decisions will yield clinically significant results for the importance of the different attributes. Subsequent development of the study involves the effect of applying such a machine learning system on the health indicators shown in the methods, in order to assess how far such a system can be applied in increasingly advanced chronicity management.

Author Contributions: Conceptualization, A.C. (Antonella Cingolani), K.K., A.L., A.P., S.K. (Sofoklis Kyriazakos), A.C. and S.P.; data curation, K.K., A.P., S.L., C.I. and S.K. (Stathis Kanavos); formal analysis, K.K., S.K. (Sofoklis Kyriazakos) and C.I.; funding acquisition, A.C. (Antonella Cingolani) and S.P.; investigation, A.C. (Antonella Cingolani), A.L., S.L., F.V.S., G.M., C.S. and S.K. (Stathis Kanavos); methodology, K.K., A.L., A.P., S.K. (Sofoklis Kyriazakos), C.I. and S.P.; project administration, S.L.; resources, A.C. (Antonella Cingolani), S.L., F.V.S., C.S. and S.P.; software, K.K., A.L., A.P., S.K. (Sofoklis Kyriazakos) and C.I.; supervision, A.C. (Antonella Cingolani), S.P., V.V. and R.C.; validation, K.K., A.L., S.K. (Sofoklis Kyriazakos) and C.I.; visualization, A.P., E.T., V.V. and R.C.; writing—original draft, A.C. (Antonella Cingolani), K.K., A.L. and A.P.; writing—review and editing, A.C. (Antonella Cingolani), K.K., A.P., S.K. (Sofoklis Kyriazakos), A.C. (Alfredo Cesario), E.T., S.P., V.V. and R.C. All authors have read and agreed to the published version of the manuscript.

Funding: This research received no external funding.

Institutional Review Board Statement: The study was conducted according to the guidelines of the Declaration of Helsinki and approved by the Institutional Review Board (or Ethics Committee) of Università Cattolica S. Cuore, protocol ID 3436.

Informed Consent Statement: Informed consent was obtained from all subjects involved in the study.

Data Availability Statement: Data available on request due to restrictions for privacy. The data presented in this study is available on request from the corresponding author. The data is not publicly available due to privacy restrictions.

Acknowledgments: The authors acknowledge Nadia Cerasaro, Silvia Parise, Anna Iannuzzi, Anna Bianchelli, and Maria Grazia Del Moro for the support as research nurses; Elena Visconti, Simona Di Giambenedetto, and Domenico Faliero as treating physicians; and all the patients involved.

Conflicts of Interest: The authors declare no conflict of interest.

References

1. Ho, H.E.; Peluso, M.J.; Margus, C.; Matias Lopes, J.P.; He, C.; Gaisa, M.M.; Osorio, G.; Aberg, J.A.; Mullen, M.P. Clinical outcomes and immunologic characteristics of Covid-19 in people with HIV. *J. Infect. Dis.* **2020**, *223*, 403–408. [CrossRef] [PubMed]
2. Bhaskaran, K.; Rentsch, C.T.; MacKenna, B.; Schultze, A.; Mehrkar, A.; Bates, C.J.; Eggo, R.M.; Morton, C.E.; Bacon, S.C.; Inglesby, P.; et al. HIV infection and COVID-19 death: A population-based cohort analysis of UK primary care data and linked national death registrations within the OpenSAFELY platform. *Lancet HIV* **2021**, *8*, e24–e32. [CrossRef]
3. Boulle, A.; Davies, M.-A.; Hussey, H.; Ismail, M.; Morden, E.; Vundle, Z.; Zweigenthal, V.; Mahomed, H.; Paleker, M.; Pienaar, D.; et al. Risk factors for COVID-19 death in a population cohort study from the Western cape province, South Africa. *Clin. Infect. Dis.* **2021**, *73*, e2005–e2015.
4. Tesoriero, J.M.; Swain, C.E.; Pierce, J.L.; Zamboni, L.; Wu, M.; Holtgrave, D.R.; Gonzalez, C.J.; Udo, T.; Morne, J.E.; Malloyet, R.H.; et al. Elevated COVID-19 outcomes among persons living with diagnosed HIV infection in New York state: Results from a population-level match of HIV, COVID-19, and hospitalization databases. *JAMA Netw Open.* **2021**, *4*, e2037069. [CrossRef] [PubMed]

5. Geretti, A.M.; Stockdale, A.J.; Kelly, S.H.; Cevik, M.; Collins, S.; Waters, L.; Villa, G.; Docherty, A.; Harrison, E.M.; Turtle, L.; et al. Outcomes of COVID-19 related hospitalization among people with HIV in the ISARIC WHO clinical characterization protocol (UK): A prospective observational study. *Clin. Infect. Dis.* **2021**, *7*, 2095–2106. [CrossRef]
6. UNAIDS. New Modelling Shows COVID-19 Should Not Be a Reason for Delaying the 2030 Deadline for Ending AIDS as a Public Health Threat. Available online: https://www.unaids.org/en/resources/presscentre/featurestories/2020/december/20201214_covid19-2030-deadline-for-ending-aids (accessed on 1 January 2022).
7. Lamontagne, E.; Doan, T.; Howell, S.; Yakusik, A.; Baral, S.; Santos, G.-M.; Ackerman, B.; Wallach, S.; Arreola, S.; Holloway, I.W.; et al. COVID-19 pandemic increases socioeconomic vulnerability of LGBTI+ communities and their susceptibility to HIV. In Proceedings of the AIDS 2020, Virtual, 6–10 July 2020.
8. Rapporto ISS COVID19 12/20. Indicazioni ad Interim per Servizi Assistenziali di Telemedicina Durante L'emergenza Sanitaria COVID-19. Available online: https://www.iss.it/rapporti-covid-19/-/asset_publisher/btw1J82wtYzH/content/rapporto-iss-covid-19-n.-12-2020-indicazioni-ad-interim-per-servizi-assistenziali-di-telemedicina-durante-l-emergenza-sanitaria-covid-19.-versione-del-13-aprile-2020 (accessed on 1 January 2022).
9. DHHS. Interim Guidance for COVID-19 and Persons with HIV. Available online: https://clinicalinfo.hiv.gov/en/guidelines/covid-19-and-persons-hiv-interim-guidance/interim-guidance-covid-19-and-persons-hiv (accessed on 1 January 2022).
10. BHIVA Guidance for the Management of Adults with HIV on Antiretroviral Treatment (ART) during the Coronavirus Pandemic. Available online: https://www.bhiva.org/file/5f56057450cc3/BHIVA-interim-ART-guidelines-COVID-19.pdf (accessed on 1 January 2022).
11. Intensive Care Society (ICS) and British HIV Association (BHIVA) Statement on Considerations for Critical Care for People with HIV during COVID-19. Available online: https://www.bhiva.org/updated-ICS-BHIVA-statement-on-considerations-for-critical-care-for-people-with-HIV-during-COVID-19 (accessed on 1 January 2022).
12. BHIVA, DAIG, EACS, GESIDA & Polish Scientific AIDS Society Statement on Risk of COVID-19 for People Living with HIV (PLWH). 2020. Available online: https://www.eacsociety.org/home/bhiva-daig-eacs-gesida-and-polish-scientific-aids-society-statement-on-risk-of-covid-19-for-people-living-with-hiv-plwh.html (accessed on 1 January 2022).
13. Marhefka, S.L.; Turner, D.; Lockhart, E. Understanding women's willingness to use e-health for HIV-related services: A novel application of the technology readiness and acceptance model to a highly stigmatized medical condition. *Telemed. e-Health* **2019**, *25*, 511–518. [CrossRef]
14. Rice, W.S.; Turan, B.; Fletcher, F.E.; Nápoles, T.M.; Walcott, M.; Batchelder, A.; Kempf, M.C.; Konkle-Parker, D.J.; Wilson, T.E.; Tien, P.C.; et al. A mixed methods study of anticipated and experienced stigma in health care settings among women living with HIV in the United States. *AIDS Patient Care STDS* **2019**, *33*, 184–195. [CrossRef]
15. Flicker, S.; Goldberg, E.; Read, S.; Veinot, T.; McClelland, A.; Saulnier, P.; Skinner, H. HIV-positive youth's perspectives on the internet and e-health. *J. Med. Internet Res.* **2004**, *6*, e32. [CrossRef]
16. García, P.J.; Vargas, J.H.; Caballero, N.P.; Calle, V.J.; Bayer, A.M. An e-health driven laboratory information system to support HIV treatment in Peru: E-quity for laboratory personnel, health providers and people living with HIV. *BMC Med. Inform. Decis. Mak.* **2009**, *9*, 50. [CrossRef]
17. Palella, F.J.; Deloria-Knoll, M.; Chmiel, J.S.; Moorman, A.C.; Wood, K.C.; Greenberg, A.E.; Holmberg, S.D.; HIV Outpatient Study Investigators. Survival benefit of initiating antiretroviral therapy in HIV-infected persons in different CD4+ cell strata. *Ann. Intern. Med.* **2003**, *138*, 620–626. [CrossRef]
18. Euroqol Research Foundation. 2021. Available online: https://euroqol.org/eq-5d-instruments/eq-5d-3l-about/ (accessed on 1 January 2022).
19. Health Psychology Research. Available online: https://www.healthpsychologyresearch.com/guidelines/hivsrq-hiv-symptom-rating-questionnaire- (accessed on 1 January 2022).
20. Swinson, R.P. The GAD-7 scale was accurate for diagnosing generalised anxiety disorder. *Evid. Based Med.* **2006**, *11*, 184. [CrossRef] [PubMed]
21. Kroenke, K.; Spitzer, R.L.; Williams, J.B. The PHQ-9: Validity of a brief depression severity measure. *J. Gen. Intern. Med.* **2001**, *16*, 606–613. [CrossRef] [PubMed]
22. Chaiyachati, K.; Hirschhorn, L.R.; Tanser, F.; Newell, M.L.; Bärnighausen, T. Validating five questions of antiretroviral nonadherence in a public-sector treatment program in rural South Africa. *AIDS Patient Care STDS* **2011**, *25*, 163–170. [CrossRef]
23. Damiani, A.; Masciocchi, C.; Lenkowicz, J.; Capocchiano, N.D.; Boldrini, L.; Tagliaferri, L.; Cesario, A.; Sergi, P.; Marchetti, A.; Luraschi, G.; et al. Building an artificial intelligence laboratory based on real world data: The experience of gemelli generator. *Front. Comput. Sci.* **2021**, *3*, 768266. [CrossRef]
24. Mosley, L. A balanced approach to the multi-class imbalance problem. *IJCV* **2010**, *1*, 1–140.
25. Schmidhuber, J. Deep learning in neural networks: An overview. *Neural Netw.* **2015**, *61*, 85–117. [CrossRef] [PubMed]
26. Breiman, L. Random forest. *Machine learning.* **2001**, *45*, 5–32. [CrossRef]
27. Ojala, M.; Garriga, G. Permutation tests for studying classifier performance. *J. Mach. Learn. Res.* **2010**, *11*, 1833–1863.
28. Lundberg, S.M.; Lee, S.I. A unified approach to interpreting model predictions. In Proceedings of the 31st International Conference on Neural Information Processing Systems, Long Beach, CA, USA, 4–9 December 2017.

29. Wood, B.R.; Young, J.D.; Abdel-Massih, R.C.; McCurdy, L.; Vento, T.J.; Dhanireddy, S.; Moyer, K.J.; Siddiqui, J.; Scott, J.D. Advancing Digital Health Equity: A Policy Paper of the Infectious Diseases Society of America and the HIV Medicine Association. *Clin. Infect. Dis.* **2022**, *72*, 6913–6919. [CrossRef]
30. Guaraldi, G.; Milic, J.; Martinez, E.; Kamarulzaman, A.; Mussini, C.; Waters, L.; Pozniak, A.; Mallon, P.; Rockstroh, J.K.; Lazarus, J.V. HIV care models during the COVID-19 era. *Clin. Infect. Dis.* **2021**, *73*, e1222–e1227. [CrossRef]
31. Enevoldsen, K.C.; Danielsen, A.A.; Rohde, C.; Jefsen, O.H.; Nielbo, K.L.; Østergaard, S.D. Monitoring of COVID-19 pandemic-related psychopathology using machine learning. *Acta Neuropsychiatr.* **2022**, 1–14. [CrossRef]
32. Pandey, R.; Gautam, V.; Pal, R.; Bandhey, H.; Dhingra, L.S.; Misra, V.; Sharma, H.; Jain, C.; Bhagat, K.; Arushi Patel, L.; et al. A machine learning application for raising WASH awareness in the times of COVID-19 pandemic. *Sci. Rep.* **2022**, *12*, 810. [CrossRef]
33. Arévalo-Lorido, J.C.; Carretero-Gómez, J.; Casas-Rojo, J.M.; Antón-Santos, J.M.; Melero-Bermejo, J.A.; López-Carmona, M.D.; Palacios, L.C.; Sanz-Cánovas, J.; Pesqueira-Fontán, P.M.; de la Peña-Fernández, A.A.; et al. SEMI-COVID-19 Network. The importance of association of comorbidities on COVID-19 outcomes: A machine learning approach. *Curr. Med. Res. Opin.* **2022**, 1–10. [CrossRef]
34. Chiu, H.R.; Hwang, C.K.; Chen, S.Y.; Shih, F.Y.; Han, H.C.; King, C.C.; Gilbert, J.R.; Fang, C.C.; Oyang, Y.J. Machine learning for emerging infectious disease field responses. *Sci. Rep.* **2022**, *12*, 328. [CrossRef] [PubMed]
35. Mgbako, O.; Miller, E.H.; Santoro, A.F.; Remien, R.H.; Shalev, N.; Olender, S.; Gordon, P.; Sobieszczyk, M.E. COVID-19, telemedicine, and patient empowerment in HIV care and research. *AIDS Behav.* **2020**, 1–4. [CrossRef] [PubMed]
36. Basch, E.; Deal, M.A.; Kris, M.G.; Scher, H.I.; Hudis, C.A.; Sabbatini, P.; Rogak, L.; Bennett, A.V.; Dueck, A.C.; Atkinson, T.M.; et al. Symptom monitoring with patient-reported outcomes during routine cancer treatment: A randomized controlled trial. *J. Clin. Oncol.* **2016**, *34*, 557–565. [CrossRef]
37. Zhou, X.; Snoswell, C.L.; Harding, L.E.; Bambling, M.; Edirippulige, S.; Bai, X.; Smith, A.C. The role of telehealth in reducing the mental health burden from COVID-19. *Telemed. e-Health* **2020**, *26*, 377–379. [CrossRef] [PubMed]
38. Wind, T.R.; Rijkeboer, M.; Andersson, G.; Riper, H. The COVID-19 pandemic: The 'black swan' for mental health care and a turning point for e-health. *Internet Interv.* **2020**, *20*, 100317. [CrossRef]

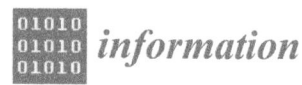

Article

An Attentive Multi-Modal CNN for Brain Tumor Radiogenomic Classification

Ruyi Qu [1,*] and Zhifeng Xiao [2,*]

1 Department of Mathematics, University of Toronto, Toronto, ON M5S 2E4, Canada
2 School of Engineering, Penn State Erie, The Behrend College, Erie, PA 16563, USA
* Correspondence: ruyi.qu@mail.utoronto.ca (R.Q.); zux2@psu.edu (Z.X.); Tel.: +1-814-898-6252 (Z.X.)

Abstract: Medical images of brain tumors are critical for characterizing the pathology of tumors and early diagnosis. There are multiple modalities for medical images of brain tumors. Fusing the unique features of each modality of the magnetic resonance imaging (MRI) scans can accurately determine the nature of brain tumors. The current genetic analysis approach is time-consuming and requires surgical extraction of brain tissue samples. Accurate classification of multi-modal brain tumor images can speed up the detection process and alleviate patient suffering. Medical image fusion refers to effectively merging the significant information of multiple source images of the same tissue into one image, which will carry abundant information for diagnosis. This paper proposes a novel attentive deep-learning-based classification model that integrates multi-modal feature aggregation, lite attention mechanism, separable embedding, and modal-wise shortcuts for performance improvement. We evaluate our model on the RSNA-MICCAI dataset, a scenario-specific medical image dataset, and demonstrate that the proposed method outperforms the state-of-the-art (SOTA) by around 3%.

Keywords: multi-modal medical image; image classification; brain tumor

1. Introduction

GLOBOCAN recently conducted a survey in 185 countries, reporting an estimation of over 300 K new brain cancer cases and above 250 K new deaths in 2020 [1]. Among the various types of malignant brain tumors, glioblastoma multiforme (GBM) is one of the most deadly types, with a low survival rate and limited treatment options. In the United States, the estimated number of GBM diagnoses is over 13 K, and the number of deaths resulting from GBM is over 10 K per year [2]. GBM has been classified as the highest-grade brain cancer (a grade five) by the World Health Organization. A combination of chemotherapy and radiotherapy is a typical treatment following the removal of the tumor by surgery. Radiotherapy can cause severe side effects since radiation could kill both normal and cancer cells. Chemotherapy, on the other hand, works by placing a chemical on the guanine DNA, preventing the replicating of new DNA and leading to cancer cell apoptosis. However, it is known that chemotherapy can be ineffective due to an enzyme named O^6-methylguanine DNA methyltransferase (MGMT). The function of MGMT is determined by its promoter methylation status. If the promoter region is methylated, the enzyme transcription is affected, leading to potentially effective chemotherapy treatment. Therefore, the MGMT promoter methylation status has become a prognostic factor, and a predictor of chemotherapy response [3].

Invasive surgeries can be utilized to determine the status of the MGMT promoter methylation. However, this approach, based on genetic analysis, is an iterative and time-consuming process that requires surgical extraction of brain tissue samples and several weeks of genetic characterization. In addition, the surgery itself may lead to side effects. An alternative that does not involve surgery is to apply computer vision techniques to

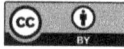

analyze the magnetic resonance imaging (MRI) data. Recent advances in deep learning have achieved extensive success in a broad spectrum of domains [4]. With the continuous efforts of MRI data collection and annotation, deep learning shows its potential in MGMT promoter methylation detection by learning and extracting biomarkers and patterns from MIR scans that are highly indicative of the methylation status. Thus, deep-learning-based approaches have the potential to offer a non-invasive, efficient, and accurate alternative with less patient suffering and more effective treatment for GBM.

MRI scans contain abundant data with a characteristic of multi-modality, which can be and should be better exploited by deep learning algorithms. However, our investigation of the literature shows that prior studies have not fully explored the usage of multi-modal MRI data to detect MGMT methylation. Among the several studies [5–8] that considered multi-modality, only a basic fusion strategy has been adopted, and there is a lack of in-depth investigation for utilizing the multi-modality feature of MRI data for brain tumor detection. Our study aims to fill this gap.

In this paper, we propose a novel deep neural network (DNN) architecture that integrates three performance boosters, including a lite attention mechanism, a separable embedding module, and a model-wise shortcut strategy. The three boosters are designed to better mine multi-modal features and capture informative patterns to make a final prediction. Our proposed model is lightweight and can effectively improve the model performance. The main contributions of this study are as follows.

- We propose an attentive multi-modal DNN to predict the status of the MGMT promoter methylation. In addition to a multi-modal feature aggregation strategy, our proposed model integrates three performance boosters, including a lite attention mechanism to control the model size and speed up training, a separable embedding module to improve the feature representation of MRI data, and a modal-wise shortcut strategy to ensure the modal specificity. These joint efforts have improved the detection accuracy of our model by 3%, compared to the SOTA method. Experiments and results are obtained on the RSNA-MICCAI 2021 dataset [9], which is a recently released dataset with the most patients and MRI scans compared to existing datasets.
- We have made the project source code publicly available at https://github.com/ruyiq/An-Attentive-Multi-modal-CNN-for-Brain-Tumor-Radiogenomic-Classification (accessed at 26 February 2020), offering a credible benchmark for future studies.

The rest of this paper is organized as follows. Section 2 reviews research work related to fusion of multi-modal medical images. Section 3 explains our proposed model and dataset. In Section 4, several experiments are conducted to evaluate the effectiveness of the proposed model. Finally, in Section 5 we conclude the paper and provide future work.

2. Related Work

2.1. Detection of MGMT Methylation Status Based on MRI Data

Table 1 lists a collection of learning-based methods trained with brain MRI scans for the classification of methylation status, which is usually treated as a binary classification problem; namely, methylation vs. non-methylation. It is observed that both traditional feature-based learning methods [5,10,11], such as SVM, RF, KNN, RF, J48, NB, and XGBoost, and deep learning models [6–8,12,13], such as CNN and RNN, have been extensively adopted to build classifiers. It is also noted that a lack of sufficient training data has been a long-lasting challenge, limiting the power of deep-learning-based models. Most prior studies have used data from the Cancer Genome Atlas (TCGA) database, which contains MRI scans from fewer than 250 patients. The recent 2021 RSNA-MICCAI dataset [9] has doubled the number of patients with data collected from multiple centers. This enhancement can boost the quantity and diversity of data used for training deep neural network (DNN) models in the area of methylation detection and potentially benefit the model performance. Meanwhile, it is essential to utilize MRI scans with different modalities, which provide more abundant image features and patterns to be learned by a model. It is found that only half of the studies [5–8] have considered the multi-modality characteristic of the data. We argue that the multi-modal image features play a crucial role in building a more accurate and robust model for MGMT methylation detection, which drives us to integrate a multi-modal feature fusion strategy into the learning pipeline. Moreover, we propose to adopt three performance boosters, including a lite attention mechanism, a modal-wise shortcut, and a separable embedding strategy, which have not been seen in prior studies.

Table 1. A review of MRI-based learning models for the detection of MGMT methylation status. The table includes the following abbreviations: dataset size (D.S.), multi-modality (M.M.), attention mechanism (A.M.), modal-wise shortcut (M.W.S.), separable embedding (S.E.), support vector machine (SVM), random forest (RF), k-nearest neighbor (KNN), naive Bayes (NB), convolutional neural network (CNN), and deep neural network (DNN).

Reference	Year	Model	D.S.	M.M.	A.M.	M.W.S.	S.E.
[10]	2016	SVM, RF	155	✗	✗	✗	✗
[11]	2017	KNN, RF, J48, NB	86	✗	✗	✗	✗
[6]	2017	ResNet	155	✓	✗	✗	✗
[7]	2018	CNN+RF	133	✓	✗	✗	✗
[8]	2018	CRNN	262	✓	✗	✗	✗
[5]	2020	XGBoost	53	✓	✗	✗	✗
[12]	2020	Custom CNN	153	✗	✗	✗	✗
[13]	2021	MGMT-Net	247	✗	✗	✗	✗
Our work	2022	Custom DNN	585	✓	✓	✓	✓

2.2. Multi-Modal Learning on MRI Data

It has been shown both theoretically [14] and empirically [15,16] that models aggregating data from multiple modalities outperform their uni-modal counterparts due to the enriched features and patterns to be learned from the multi-modal data. The usage of multi-modal learning has seen success in a wide range of learning tasks such as object detection [17], semantic segmentation [18], video action recognition [19], and detection of disease [20,21].

MRI data also present multiple modalities that can be extensively utilized for training DNN models. Several studies have developed various techniques to pursue better predictive performance. Myronenko et al. applied AutoEncoder, which fuses the inputs from different modalities [15] to achieve a better performance in 3D MRI brain tumor segmentation. Tseng et al. proposed a deep encoder–decoder structure with cross-modality convolution layers for 3D image segmentation [16]. Shachor et al. proposed an ensemble network architecture to address the classification task by fusing several data sources [22]. The designed network consists of three different modality-specific encoders to capture features of different levels. The proposed method focuses on two-view mammography, which could be extended to multiple views and/or multiple scans. Nie et al. proposed the use of fully convolutional networks (FCNs) for the segmentation of isointense phase brain MR images. They trained one network for each modality image and then fused their high-layer features for final segmentation, which uses different modality paths to obtain the modality-specific features and then fuses the features to make final decisions [23]. Kamnitsas et al. fused the input modality-wise information directly [24]. They proposed a dual pathway, 11-layer deep, 3-dimensional convolutional neural network for brain lesion segmentation. They also devised an efficient and effective dense training scheme, which joins the processing of adjacent image patches into one pass.

The aforementioned studies mainly use multi-modal MRI data to build DNN models for the segmentation task. To the best of our knowledge, the usage of multi-modal MRI data for the detection of MGMT methylation has not been seen. Moreover, the proposed learning pipeline integrates three performance boosters to utilize better the extracted multi-modal MRI features, which have not appeared in any prior studies we have investigated.

3. Materials and Methods

3.1. Dataset

In this research, we focus on the RSNA-MICCAI dataset [9], a multi-center brain tumor MRI dataset that comes with two tasks; namely, tumor segmentation and MGMT detection. In this study, we only tackle the second one. In the dataset, each patient's data is stored in a dedicated folder with a five-digit identification number. Each sample folder consists of four sub-folders corresponding to the four modalities of the MRI scans, including fluid attenuated inversion recovery (FLAIR), T1-weighted pre-contrast (T1w), T1-weighted post-contrast (T1Gd), and T2-weighted (T2), obtained from the video cut frames acquired by imaging. Each modality (i.e., scan type) specifies a focus during imaging. For instance, FLAIR captures the effect after cerebrospinal fluid (CSF) suppression, where liquid signals such as water are suppressed to highlight other parts. T2-weighted, on the other hand, highlights the difference in lateral tissue relaxation, and the combination of different effects provides a comprehensive description of the lesion from multiple perspectives. Each sample in the dataset is described by a quadruple of these four different imaging modalities. Figure 1 shows the four modalities of a positive sample (Figure 1a–d) and a negative sample (Figure 1e–h).

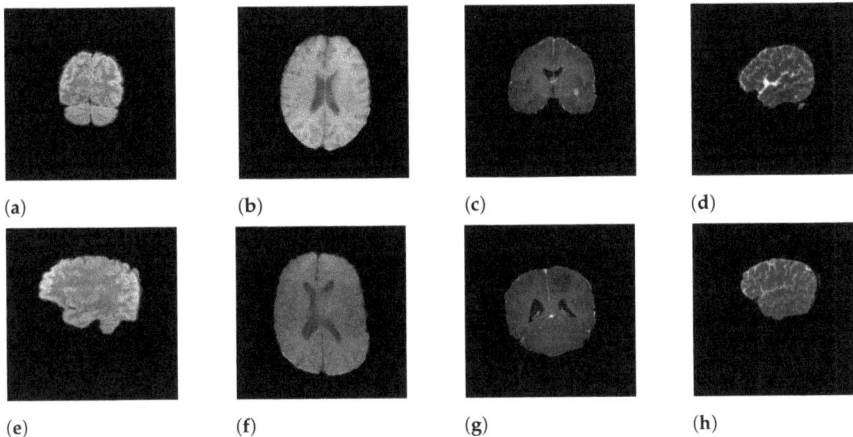

Figure 1. Samples of MRI scans: (**a–d**) represent the FLAIR, T1w, T1Gd, and T2 modalities of a positive sample, and (**e–h**) represent the FLAIR, T1w, T1Gd, and T2 modalities of a negative sample.

RSNA-MICCAI has 585 annotated samples, each corresponding to four modalities containing samples ranging from a few tens to a few hundred. Each modality of a patient consists of a sequence of MRI scans within a period of time. Figure 2 shows such an MRI sequence of FLAIR scans (74 in total) for patient ten in the dataset. Compared with other datasets used in prior studies in Table 1, RSNA-MICCAI contains a larger amount of data and is a clearly labeled dichotomous dataset, which can better characterize the patient in different imaging modalities and have better generalization. The number of positive MRI scans is 3070, or 57.5%, and the number of negative samples is 2780, or 52.5%. The classes of the dataset are relatively balanced. Table 2 reports the statistics of the number of MRI scans for each modality. It is observed that the average number of scans for modality per patient is in the range 127 and 171, which provides abundant information for pattern learning.

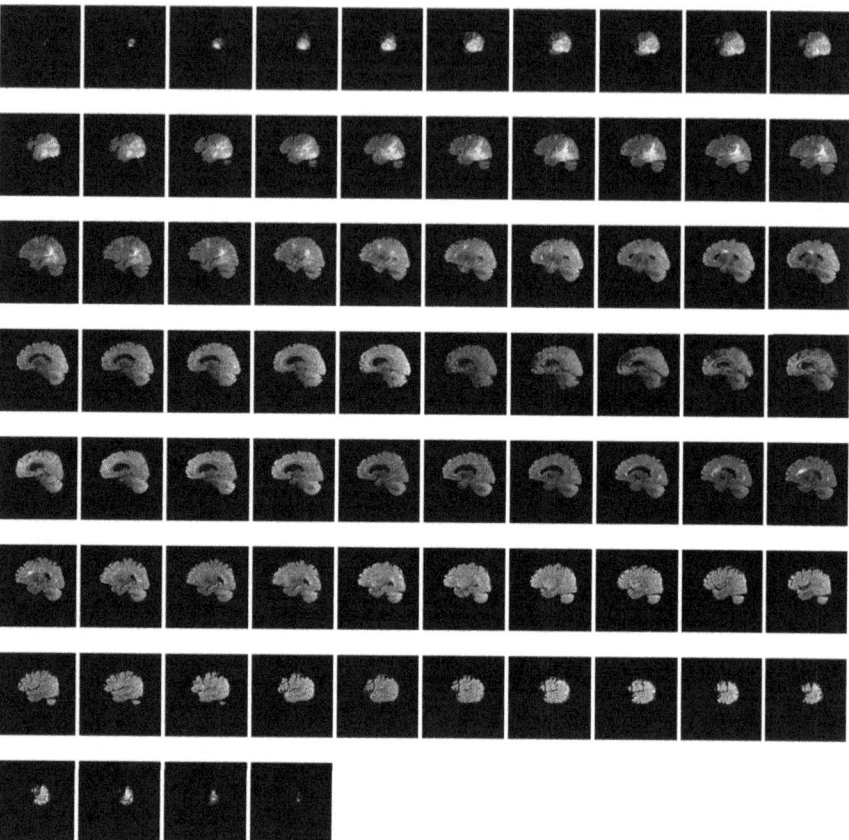

Figure 2. A sequence of FLAIR scans for patient 10 in the dataset.

Table 2. Number of files for each scan type.

Scan Type	FLAIR	T1w	T1wCE	T2w
# files	74,248	77,627	96,766	100,000
Avg. # files per case	127	133	165	171

Figure 3 shows an intensity visualization of MRI scans for three random patients. The charts are grouped by the four modalities. For each sub-chart, the x-axis represents the time step, and the y-axis denotes an intensity score, which reflects the amount of information expressed by the MRI scan at a time step. The intensity defines the shade of gray of tissues or fluid, and different levels of intensity are encoded by different colors in the MRI scan. The higher the intensity, the more white area in the scan; the lower the intensity, the more black in the scan. Thus, gray encodes intermediate signal intensity. Intuitively, images with higher intensity carry more expressive patterns that can be learned, and these images often appear in the middle of the MRI sequence, as shown in Figure 2. It is also observed that even for the same patient, the times of peak intensity for the four modalities vary. This finding allows us to better pre-process the data by selecting the most informative scans (namely, the ones with the highest intensity scores) for each modality to train our model.

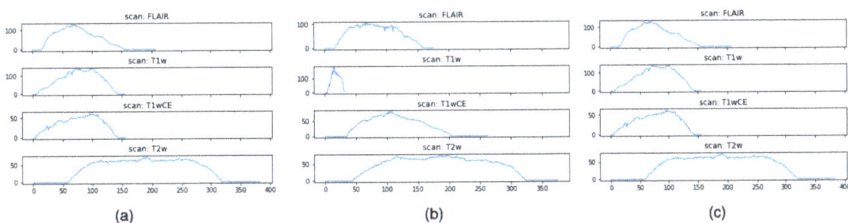

Figure 3. Intensity visualization. Subfigures (a–c) represent the intensity charts of the four modalities for three randomly selected samples.

3.2. Learning Framework

Figure 4 illustrates the learning framework. To ensure the model effect and retain the original input details, the output of attention is fused with the input through shortcut connection and weighted summation, and the fused features are mapped to a more divisible space by a smaller DNN module. Finally, the classification results are obtained by using the LSTM structure. In this paper, four sub-structures, including multi-modal feature aggregation, lite attention mechanism, separable embedding, and modal-wise shortcut, are applied together to enhance the overall performance of classification.

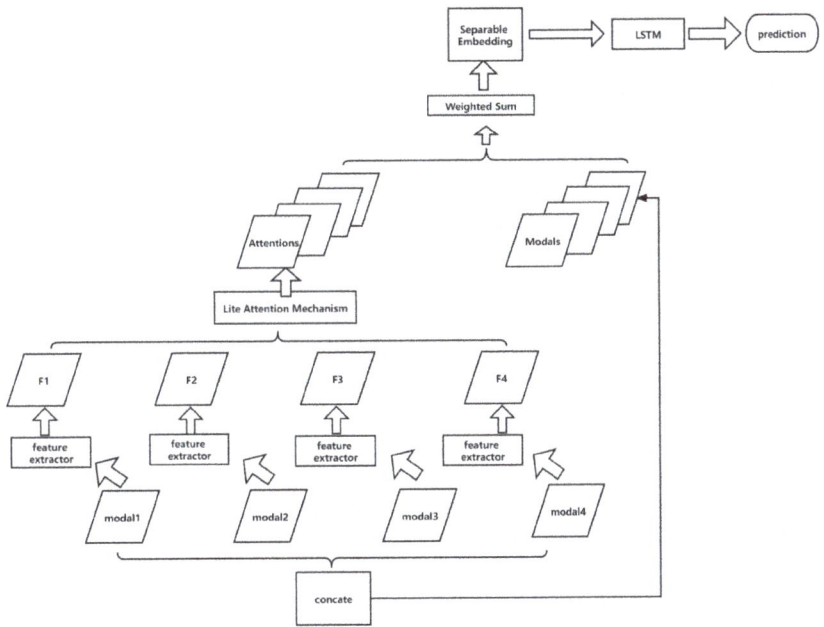

Figure 4. The learning framework.

3.3. Multi-Modal Feature Fusion

The data of each modality are considered for modality-by-modality feature extraction due to the significant differences in imaging principles. Each sample corresponds to four images, namely fluid attenuated inversion recovery (FLAIR), T1-weighted pre-contrast (T1w), T1-weighted post-contrast (T1Gd), and T2-weighted (T2), corresponding to modal1, modal2, modal3, and modal4 inputs in the above figure.

The feature maps F1, F2, F3, and F4, obtained through feature extraction from each modality, are fused by the attention module to obtain the attentions that can fully describe the overall information across the modalities.

Here, the specific form of feature extractor needs to be selected. Since the images of each modality are 256*256 single-channel images with small scales, an overly complex feature extraction process will greatly destroy the original information and make the subsequent operation difficult. It is found that a simple single-layer convolution can be used to obtain a balance between extracting features and preserving the original information. Since the data of each modality have a different distribution, the feature extractor of each branch does not share the weights.

To extract information from multiple perspectives, the subsequent attention module still adopts the multi-head model. The number of heads is chosen to be 4, which is explained below in Section 3.5.

3.4. Lite Attention Mechanism

Since each sample has four modalities, the data of each modality have a different emphasis due to their different methods of acquisition. It is necessary to analyze each data characteristic to decide how to fuse features from different modalities. The two commonly used methods are as follows:

1. Fuse multi-modal data in the form of sequences and use recurrent neural network (RNN) models for feature extraction. This operation requires traversing the input from the first time-step to the last one, which is computationally expensive [25]. Even though improved RNN variants such as LSTM [26] and GRU [27] can effectively reduce the difficulty of parameter updates in training, the sequential arrangement of different modal data introduces unnecessary sequential priors, which can force the model to learn an unreasonable one-way information flow while understanding the inter-modal relationships to fit the main features, affecting the effectiveness of feature extraction [28,29].
2. Use the attention mechanism to fuse the features extracted from different modalities. Attention can easily obtain global feature information compared to the sequential models such as LSTM and GRU mentioned above, which can better obtain contextual relationships and obtain an overall understanding of the input.

The attention mechanism was first proposed by the Google machine translation team in 2017. It completely breaks away from the previous framework based on a recurrent neural network and dynamically extracts the feature part that it cares most for from each current input and fuses it to control the impact of all time-step features on the current output through different weights [30]. A brief description of the attention mechanism is given as follows. In each time step, the input obtained by the model consists of three parts: the current query, different feature values, and the corresponding keys of the features. The query is the object that the model needs for the current time-step, which may be a concrete input or an abstract representation of the features extracted in the previous step. To fully determine the important differences of features, an attention mechanism uses the dot product of the query and key to calculate the weights of corresponding features. At this point, the similarity between the query and key is measured by the dot product [31]. This way of calculating attention weights is called dot-product attention. As such, we obtain the following Equation (1) for calculation, where k_i and v_i are the input key and values. The query at this point is denoted as q.

$$Attention(q, k, v) = \sum_{i=1}^{N} q^T k_i v_i \tag{1}$$

When the length of the vector becomes longer, the scale of its dot product result also becomes larger. After the calculation through softmax, it reaches the saturation zone, making the gradient smaller, which is not conducive to the model optimization. Therefore, before performing softmax, the inner product value is divided by the square root of the length d, as shown in Equation (2).

$$Attention(Q, K, V) = Softmax\left(\frac{QK^T}{\sqrt{d}}\right)V \qquad (2)$$

After a further examination of the equations above, it can be found that to perform the dot product operation, the key used by the model, i.e., k_i, and the query, i.e., q, need to have the same dimensionality. The additive attention method is proposed to perform the weight calculation on different occasions adequately. This method concatenates the input query of length u and the key of length k. The resulting (query, key) pair is fed into a feedforward neural network with a single hidden layer, and the value describing the degree of similarity between the two is obtained by the sigmoid function and used as the weight [32].

In the above dot-product attention process, to calculate the weight corresponding to the i-th input, two vectors of length d, query and k_i, for the case of N time steps or N different modalities, the number of parameters to be retained and trained is $(N+1)d$. To fully guarantee the relative importance of different inputs, the specific value of d cannot be too small since it is challenging to train the model effectively in the case of insufficient data.

In this study, we propose a lite attention mechanism, which is a light weighted improvement of the original attention mechanism, by directly modeling the weights of different modalities, i.e., rewriting the attention formula to the following:

$$Attention(v) = \sum_{i=1}^{N} w_i v_i \qquad (3)$$

For the training process of w_i, the number of parameters is reduced from $(N+1)d$ to N, which significantly improves the training speed and generalization performance [33,34]. It does not cost much to train w_i. We do not use a softmax function for normalization and nonlinear processing before the weighted summation but achieve better results. Our conjecture is that the simple scale variation corresponding to normalization can be adjusted by the subsequent DNN embedding, while the parameters corresponding to formally relative simpler binary classification problems can be directly derived by incorporating the relationship of nonlinear mapping into the model structure.

3.5. Modal-Wise Shortcut

The features of each modal, after feature extraction and processing by the attention modules, are represented with a highly task-relevant tensor, but the following fusion process leads to a loss of image details that may be informative to the task, which may further result in severe performance degradation for the prediction. Our solution is to add a shortcut between the original input and the output of the attention module; namely, a residual connection [4] for each modal. Bypassing all the convolution and weighted summation, we keep and pass all the original detailed features in the network without any loss, which significantly reduces the possibility of model degradation.

The feature map that is finally fed into the DNN embedding d_i can be represented as follows:

$$d_i = Attention_i + modal_i \qquad (4)$$

where $Attention_i$ is the ith feature map generated by the lite attention mechanism module, while $modal_i$ is the original input for the ith modal. Fusing these two, we obtain d_i, the new feature representation of the ith modal. To ensure the feasibility of the operation, the number of feature maps output by multi-head attention is set to be the same as the number of modals; namely, four. This step is processed separately for each modal to avoid cross-modal information interference, and the final improvement fully demonstrates the effectiveness of this operation.

3.6. Separable Embedding

A prior study named CLDNN [35] shows that mapping and projecting the extracted features into a new separable space before feeding them into the detection head can effectively boost the model's accuracy. Inspired by this empirical finding, we adopt a separable embedding strategy in our study. Specifically, a separate CNN is utilized again to fuse the tensor produced from the previous module. We have evaluated two CNN backbones to fill this role and report their effects in the next section. The output of this module is given as follows.

$$f_i = CNN_{SE}(d_i) \tag{5}$$

where CNN_SE refers to the CNN that performs separable embedding; d_i and f_i refer to the input and output tensors of this module.

3.7. LSTM and Detection Head

The output of the separable embedding for each time step is then collected to form a collection of sequential tensors ordered by the time step of the MRI scans. The tensor sequence is then fed into a long short-term memory (LSTM) network, followed by a fully connected layer and a sigmoid function layer as the detection head that outputs a value in [0,1], indicating the probability of MGMT promoter methylation.

4. Experiments and Results

All experiments were implemented using Python. The adopted deep learning framework is Pytorch 1.8.0. Experiments were run on a Windows workstation with an i7-10875h CPU and a GTX2080TI GPU. Ten quartets were extracted from each original sample in the RSNA-MICCAI dataset as a new dataset, and a total of 5850 samples were obtained. The training and test sets were randomly divided according to the ratio of 8:2.

4.1. Evaluation Metrics

The primary metric of RSNA-MICCAI is the accuracy of the classification. We need to accurately determine whether the input image is obtained from malignant brain tumor imaging. Under the current scenario, the model should enhance the classification of positive samples that threaten the lives of patients. At the same time, misclassifying a true negative sample as a positive sample can lead to unnecessary surgery and post-operative torment for the patient. We need to improve the accuracy of both situations. To optimize both objectives simultaneously, the accuracy rate is used as the evaluation metric. The model with minor misclassification and omission is chosen.

$$Acc = \frac{TP + TN}{TP + TN + FP + FN} \tag{6}$$

in which TP (true positive) is the number of true positive samples; TN (true negative) is the number of true negative samples; FP (false positive) represents the number of false positive samples; and FN (false negative) is the number of false negative samples.

4.2. Baseline

We consider the following baselines in this study.

- ResNet by He et al. [4] is an effort to understand how deepening a neural network can increase the expressiveness and the complexity of the network. It is found that for DNN, if a newly added layer can be treated as an identity function, the deepened network is as effective as the original one. This finding drives the development of the residual block, which adds a shortcut connection to the layer output before the activation function. The simple design allows a DNN to be trained more easily and efficiently. ResNet was the winning solution for the ImageNet Large-Scale Visual Recognition Challenge in 2015 and has been applied to numerous computer vision tasks with SOTA performance. Therefore, we consider ResNet a decent baseline. Our empirical result shows that ResNet34 presents the highest accuracy. We thus use ResNet34 to represent the baseline result.

- The EfficientNet [36] paper makes two major contributions. First, a simple and mobile-size neural architecture was proposed. Second, a compound-scaling method was proposed to increase the network size to achieve maximum performance gains. It is suggested that to pursue better performance, the key is to balance all three dimensions, including network depth, width, and resolution, during ConvNet scaling. Thus, the authors of EfficientNet adopted a global scaling factor to uniformly scale the depth, width, and resolution of the network. The scaling factor makes it possible to apply grid searching to find the parameters that lead to the best performance. EfficientNet offers a generic neural architecture optimization technique applied to existing CNNs such as ResNet. It has shown superior performance in numerous tasks with SOTA results, which is why we chose it as a strong baseline.

- The gold-medal-winning strategy was developed by Firas Baba, who open-sourced the code at https://github.com/FirasBaba/rsna-resnet10 (accessed at 24 January 2020). The final model of the winning team is a 3D CNN using the ResNet10 backbone with the following design choices: BCE Loss, Adam optimizer, 15 epochs, a learning rate of 0.00001 (from epoch 1 to 10) and 0.000005 (from epoch 10–15), image size 256 by 256, batch size 8. Each epoch took around 80 s on an RTX 3090. The author also reported the best central image trick, which is a strategy to select the biggest MRI scan that contains the largest brain cutaway view for training. In this study, we refer to the model developed by Firas Baba as the SOTA since it was in first place on the contest leader board.

4.3. Training Setting

The 3×3 convolution is used as the feature extractor for each modality, and each modality uses its own feature extractor to obtain different features without sharing weights. We choose Adam as the optimizer with a learning rate of 0.0001, and beta1 and beta2 values of 0.9 and 0.999, respectively. We set eps=1×10^{-8} to prevent the denominator from being 0. Other parameter configurations are weight decay to be 0, batch size to be 8, and binary cross-entropy with logits to be the loss function of the binary classification problem. Several hyperparameters, including the learning rate, the batch size, and eps are tuned via a five-fold cross validation to obtain the optimal values given a list of value choices for each hyperparameter.

We also choose albumentation for data augmentation for the training dataset, with the following configurations:

1. Horizontal flip with a probability of 0.5;
2. Random affine transformation configured as shift-limit = 0.0625, scale_limit = 0.1, rotate_limit = 10 with a probability of 0.5;
3. Random contrast transformation with 0.5 probability.

4.4. Performance Evaluation

The accuracy of the evaluated models on the training set and the validation set is demonstrated in Figure 5. Under all configurations in this experiment, after 50 epochs of training, the models converge, and accuracy becomes stable.

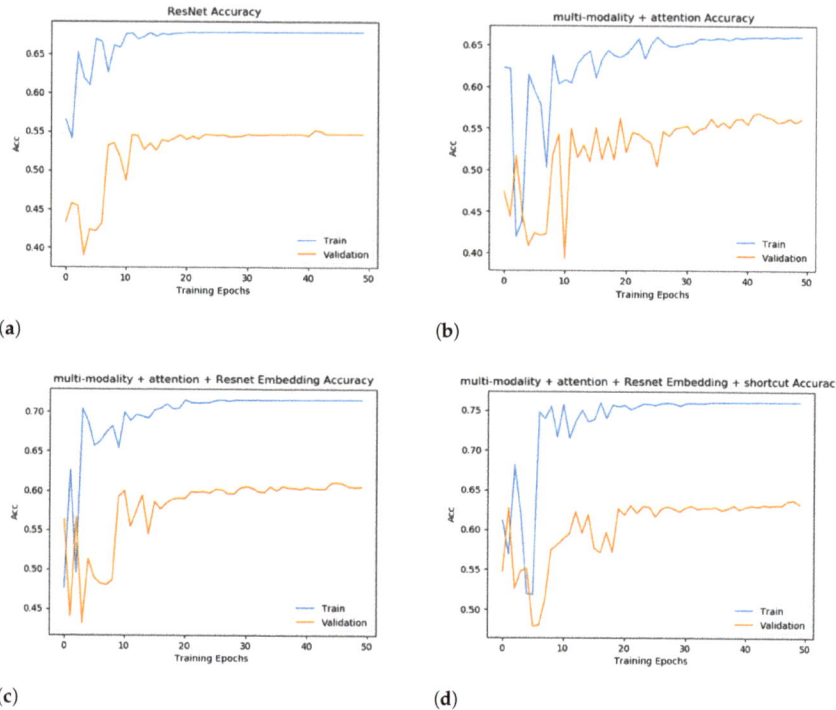

Figure 5. Training and validation accuracy to show an ablation study. Subfigures (**a**–**d**) represent the four evaluated models with a booster added incrementally to the previous model.

Figure 5b shows the performance of adding the attention module only. The accuracy is only improved to 56.74%. However, the accuracy curve converges slower and a noticeable scale of oscillation appears in 20–30 epochs, which indicates that without adding other modules to the fusion of the extracted features the model is not able to obtain effective information. The training effect is poor, and the accuracy is not particularly satisfactory.

After adding two different separable embedding modules to the model, ResNet34 and EfficientNet [36], it can be observed that both accuracy and the convergence speed are greatly optimized, which fully illustrates the necessity of separable embedding. Specifically, the improvement of the performance by adding ResNet34 is more obvious and the convergence speed is also faster. The accuracy is improved by 4.35%, which is 61.09%. We chose ResNet34 as the separable embedding module for further experiments.

Finally, we added the shortcut model to the multi-modality + attention + Resnet34 embedding model, using weighted summation to fuse the original information and extracted features. It can be observed that adding the shortcut model further improves the metrics by more than 2%, reflecting the effect of direct-concatenation for training the model. The performance of different models and training plans is provided in Table 3. Overall, the strategy of multi-modality + attention + Resnet34 Embedding + shortcut largely outperforms the baseline. Combining the above four submodules substantially improves the accuracy by more than 10%, but the absence of any one of them brings about a significant metric degradation. We also replicated the SOTA model, which utilized a 3D CNN + ResNet10 neural architecture. The SOTA had an accuracy of 60.74%, which is 3-point worse than our model.

Table 3. Performance of different models. Abbreviations: separable embedding (S.E.), training duration per epoch (T.D.P.E).

Method	S.E	Acc	T.D.P.E (s)
ResNet34	NA	53.12%	65.4
EfficientNet	NA	54.80%	52.3
3D CNN + ResNet10 (SOTA)	NA	60.74%	73.1
multi-modality + attention	NA	56.74%	67.3
multi-modality + attention	EfficientNet	59.03%	72.2
multi-modality + attention	Resnet34	61.09%	78.8
multi-modality + attention + shortcut	Resnet34	63.71%	79.3

We also report the average training duration per epoch (T.D.P.E.) in the last column of Table 3. It is observed that the average T.D.P.E. for all models ranges from 52.3 to 79.3 s on our deep learning workstation. The training has been relatively efficient mainly due to the following: (1) the MRI scans have been down-scaled to 256 by 256 pixels and (2) the fast processing speed offered by the RTX 3090. It is also noted that the best performing model only added a reasonable amount of time compared to the SOTA (79.3 vs. 73.1), which validates the efficient design of the lightweight attention module.

It is observed in Figure 5a–d that overfitting occurs in all evaluated models. Our observation is aligned with other contest participants (see a post at https://www.kaggle.com/c/rsna-miccai-brain-tumor-radiogenomic-classification/discussion/281347 accessed at 20 February 2022). It is mentioned that many teams obtained higher training scores than validation scores. In machine learning, overfitting is mainly caused by the nature of data [37]. Specifically, the data points of training and test sets do not follow the same distribution. As such, the models trained on the training set have learned knowledge and patterns that do not apply well to the samples on the test set. For this study, the quantity of MRI scans is increased compared to prior datasets. However, most scans only contain a partial area of the brain, which does not offer many expressive patterns to be learned by a model. We adopted the following strategies to handle overfitting. First, we applied several data augmentation strategies to enhance the diversity of the dataset (see Section 4.3). Second, we conducted cross-validation to examine the robustness of model performance. Despite these efforts, a performance gap in the range 10–15% still exists between the training and validation accuracy scores, even for our best-performing model.

5. Conclusions

Malignancy analysis of brain tumors is crucial for the lives of patients and early prevention. For early screening and reducing patients' suffering, accurate classification is needed. However, the effectiveness of existing models cannot be guaranteed. In this paper, we proposed a new classification model based on multi-modal feature aggregation, lite attention mechanism, separable embedding, and modal-wise shortcut. The combined effects of these boosters increased the prediction accuracy to 63.71% on the RSNA-MICCAI dataset, outperforming the SOTA by 3%.

This work has the following limitations, which also suggest future directions. First, our proposed method only considers the temporal association between same-modality data, while the relationship between different modality data is not examined. This inter-modality relation is worthy of further investigation. Second, in addition to the modal-wise attention used in this study, image-wise attention can also be considered since some critical areas of an MRI scan could carry informative patterns that should be learned and used to make a better prediction. Lastly, a joint model that handles tumor segmentation and MGMT detection is expected.

Author Contributions: Conceptualization and methodology, R.Q. and Z.X.; software, validation, and original draft preparation, R.Q.; review and editing, and supervision, Z.X. All authors have read and agreed to the published version of the manuscript.

Funding: This research received no external funding.

Institutional Review Board Statement: Not applicable.

Informed Consent Statement: Not applicable.

Data Availability Statement: The dataset supporting the conclusions of this article are available at https://www.kaggle.com/c/rsna-miccai-brain-tumor-radiogenomic-classification (accessed on 20 November 2021).

Conflicts of Interest: The authors declare no conflict of interest.

References

1. Sung, H.; Ferlay, J.; Siegel, R.L.; Laversanne, M.; Soerjomataram, I.; Jemal, A.; Bray, F. Global cancer statistics 2020: Globocan estimates of incidence and mortality worldwide for 36 cancers in 185 countries. *CA Cancer J. Clin.* **2021**, *71*, 209–249. [CrossRef] [PubMed]
2. Ostrom, Q.T.; Patil, N.; Cioffi, G.; Waite, K.; Kruchko, C.; Barnholtz-Sloan, J.S. CBTRUS statistical report: Primary brain and other central nervous system tumors diagnosed in the United States in 2013–2017. *Neuro-Oncology* **2020**, *22*, iv1–iv96. [CrossRef] [PubMed]
3. Zhou, T.; Ruan, S.; Canu, S. A review: Deep learning for medical image segmentation using multi-modality fusion. *Array* **2019**, *3–4*, 100004. [CrossRef]
4. He, K.; Zhang, X.; Ren, S.; Sun, J. Deep Residual Learning for Image Recognition. In Proceedings of the 2016 IEEE Conference on Computer Vision and Pattern Recognition, Las Vegas, NV, USA, 27–30 June 2016; Volume 30, pp. 770–778.
5. Le, N.Q.K.; Do, D.T.; Chiu, F.Y.; Yapp, E.K.Y.; Yeh, H.Y.; Chen, C.Y. XGBoost Improves Classification of MGMT Promoter Methylation Status in IDH1 Wildtype Glioblastoma. *J. Pers. Med.* **2020**, *10*, 128. [CrossRef]
6. Korfiatis, P.; Kline, T.L.; Lachance, D.H.; Parney, I.F.; Buckner, J.C.; Erickson, B.J. Residual Deep Convolutional Neural Network Predicts MGMT Methylation Status. *J. Digit. Imaging* **2017**, *30*, 622–628. [CrossRef] [PubMed]
7. Li, Z.C.; Bai, H.; Sun, Q.; Li, Q.; Liu, L.; Zou, Y.; Chen, Y.; Liang, C.; Zheng, H. Multiregional radiomics features from multiparametric MRI for prediction of MGMT methylation status in glioblastoma multiforme: A multicentre study. *Eur. Radiol.* **2018**, *28*, 3640–3650. [CrossRef]
8. Han, L.; Kamdar, M.R. MRI to MGMT: Predicting methylation status in glioblastoma patients using convolutional recurrent neural networks. In *Pacific symposium on Biocomputing 2018, Proceedings of the Pacific Symposium, Coast, HI, USA, 3–7 January 2018*; World Scientific: Singapore, 2018; pp. 331–342.
9. Baid, U.; Ghodasara, S.; Mohan, S.; Bilello, M.; Calabrese, E.; Colak, E.; Farahani, K.; Kalpathy-Cramer, J.; Kitamura, F.C.; Pati, S.; et al. The rsna-asnr-miccai brats 2021 benchmark on brain tumor segmentation and radiogenomic classification. *arXiv* **2021**, arXiv:2107.02314.
10. Korfiatis, P.; Kline, T.L.; Coufalova, L.; Lachance, D.H.; Parney, I.F.; Carter, R.E.; Buckner, J.C.; Erickson, B.J. MRI texture features as biomarkers to predict MGMT methylation status in glioblastomas. *Med. Phys.* **2016**, *43*, 2835–2844. [CrossRef]
11. Kanas, V.G.; Zacharaki, E.I.; Thomas, G.A.; Zinn, P.O.; Megalooikonomou, V.; Colen, R.R. Learning MRI-based classification models for MGMT methylation status prediction in glioblastoma. *Comput. Methods Programs Biomed.* **2017**, *140*, 249–257. [CrossRef]
12. Chen, X.; Zeng, M.; Tong, Y.; Zhang, T.; Fu, Y.; Li, H.; Zhang, Z.; Cheng, Z.; Xu, X.; Yang, R.; et al. Automatic Prediction of MGMT Status in Glioblastoma via Deep Learning-Based MR Image Analysis. *Biomed Res. Int.* **2020**, *2020*, 9258649. [CrossRef]
13. Yogananda, C.; Shah, B.R.; Nalawade, S.; Murugesan, G.; Yu, F.; Pinho, M.; Wagner, B.; Mickey, B.; Patel, T.R.; Fei, B.; et al. MRI-based deep-learning method for determining glioma MGMT promoter methylation status. *Am. J. Neuroradiol.* **2021**, *42*, 845–852. [CrossRef] [PubMed]
14. Huang, Y.; Du, C.; Xue, Z.; Chen, X.; Zhao, H.; Huang, L. What Makes Multi-modal Learning Better than Single (Provably). *Adv. Neural Inf. Process. Syst.* **2021**, *34* .
15. Myronenko, A. 3D MRI Brain Tumor Segmentation Using Autoencoder Regularization. In Proceedings of the International Conference on Medical Image Computing and Computer Assisted Intervention Workshop(MICCAI), Shenzhen, China, 13–17 October 2019 ; pp. 311–320. [CrossRef]
16. Tseng, K.L.; Lin, Y.L.; Hsu, W.; Huang, C.Y. Joint Sequence Learning and Cross-Modality Convolution for 3D Biomedical Segmentation. In Proceedings of the IEEE Computer Society Conference on Computer Vision and Pattern Recognition (CVPR), Honolulu, HI, USA, 21–26 July 2017; pp. 311–320. [CrossRef]
17. Wang, A.; Lu, J.; Cai, J.; Cham, T.J.; Wang, G. Large-margin multi-modal deep learning for RGB-D object recognition. *IEEE Trans. Multimed.* **2015**, *17*, 1887–1898. [CrossRef]

18. Liu, W.; Luo, Z.; Cai, Y.; Yu, Y.; Ke, Y.; Junior, J.M.; Gonçalves, W.N.; Li, J. Adversarial unsupervised domain adaptation for 3D semantic segmentation with multi-modal learning. *ISPRS J. Photogramm. Remote Sens.* **2021**, *176*, 211–221. [CrossRef]
19. Wang, Z.; She, Q.; Smolic, A. TEAM-Net: Multi-modal Learning for Video Action Recognition with Partial Decoding. *arXiv* **2021**, arXiv:2110.08814.
20. Ning, Z.; Xiao, Q.; Feng, Q.; Chen, W.; Zhang, Y. Relation-induced multi-modal shared representation learning for Alzheimer's disease diagnosis. *IEEE Trans. Med. Imaging* **2021**, *40*, 1632–1645. [CrossRef]
21. Rani, G.; Oza, M.G.; Dhaka, V.S.; Pradhan, N.; Verma, S.; Rodrigues, J.J. Applying deep learning-based multi-modal for detection of coronavirus. *Multimed. Syst.* **2021**, 1–12. [CrossRef]
22. Shachor, Y.; Greenspan, H.; Goldberger, J. A mixture of views network with applications to multi-view medical imaging. *IEEE Trans. Med. Imaging* **2020**, *374*, 1–9. [CrossRef]
23. Nie, D.; Wang, L.; Gao, Y.; Shen, D. Fully convolutional networks for multi-modality isointense infant brain image segmentation. In Proceedings of the 2016 IEEE 13th International Symposium on Biomedical Imaging (ISBI), Prague, Czech Republic, 13–16 April 2016; pp. 1342–1345. [CrossRef]
24. Kamnitsas, K.; Ledig, C.; Newcombe, V.F.; Simpson, J.P.; Kane, A.D.; Menon, D.K.; Rueckert, D.; Glocker, B. Efficient multi-scale 3D CNN with fully connected CRF for accurate brain lesion segmentation. *Med. Image Anal.* **2017**, *36*, 61–78. [CrossRef]
25. Cho, K.; Merrienboer, B.V.; Gulcehre, C.; Bahdanau, D.; Bougares, F.; Schwenk, H.; Bengio, Y. Learning Phrase Representations using RNN Encoder-Decoder for Statistical Machine Translationn. *Comput. Sci. Comput. Lang.* **2014**, *36*, 61–78. [CrossRef]
26. Sainath, T.N.; Vinyals, O.; Senior, A.; Sak, H. Convolutional, Long Short-Term Memory, fully connected Deep Neural Networks. In Proceedings of the 2015 IEEE International Conference on Acoustics, Speech and Signal Processing (ICASSP), South Brisbane, QLD, Australia, 19–24 April 2015. [CrossRef]
27. Zaremba, W.; Sutskever, I.; Vinyals, O. Recurrent Neural Network Regularization. *Neural Evol. Comput.* **2014**, arXiv:1409.2329. .
28. Bahdanau, D.; Cho, K.; Bengio, Y. Neural Machine Translation by Jointly Learning to Align and Translate. *Comput. Sci. Comput. Lang.* **2014** , arXiv:1409.0473.
29. Cho, K.; van Merrienboer, B.; Bahdanau, D.; Bengio, Y. On the properties of neural machine translation: Encoder-decoder approaches. *Comput. Sci. Comput. Lang.* **2014**, arXiv:1409.1259.
30. Vaswani, A.; Shazeer, N.; Parmar, N.; Uszkoreit, J.; Jones, L.; Gomez, A.N.; Kaiser, L.; Polosukhin, I. Attention is All you Need. In Proceedings of the Conference on Neural Information Processing Systems (NeurIPS), Red Hook, NY, USA, 4–9 December 2017 ; Volume 30, pp. 1–12.
31. Devlin, J.; Chang, M.; Lee, K.; Toutanova, K. BERT: Pre-training of Deep Bidirectional Transformers for Language Understanding. *arXiv* **2018**, arXiv:1810.04805.
32. Lan, Z.; Chen, M.; Goodman, S.; Gimpel, K.; Sharma, P.; Soricut, R. ALBERT: A Lite BERT for Self-supervised Learning of Language Representations. *Neural Evol. Comput.* **2019**, arXiv:1909.11942.
33. Zhang, Z.; Hanand, X.; Liu, Z.; Jiang, X.; Sun, M.; Liu, Q. ERNIE: Enhanced Language Representation with Informative Entities. In Proceedings of the 57th Annual Meeting of the Association for Computational Linguistics, Florence, Italy, 28 July–2 August 2019. https://arxiv.org/abs/1905.07129.
34. Liu, Y.; Ott, M.; Goyal, N.; Du, J.; Joshi, M.; Chen, D.; Levy, O.; Lewis, M.; Zettlemoyer, L.; Stoyanov, V. RoBERTa: A Robustly Optimized BERT Pretraining Approach. *arXiv* **2019**, arXiv:1907.11692
35. Sainath, R.Z.C.T.; Parada, C. *Feature Learning with Raw-Waveform CLDNNs for Voice Activity Detection*; Interspeech: Baixas, France, 2016.
36. Tan, M.; Le, Q.V. Efficientnet: Rethinking model scaling for convolutional neural networks. *arXiv* **2019**, arXiv:1905.11946.
37. Dietterich, T. Overfitting and undercomputing in machine learning. *Acm Comput. Surv. (CSUR)* **1995**, *27*, 326–327. [CrossRef]

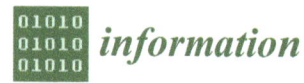

Article

Motivating Machines: The Potential of Modeling Motivation as MoA for Behavior Change Systems

Fawad Taj [1,2,*], Michel C. A. Klein [1] and Aart Van Halteren [1,3]

[1] Social AI, Department of Computer Science, Vrije Universiteit Amsterdam, 1081 HV Amsterdam, The Netherlands; michel.klein@vu.nl (M.C.A.K.); a.t.van.halteren@vu.nl (A.V.H.)
[2] Department of Computer Science, University of Swabi, Swabi 94640, Pakistan
[3] Philips Research, High Tech Campus 34, 5656 AE Eindhoven, The Netherlands
* Correspondence: fawadtaj1@gmail.com

Abstract: The pathway through which behavior change techniques have an effect on the behavior of an individual is referred to as the Mechanism of Action (MoA). Digitally enabled behavior change interventions could potentially benefit from explicitly modelling the MoA to achieve more effective, adaptive, and personalized interventions. For example, if 'motivation' is proposed as the targeted construct in any behavior change intervention, how can a model of this construct be used to act as a mechanism of action, mediating the intervention effect using various behavior change techniques? This article discusses a computational model for motivation based on the neural reward pathway with the aim to make it act as a mediator between behavior change techniques and target behavior. This model's formal description and parametrization are described from a neurocomputational sciences prospect and elaborated with the help of a sub-question, i.e., what parameters/processes of the model are crucial for the generation and maintenance of motivation. An intervention scenario is simulated to show how an explicit model of 'motivation' and its parameters can be used to achieve personalization and adaptivity. A computational representation of motivation as a mechanism of action may also further advance the design, evaluation, and effectiveness of personalized and adaptive digital behavior change interventions.

Keywords: AI-powered behavioral change support systems; motivation; computational modeling; behavior change techniques; AI in health; pervasive health system

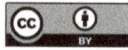

1. Introduction

In medical sciences, the mechanism of action of a particular medicine enables physicians to understand the correct dosing better. It helps identify which patients are likely to respond to that medicine. There are also different models and evidence-based theories available for health behavior change. These theories/models identify the key constructs and processes of behavior change. However, serious discussion and research are still going on about these constructs and their mechanism of action. The fundamental disagreement is on the causality of Behavior Change Techniques (BCTs) for various theoretical psychological constructs. For example, one might argue that BCT "information about health consequences" changes behavior by changing one's belief about health consequences. The most common term used for this connection between BCTs and the modifiable factors is a Mechanism of Action (MoA), defined broadly as 'the processes through which a behavior change technique affects behavior. In comparison, others call it the process of operational manipulation of psychological constructs [1].

One of the challenges identified in the international workshop on developing and evaluating digital interventions is that digital behavior change interventions often lack clarity around the mechanism through which they have their effect [2]. It is recommended to develop and specify the circumstances in which the proposed mechanism of action would generate a targeted effect and represent the resulting knowledge as a behavior change ontology [2]. Moreover, the limited collaboration between technology designers and health behavior experts typically leads to poorly developed technologies or applications in which the choice of health behavior theories is not suitable. The theory and models chosen are not sufficiently versatile to cover all aspects of the target behavior [3]. We consider digital health change intervention as the interventions that use digital technologies to promote and facilitate behavior change through specific context and information, for example, mobile apps, web-based, etc. Due to the latest advancement in digital technologies and their capacity to collect extensive user data, these interventions consider variations in an individual's characteristics, contexts, and changes over time [4].

To account for the knowledge of health psychology, recently, the Human Behavior Change Project established a link between the BCTs and their mechanism of action [5,6]. For example, the BCTs goal-setting, feedback and reward, work by manipulating the motivation of the target. So, if motivation is chosen as the theoretical construct to be targeted in any intervention development phase, the effective and agreed BCTs can be selected from this project [6]. To effectively use BCTs in digital interventions, the parameters of the BCTs and the mediating factors need to be explicitly defined. The 'motivation' cannot work as a black box (every human is different). By creating an explicit model of the underlying MoA, in this case 'motivation', we can accommodate individual characteristics and provide the mediating feedback loop to both BCTs and the targeted behavior.

Therefore, in this paper, we present an extended version of the temporal causal network model of motivation [7] that will describe how the high-level BCTs can be made adaptive and personalized via a lower-level process of 'motivation.' The temporal causal network modeling technique gives us the flexibility to represent any complex problem having time and causality dimensions between states more efficiently and easily. The low-level process (motivation) and its components are modeled based on the observations from the neuro-reward system and represented through the temporal causal network modeling technique. More detail about the temporal modeling technique and the representation of 'motivation' is provided in Section 3.1. Furthermore, Figure 1 depicts how the model will be used in the intervention and how different BCTs can be used to affect various components of the model. So, rather than studying the manipulating effect of psychological constructs, we are modeling the mediating role of motivation and its core components for BCTs and the targeted behavior. This model will serve different purposes and illustrates the work's novelty. Firstly, using this model allows digital intervention designers to report the mechanism of action in their interventions properly. Secondly, the intervention can be made more adaptive and personalized. For example, goal-setting and feedback can be customized based on the model outputs for different personalities like introversion, extraversion, neuroticism, conscientiousness, etc.

To summarize, the objectives of this article are:

- To propose a formal description of the dynamics of motivation and a computational implementation to show its working as a 'mechanism of action' component in digital behavior change intervention.
- To illustrate the relevance of the model for the study of digital behavior change interventions, specifically for generating and maintaining motivation, and how this can be used for personalization and adaption of interventions.

The paper is organized as follows: Section 2 shows the role of motivation in health behavior change and, more specifically, how we can generate and maintain motivation. Section 3 explains the term 'mechanism of action' and explains different possible ways that can be used to define/present a psychological construct as a mechanism of action. Section 4 describes the extended version of the motivation model for digital health behavior change based on the neuro reward pathway. Motivation is a mechanism of action with its mathematical formulation for health behavior change. Section 5 further represents an example intervention with simulation for increasing physical activity behavior in office employees. The paper concludes with remarks and future work.

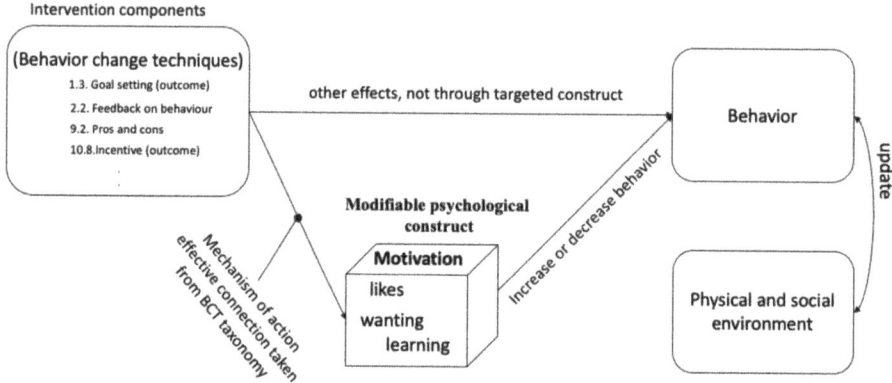

Figure 1. The model postulates the 'motivation' as the mechanism of action for a behavior change intervention.

2. Health Behavior Change and Motivation

This section of the article aims to understand the motivation construct from a neurosciences perspective and its possible role in health behavior change. Most cognitive health theories describe the potential relationships between psycho-social factors and healthy behaviors. For example, the Social Cognitive Theory, Health Belief model, and Theory of Planned Behavior are examples of theories that describe the role of individual beliefs, experiences, social factors, and environmental factors on individual health behaviors. Conversely, the widely used Transtheoretical model (TTM) and Health Action Process (HAPA) define the stages through which individuals go through to change their behavior [8,9]. Similarly, self-determination theory (SDT) explains the process of intrinsic motivation with three basic psychological needs: autonomy, competence, and relatedness [10].

Motivation in the neurosciences refers to neurotransmitters, or brain networks, which are collectively involved in different processes like releasing a chemical named dopamine, reward/punishment anticipation processing, reinforcement (learning), storing and updating a reward value, and decision-making drive human behavior. Together, these processes and chemical reactions control motivational behavior that leads to achieving a specific goal or reward. The details of all these brain networks and processes are discussed in Section 4 below. Here the mechanism of motivation concerning health behavior change is explained as two separate processes, i.e., motivation generation; how value-based anticipation of stimulus can generate 'motivation', and what can be the possible techniques for it? Similarly, to sustain a healthy behavior, how is motivation maintained or regulated, and what are the possible techniques?

2.1. Motivation Generation

Humans do or refrain from doing particular behaviors based on the calculated value of reward or punishment. To elicit approach behavior (motivation), the first step is to make the anticipation of reward from that behavior or actions. Anticipating reward means any object, event, or activity can be a reward if it motivates us, causes us to learn, or elicits pleasurable feelings. Humans are pre-programmed with certain behaviors like food or sex because they are naturally rewarding and necessary for the survival of a species. In the case of secondary reward, a specific brain area first registers the stimulus as a reward or punishment, then stores its relative value for future decision making. Before exploring different techniques that can make the stimulus rewarding and elicit pleasure feelings, there are two essential aspects of the reward mechanism in neurosciences, i.e., liking vs. wanting, and action control systems that need to be understood. The reason for presenting the differentiation between these two aspects is to be able to select an appropriate technique that can either activate liking or wanting sub-systems. Moreover, both 'wanting' and 'liking' are interchangeably used for rewards, whereas the brain circuity for both mechanisms is dissociable [11].

2.1.1. Liking vs. Wanting

It is now a widely accepted fact in neurosciences that 'wanting' is a dissociable factor from 'liking' for the same reward [11]. The more extensive brain network of the 'wanting' and the smaller one of the 'liking' systems are described in Section 4 below. Initially, it was hypothesized that brain dopamine depletion would reduce 'liking' for rewards. Still, it is experimentally proven that a lack of dopamine demolishes all motivation (wanting) while the liking remains the same [11]. This difference is vital in behavior change because the stimulus or any intervention components may influence one or another system. For example, maybe you are hungry, and your wanting-system wants to eat something, but there is broccoli available that you do not like. It is also important to mention that 'wanting' does not mean the cognitively processed desire; instead, it is a particular form of desire triggered by reward-related cues [11]. That is why recovering addicts have a genuine desire to quit drugs, but the nonconscious 'wanting' triggers when exposed to drug cues. That is why usually the best motivation is the one which is through activation of the wanting-system (either cognitively processed or subconsciously by reward cues) and pleasurable enjoying.

2.1.2. Action Control Systems

After intercepting a reward, the human brain reward system uses three different action control systems. First, (i) the innate actions system, which is the evolutionary response to a stimulus. Conversely, (ii) habitual actions develop over time through learning via interaction with different stimuli, and (iii) goal-directed actions are more cognitively processed actions toward achieving desired outcomes [12]. Generating motivation for healthy behavior change usually utilizes a goal-direction action system to achieve the desired behavior and possibly triggers other action systems that may be more effective for changing specific behaviors. The effectiveness of behavior change intervention through any action system depends on choosing the right targeted action system in the right circumstances [12]. For example, the relative effectiveness of triggering the habitual action system for smoking cessation (behavior) in a personalized intervention (population) would be greater using the social influence-based intervention.

2.2. Motivation Maintenance

This section will discuss if motivation is generated, then why it fades out and how we can maintain it. Another essential process in the neuroscientific explanation of 'motivation', i.e., reward prediction error (RPE), can be used to keep the level of motivation. RPE is the difference between received and expected rewards. This error helps humans learn about the stimulus and use it for future decision-making. Continuous interaction with the stimulus will cause learning of the reward/punishment outcome of the stimuli via reward prediction error. RPE can be used to regulate and maintain motivation, e.g., positive reward prediction means more learning of the stimulus outcome and more chances of performing the behavior often, whereas the negative reward prediction error means less learning of the stimulus-outcome association.

As mentioned earlier, the expected value of a reward is obtained through the attributes of the incentive, such as amount, type, and delay [13]. So, different techniques can be used to regulate motivation by manipulating the attribute of the reward itself. For example, increasing the incentive on a particular behavior will generate a surprise factor and cause a positive reward prediction error. Similarly, humans like instant gratification; if the unexpected reward is given before the expected time it will also cause a surprise factor and release enough dopamine to fasten the learning process. Moreover, the same type or always-expected reward will eventually be learned and will not be effective in the long term, the value of the behavior will decrease, and the frustration will grow.

2.3. Behavior Change Techniques for Motivation Generation and Maintenance

Based on Bandura's self-efficacy theory, BCTs are usually selected based on the targeted theoretical constructs; for example, *instructions on the problem* or *increasing problem-solving skills* are often used to increase self-efficacy. In this section, we will discuss some of the techniques mentioned in Table 1, taken from behavior change taxonomy [14], that can change behavior through 'motivation'. Furthermore, the techniques are discussed in the context of the two sub-processes discussed above, and the possible roles of these techniques in manipulating any of the sub-process. For example, for motivation generation, whether specific techniques would increase the reward value (or) increase pleasure feelings, etc. In the BCT taxonomy [14], the technique "10.8. incentive (outcome)", besides the effect on other psychological processes like intention and beliefs, it also has an impact on motivation. It is argued that if an external reward is promised to be delivered after achieving a specific behavior outcome, it will generate motivation by influencing the values of the outcome of the action, e.g., the monetary incentive for the employee who comes to the office by bike can ultimately have better health [15]. The motivation for cycling may be low due to the cost (fatigue) of cycling to the office and the low rewarding value. The achievement of incentive does have rewarding value itself. Still, the pleasure anticipation (expectation) in reaction to the stimulus will increase the value of cycling and ultimately give feelings of higher reward due to health improvement.

Table 1. List of the Behavior Change Techniques (BCTs) and their respective mediating purpose in our model. These BCTs are supposed to change behavior through motivation [6].

(Code). Behavior Change Techniques	Purpose	Reward System Components
1.3. Goal setting (outcome)	For planning, reduce gratification, frustration	Maintain reward prediction error
9.2. Pros and Cons	Increase wanting (pros) and not wanting (cons)	Wanting
10.8. Incentive (outcome)	Increase outcome value	Liking
10.10. Reward (outcome)	Increase outcome value	Liking

Similarly, the BCT "9.2 pros and cons" can increase motivation by reducing the cost of ignoring unhealthy behavior consequences. Likewise, with the negative reward prediction error due to the same type or always-expected reward, the motivation will decrease, and the frustration will grow. The best strategy could be to use "1.3 goal setting (outcome)". This strategy can activate cognitive control for self-regulation by providing reasonable goals and plans to overcome immediate impulses and low execution process capacity.

3. Why and How to Model 'Mechanism of Actions'

This section aims to show the number of possible methods for representing different psychological constructs or processes that usually or possibly can act as mechanisms of action between behavior change techniques and targeted behavior. The term 'MoA' evolved with the increasing need to improve the effectiveness of behavior change interventions. The major problem is that the MoAs are not mentioned for the active ingredient, i.e., BCT, in any intervention [3]. So, a clear understanding of the processes through which individual BCTs have their effects (i.e., their Mechanisms of Action) will allow us to make more effective interventions by making intervention personalized and making replicable components in any intervention. These mechanisms of actions are defined as a range of theoretical constructs that represent the processes through which a BCT affects behavior, and these constructs specified in theories of behavior and behavior change that can be seen to 'mediate' intervention effects, such as 'beliefs about capabilities', 'knowledge', and 'behavioral regulation'. They can be characteristics of the individual (i.e., intrapersonal psychological processes) and characteristics of the social and physical environment (e.g., social support). Moreover, another challenge for digital intervention is to represent these MoAs as an explicit model and the acquired knowledge as behavior change taxonomy of that construct. Below, we discuss some possibilities to model these constructs as MoA when the respective effective BCTs are chosen in any behavior change intervention.

3.1. Temporal Causal Network Models

The mechanism of a particular construct at the psychological or neural level could be defined as a temporal causal network model. Each node on the network represents the behavioral constructs, and the arrow shows the causal impact of one construct on another. For example, in [7], a temporal causal network model for the motivation generation and maintenance process is presented based on the dopaminergic reward pathway. The model shows the casual relationship between external incentives and internal body feeling for change in a targeted behavior. The external incentive state has a causal impact on the feeling state, and feeling better about the action increases motivation. Using this type of model to change sedentary behavior is given in [16]. Similarly, emotion regulation techniques are modeled as a temporal causal network, which shows how and when specific strategies can be activated for more effective behavior change intervention [17]. So, according to our agent-based framework, any causal model for any theoretical construct that explains the causality among the behavior change components and its parameters can be plugged in as a mechanism of action [18]. This paper considers our previously published temporal causal network model for motivation [7], extending it and integrating it as the mechanism of action for digital health behavior change intervention.

3.2. Multidimensional Generalization Space

Based on [4], a state-space representation is another important way to represent when, where, for whom, and in what state intervention will produce a targeted effect for that person. The "state" is the social-psychological or environmental constructs defined based on the target populations represented as multiple variables that determine the "space" when a MoA may produce the effect [4]. For example, feedback on behavior (e.g., showing daily average steps taken) could only inspire a physical activity if the state space of the person is appropriately receptive to this intervention. The probability of a person taking 10,000 daily steps increases if the motivation is high (motivation high = yes) and if their outcome expectation is high.

3.3. Computational Agent/System Models

Computational models are often represented and validated using different statistical and mathematical models, which means the explicit specification of constructs and how constructs interact with one another. For example, in [19], the author presented a computational model based on social cognitive theory for influences on physical activity. Social cognitive theory is also modeled as dynamical systems using fluid analogies and control systems principles drawn from engineering [20]. Similarly, in [21], a computational model of behavior change, based on existing psychological theories (the transtheoretical model, social cognitive theory, the theory of planned behavior, and attitude formation theory), is proposed that describes formal relations between the psychological constructs and their role in different stages of behavior change.

4. Model Description and Formalization

This section provides an extended version of the temporal-causal network model of motivation [7], with a complete description and formalization. The earlier published model is based on the underlying neuroscientific processes (dopamine pathway and its subsystems: mesolimbic dopamine system and mesocortical dopamine system) of motivation and explains how reward is anticipated and how the brain's relative valuation system processes it. The model represents processes and psychological constructs with several different states. For example, one state represents the sensory representation of the stimulus, and the other represents its rewarding value (positive feelings). This positive feeling state influences the action state, which means the human would approach or act toward attaining the reward (called motivation generated). Furthermore, the model encoded the process of motivation maintenance through reward prediction error (RPE). RPE means the certain amount of dopamine released on either received reward is better or worse than expected. RPE plays an important role in learning (action-outcome) and provides a basis for an explanation for decreasing/increasing motivation.

Dopamine not only plays a role as the mechanism of action in motivation but also in other different human cognitive processes like movement, attention, sleep, etc. Similarly, we want to use this model as a MoA for effective, adaptive, and personalized behavior change techniques in health behavior change intervention. We now understand how motivation is generated and maintained from the neurological level, and how this mechanism needs to be exploited for healthy behavior. We aim to use to model to determine what can be done so that the user does or refrains from target behavior by *value-based reward anticipation* and how we can maintain their motivation for target behavior by *reward prediction error*. These two motivation processes need to be optimized for an effective health behavior change intervention. Before we can introduce the formal description of the model, the following questions need to be answered:

1. What strategies can be used to increase the rewarding value of a stimulus? Increasing the anticipated value of the stimulus (any behavior, goal, etc.) will be assumed that motivation is generated, and the behavior will be performed more often because of the enriching value.
2. What strategies can be used to keep the RPE as positive as possible, as the association between stimulus-reward will be learned when the RPE is positive. In the case of negative RPE, the learning would get slow or stop, and eventually, the chances are that an agent will switch to perform other behavior for greater reward.

Different behavior science, health psychology, and neuroscience literature are approached to find answers to the above questions. The collected literature helped us define a simple motivation framework, given below, which structures our understanding of the phenomena associated with reward-seeking and motivation. The proposed formalization describes the computation of the valuation system (costs and benefits), and outcome values are formulated to define a human's current motivation state. We will use this process of *value-based reward anticipation* to **generate** motivation. This will be described in the next Section 4.1. Section 4.2 will look into the *reward prediction error* process for **maintaining** or improving the current motivation level.

4.1. Value-Based Reward Anticipation for Motivation Generation

To answer the first question, the net expected reward is calculated according to the utility function, taken from neurocomputational science literature [22], see Equation (1). The equation will determine the rewarding value for the action to be taken at a certain point in time (t). The net rewarding value is the subtraction of the expected reward (pleasure, health, food, etc.) from the costs (negative consequences, fatigue, etc.) associated with that action. The cost and expected values are subjective, and it means everyone would have different reward expectations for the same behavior. The calculated expectations of rewards (or punishment) during value-based decisions are updated based on experiences in the surrounding world.

$$\text{Net expected reward}_{(t)} = \sum \text{reward}_{(t)} - \sum \text{costs}_{(t)} \qquad (1)$$

In the original temporal causal network model, we considered this expected reward ($\sum$reward) in Equation (1) as the expectation of pleasure associated with the action, called "*liking*" or the *positive feelings*. Let us assume that we are only measuring *liking* or *positive feelings* as an expected reward, and the total costs are a weighted sum of all different subjective costs. Then Equation (1) can be expanded as given below:

$$\text{Net expected reward}_{(t)} = \text{liking}_{(t)} - (\text{costs}_{1(t)} + \text{costs}_{2(t)} + \text{costs}_{3(t)} \ldots) \quad (2)$$

As mentioned earlier in Section 2.1.1, this net reward value determines the motivation or the "wanting". So, motivation is directly proportional ($\propto$) to the outcome of net reward [22]. We can rewrite the Equation (2) as follows:

$$\text{Motivation}_{(t)} \propto \text{liking}_{(t)} - \gamma_1 \times \text{costs}_{1(t)} - \gamma_2 \times \text{costs}_{2(t)} - \gamma_3 \times \text{costs}_{3(t)} \ldots \quad (3)$$

A new term is introduced in Equation (3); the term temporal discounting (γ) is the inclination for a person to see a desired outcome in the future as less important than one in the present. It is considered a good characteristic in prediction for the maintenance of healthy behavior. For example, the temporal discounting rate is strongly associated with body mass [23]. Despite the potentially high cost of different behavior, they develop over a more extended period and are thus not immediately noticed, for example, weight gain. This type of cost is usually discounted and sometimes to a negligible level. As the cost and expected reward are subjective matters, similarly, every cost variable has different discounting rates.

This formalization of motivation and the different involved factors can be used to generate motivation.

4.2. Reward Prediction Error for Motivation Maintenance

To maintain motivation, we exploit the reward prediction error. The association between behavior and the outcome is learned over time. The strength of this connection is dependent on the reward prediction error and is represented as follows:

$$\text{RPE}_{(t)} = \beta \, (\text{Received Reward}_{(t)} - \text{Net expected reward}_{(t)}) \quad (4)$$

where Received Reward$_{(t)}$ denotes a received reward at time t for a certain action or behavior, and net expected reward shows the predicted/expected reward at time t. This error value is responsible for dopamine release, and it determines the learning of the action-outcome connection, whereas β is a learning rate parameter that determines how much weight of the error is registered or, in simple words, it shows the neuron's firing rate. Every human is different; that is why with the same trail of the experiment, some learn more quickly than others.

To summarize, we will use Equation (2) to generate motivation and Equation (4) to regulate or maintain the motivation. Figure 2 shows the schematic representation of the whole motivation process and the links of its components with other components in behavior change intervention.

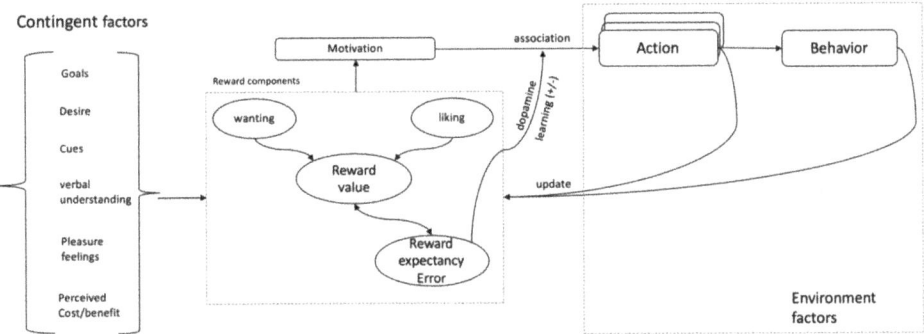

Figure 2. The schematic representation whole process of 'motivation' and its links with reward components.

5. Motivation-Based Intervention Example and Simulations

This section will illustrate integrating the above motivation model in digital health behavior change intervention. Different scenarios are simulated to show the two processes, i.e., motivation generation and motivation maintenance, with the help of the formalization of the respective process introduced above. The assumption is that chosen behavior change techniques will influence personal and environmental factors. The target population's likelihood of regularly achieving their goals means that the relevant individual changed their behavior if all plans were completed.

An intervention scenario is created for an office environment. The intervention components, i.e., target behavior, BCTs, MOA, and environment, are defined according to an agent-based framework [18], shown in Table 2. The framework is based on ontology for behavior change interventions (BCIO) [24], which defines the intervention components and explains their connection.

Table 2. Our model defines the intervention components and their relations to specific motivation processes.

Motivation Processes	Targeted Behavior	Sub-Processes in the Motivation Model	BCTs	MoA	Environmental Observations
Motivation Generation	Physical Activity	Value-Based Reward Anticipation	10.8 Incentive (outcome) 5.1 Information about health consequences	Motivation	Step count, feelings (hedonic pleasure)
Motivation Maintenance		Reward-Prediction Error	1.3 Goal setting (outcome)		

Let's suppose a scenario given below:

"The office management announced a 3-month program for employees to make them physically active. The organization targeted motivation as a core psychological construct for changing behavior. The employees are asked to subscribe, and they are provided digital wearable devices that can count their daily physical activities. The program is designed to use performance-based incentives to activate the dopamine reward pathway. When the stimuli (physical activity) are cognitively processed, it becomes a goal. The first technique to generate motivation is to give incentives for goal achievement. For this reason, after every 15 days, the incentive will be given according to the choices towards the goal. The goal is to increase the rewarding value of physical activity and overcome its costs. Furthermore, the reward prediction error will be calculated to maintain motivation to change strategies and determine the motivation level. Every component and process of the intervention is described in the concerned sector below."

Table 2 shows all the components of an intervention scenario and how specific motivation processes correspond to the different computations and relevant, effective behavior change techniques. For example, to generate motivation, an incentive will be given. The observation would be to check whether the activity for the participant is rewarding (pleasurable) or not. Similarly, in the case of motivation regulation, the reward prediction error would be observed, and strategies will be changed accordingly.

According to our model of motivation, there is some further explanation of the scenario. Participants will be given a daily goal (steps to be taken). They will have to achieve the goal and be awarded daily points based on the performance (goal achievement). On every 15th day of the intervention, the participants will get a badge based on their points in the past 15 days. We assumed two costs associated with the target behavior (physical activity), i.e., health consequences and fatigue, for demonstration purposes.

Different personalities will take this cost differently because it is a subjective matter, and everybody has a different discounting rate. Moreover, the values of each variable are determined between 0 and 0.9 (0 being the smallest and 0.9 being the highest). Based on those parameters, motivation generation and maintenance are simulated below. Each section demonstrates what parameters are observed and how these parameters can be tuned with different behavior change techniques for effectiveness and personalization of the intervention.

5.1. Motivation Generation

The hypothesis that motivation is generated through value-based reward anticipation can be observed by the intensity of the behavior for which an incentive is given. According to Equation (2), motivation is directly proportional to the difference between the expected reward and the cost of getting this reward. So this means that there could be several reasons that cause the difference in motivation level, and different techniques can be used to overcome these reasons. Firstly, let us consider how incentives can change the behavior, as the technique "10.8 incentive (outcome)" is the promise of external reward for performing a specific behavior. We keep the delay discounting and cost associated with the behavior constant (delay discounting 0.9, $cost_1$ 0.9, $cost_2$ 0.6), because we are giving them an incentive to increase the pleasure feeling; in other words, we are making the behavior rewarding for them. According to Equation (3), if the participant starts liking the incentive, it will increase their motivation to perform the behavior more often and achieve the reward again and again. Figure 3a shows how giving incentives during the intervention program increases the pleasure feeling (liking) and how motivation started building. This simulation gives us two insights; first, we can use incentives or other techniques to increase the pleasant feeling. Second, we can make these techniques adaptive according to different personalities. Next comes the subjectivity issue; maybe some employees will not consider points and badges as rewarding compared to the cost associated with them. We will show it with a difference in delay discounting value to simulate variability in different personalities. The health consequences of not living an active life are high (0.9), and doing daily physical activity has a moderate level of fatigue cost (0.6). Using the technique "5.1 information about health consequences," we can target the delay discounting of the associated costs. In Figure 3b, suppose all of them like it equally, but the difference in their discount rate for the related costs would make a difference in their motivation level. The employee with the highest discount rate does not know or care about the health consequences and fatigue associated with actions. So, giving awareness or information about health consequences can target the delay discounting parameter.

5.2. Motivation Maintenance

The process of motivation maintenance means maintaining the level of motivation generated earlier. This is done by calculating reward prediction error on different intervals in the model. The RPE value in the model represents the difference between received and expected rewards for performing some actions. If their expectation is met, a certain amount of dopamine gets released. The dopamine release shows the learning of the reward anticipation from that action. When this association is learned enough, the dopamine is released with stimulus cues only, not the reward itself. By performing this action more often because of the reward, it is assumed that the behavior gets habituated.

Positive Reward Prediction Error

The scenario to understand RPE calculation is depicted in Figure 4. In our design, RPE is calculated using Equation (4). The expected reward on the fifteenth day was 150 points; the positive reward prediction arose because it was the first time. Later, on the 30th day, the expected and received reward were the same and did not cause any dopamine spike because the participant learned the behavior and its outcome. The participants will wish for a bronze medal again on day 45th, and surprisingly, getting a gold badge will produce high dopamine spikes. On the 75th day, the participant expected a gold medal again (worth 300 points), but surprisingly he got no reward which means he does not meet the actual reward expectation; according to Equation (4), 0 − 100 = −100. This negative reward prediction error would cause the update of the reward value of the action to 0 and would be less likely to perform again.

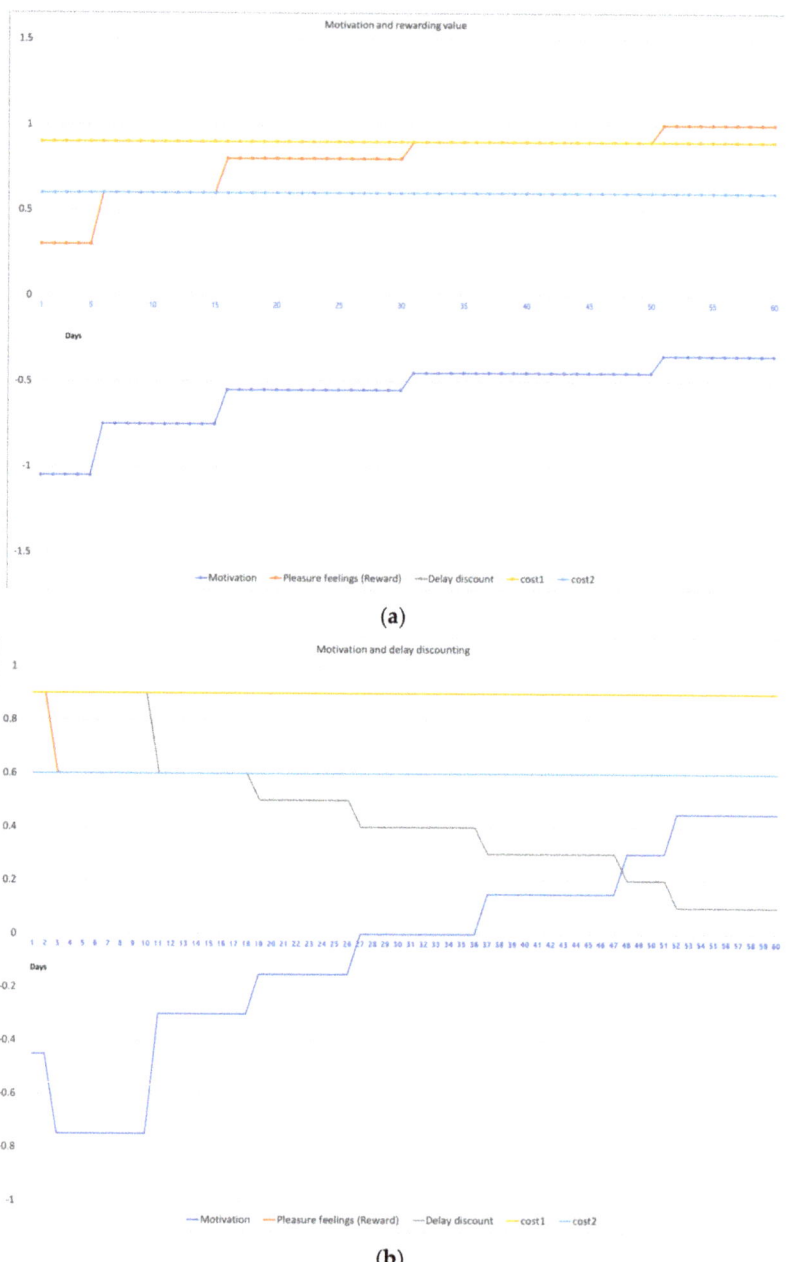

Figure 3. Motivation concerning different model parameters/processes through different BCTs (**a**) shows the effect of increasing liking for the activity by triggering a value-based reward system, and; (**b**) shows the effect of targeting the delay discounting characteristic of the participants.

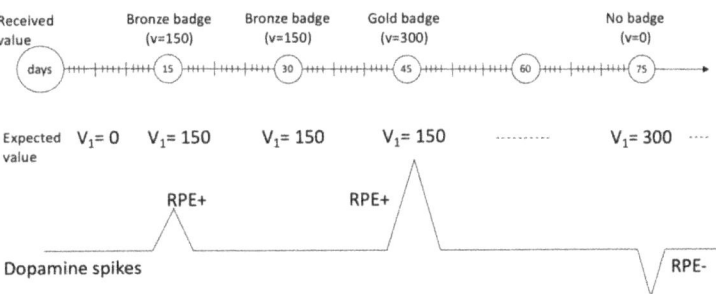

Figure 4. The timeline for incentive and the corresponding reward prediction errors.

For this reason, goal-setting techniques are primarily used to regulate motivation in different types of behavior change interventions [3]. The goal-setting helps develop a plan for maximizing the reward [12]. In addition to long-term goals (desired outcomes), it is also essential to generate short-term goals that are vivid and detectable, which allow people to monitor their progress. For this reason, small adaptive goals for daily step count and feedback based on their performance would help them monitor their progress and increase the rewards of the actions. Due to faster communication and efficient and ubiquitous seniors, these operations are pretty straightforward and precise in digital interventions.

6. Conclusions

Digital behavior change interventions usually do not report the explicit action of their techniques. If the techniques are mentioned, the mechanism of action through which these techniques have achieved their effects is not explicit. With recent consensus among health and social science researchers about the behavior change constructs and their effect pathways, we can develop theories and models that can easily be integrated into digital interventions. In this article, it has been shown how motivation can be explicitly modeled and integrated within an intervention as a mechanism of action for different behavior change techniques. Various parameters and aspects of the neuro-reward system formulated the model and presented it for motivation generation and maintenance.

An example intervention is defined and simulated to show how we can generate and maintain motivation and how the model's integration can help us achieve personalization and adaptivity through behavior change techniques. This type of research is novel and emerging. In addition to the personalization, models such as the ones presented in this paper could help digital intervention designers to properly report and use behavior change techniques by making their mechanism of action explicit.

7. Limitations and Future Work

The model proposed in this study is based on neurological observations. These observations are validated in the neurosciences to show the working of the release of different neuro-chemicals. In our work, we used these observations to propose a model of health behavior change. This type of usage requires additional validation. Preferably, a long-term experiment is performed in which data is collected about all the factors discussed in the model. In the future, we are working on designing an experiment where we can collect the relevant data to validate this model and report the result.

Another limitation is that we did not evaluate the use of this model as part of an actual intervention. We are currently working on developing such an intervention and its evaluation in a feasibility study. This intervention will use the model presented in this paper as a reasoning engine, continuously evaluating the user's current behavior and factors and using this to apply the best behavior change technique. The system will operate on mobile, web, or both. It collects real-time data from the user and uses this as input for the model, determining which necessary behavior change can be applied.

Finally, this paper only uses "Motivation" as a mechanism of action. It would also be helpful to develop models of other mechanisms of action, to evaluate the generalizability of the approach that we have presented.

Author Contributions: Conceptualization, F.T. and M.C.A.K.; Methodology, F.T.; Supervision, M.C.A.K. and A.V.H.; Visualization, F.T.; Writing—original draft, F.T.; Writing—review & editing, M.C.A.K. and A.V.H. All authors have read and agreed to the published version of the manuscript.

Funding: This research received no external funding.

Institutional Review Board Statement: Not applicable.

Informed Consent Statement: Not applicable.

Data Availability Statement: Not applicable.

Conflicts of Interest: The authors declare no conflict of interest.

References

1. Peters, G.-J. Constructs, Operationalisations, Mediators, and Why Behavior Change Techniques Cannot Change Behavior. Available online: https://behaviorchange.eu/2018/06/constructs-operationalisations-mediators-and-why-behavior-change-techniques-cannot-change-behavior/ (accessed on 20 April 2022).
2. Michie, S.; Yardley, L.; West, R.; Patrick, K.; Greaves, F. Developing and Evaluating Digital Interventions to Promote Behavior Change in Health and Health Care: Recommendations Resulting From an International Workshop. *J. Med. Internet Res.* **2017**, *19*, e232. [CrossRef] [PubMed]
3. Taj, F.; A Klein, M.C.; van Halteren, A. Digital Health Behavior Change Technology: Bibliometric and Scoping Review of Two Decades of Research. *JMIR mHealth uHealth* **2019**, *7*, e13311. [CrossRef] [PubMed]
4. Hekler, E.B.; Michie, S.; Pavel, M.; Rivera, D.; Collins, L.; Jimison, H.B.; Garnett, C.; Parral, S.; Spruijt-Metz, D. Advancing Models and Theories for Digital Behavior Change Interventions. *Am. J. Prev. Med.* **2016**, *51*, 825–832. [CrossRef] [PubMed]
5. Michie, S.; Thomas, J.; John, S.-T.; Mac Aonghusa, P.; Shawe-Taylor, J.; Kelly, M.P.; Deleris, L.A.; Finnerty, A.N.; Marques, M.M.; Norris, E.; et al. The Human Behaviour-Change Project: Harnessing the power of artificial intelligence and machine learning for evidence synthesis and interpretation. *Implement. Sci.* **2017**, *12*, 121. [CrossRef] [PubMed]
6. Connell, L.E.; Carey, R.N.; de Bruin, M.; Rothman, A.J.; Johnston, M.; Kelly, M.P.; Michie, S. Links Between Behavior Change Techniques and Mechanisms of Action: An Expert Consensus Study. *Ann. Behav. Med.* **2018**, *53*, 708–720. [CrossRef] [PubMed]
7. Taj, F.; Klein, M.C.A.; van Halteren, A. Computational model for reward-based generation and maintenance of motivation. In *Brain Informatics*; Lecture Notes in Computer Science (including Subseries Lecture Notes in Artificial Intelligence and Lecture Notes in Bioinformatics); Springer: Cham, Switzerland, 2018; Volume 11309, pp. 41–51.
8. Prochaska, J.O.; Velicer, W.F. The Transtheoretical Model of Health Behavior Change. *Am. J. Health Promot.* **1997**, *12*, 38–48. [CrossRef] [PubMed]
9. Schwarzer, R.; Luszczynska, A. How to Overcome Health-Compromising Behaviors. *Eur. Psychol.* **2008**, *13*, 141–151. [CrossRef]
10. Bouffard, L. Review of Ryan, R.M.; Deci, E.L. (2017). Self-determination theory. Basic psychological needs in motivation, development and wellness. New York, NY: Guilford Press. *Rev. Québécoise Psychol.* **2017**, *38*, 231.
11. Berridge, K.C.; Robinson, T.E. Liking, wanting, and the incentive-sensitization theory of addiction. *Am. Psychol.* **2016**, *71*, 670–679. [CrossRef] [PubMed]
12. Vlaev, I.; Dolan, P. Action Change Theory: A Reinforcement Learning Perspective on Behavior Change. *Rev. Gen. Psychol.* **2015**, *19*, 69–95. [CrossRef]
13. Diederen, K.M.J.; Fletcher, P.C. Dopamine, Prediction Error and Beyond. *Neuroscientist* **2020**, *27*, 30–46. [CrossRef] [PubMed]
14. Michie, S.; Richardson, M.; Johnston, M.; Abraham, C.; Francis, J.; Hardeman, W.; Eccles, M.P.; Cane, J.; Wood, C.E. The behavior change technique taxonomy (v1) of 93 hierarchically clustered techniques: Building an international consensus for the reporting of behavior change interventions. *Ann. Behav. Med.* **2013**, *46*, 81–95. [CrossRef] [PubMed]
15. Locke, E.A.; Latham, G.P. Goal setting theory. In *Motivation: Theory and Research*; Routledge: London, UK, 2012; pp. 23–40.
16. Taj, F.; Ullah, N.; Klein, M. Computational model for changing sedentary behavior through cognitive beliefs and introspective body-feelings. In Proceedings of the 14th International Joint Conference on Biomedical Engineering Systems and Technologies, Online Streaming, 11–13 February 2021; pp. 443–450.
17. Ullah, N.; Klein, M.; Treur, J. Food Desires, Negative Emotions and Behaviour Change Techniques: A Computational Analysis. *Smart Cities* **2021**, *4*, 48. [CrossRef]
18. Taj, F.; Klein, M.; van Halteren, A. An agent-based framework for persuasive health behavior change intervention. In *Health Information Science*; Lecture Notes in Computer Science (including Subseries Lecture Notes in Artificial Intelligence and Lecture Notes in Bioinformatics); Springer: Cham, Switzerland, 2020; Volume 12435, pp. 157–168.

19. Mollee, J.S.; van der Wal, C.N. A computational agent model of influences on physical activity based on the social cognitive theory. In Proceedings of the International Conference on Principles and Practice of Multi-Agent Systems, Nagoya, Japan, 18–20 November 2013; pp. 478–485.
20. Riley, W.; Martin, C.; Rivera, D.; Hekler, E.; Buman, M.; Adams, M.; Pavel, M. The development of a control systems model of social cognitive theory. *Ann. Behav. Med.* **2014**, *47*, S149.
21. Klein, M.; Mogles, N.; van Wissen, A. Why won't you do what's good for you? Using intelligent support for behavior change. In Proceedings of the International Workshop on Human Behavior Understanding, Amsterdam, The Netherlands, 16 November 2011; pp. 104–115.
22. Verharen, J.P.H.; Adan, R.A.H.; Vanderschuren, L.J.M.J. How Reward and Aversion Shape Motivation and Decision Making: A Computational Account. *Neuroscientist* **2019**, *26*, 87–99. [CrossRef] [PubMed]
23. Jarmolowicz, D.P.; Cherry, J.C.; Reed, D.; Bruce, J.M.; Crespi, J.M.; Lusk, J.L.; Bruce, A.S. Robust relation between temporal discounting rates and body mass. *Appetite* **2014**, *78*, 63–67. [CrossRef] [PubMed]
24. Larsen, K.R.; Michie, S.; Hekler, E.B.; Gibson, B.; Spruijt-Metz, D.; Ahern, D.; Cole-Lewis, H.; Ellis, R.J.B.; Hesse, B.; Moser, R.P.; et al. Behavior change interventions: The potential of ontologies for advancing science and practice. *J. Behav. Med.* **2016**, *40*, 6–22. [CrossRef] [PubMed]

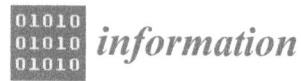

Article

Investigating the Feasibility of Assessing Depression Severity and Valence-Arousal with Wearable Sensors Using Discrete Wavelet Transforms and Machine Learning

Abdullah Ahmed [1,*], Jayroop Ramesh [2,*], Sandipan Ganguly [3], Raafat Aburukba [2], Assim Sagahyroon [2] and Fadi Aloul [2]

1. Department of Electrical and Computer Engineering, University of Massachusetts Amherst, Amherst, MA 01003, USA
2. Department of Computer Science and Engineering, American University of Sharjah, Sharjah 26666, United Arab Emirates
3. Department of Computer Science, University College London, London WC1TE 6BT, UK
* Correspondence: amahmed@umass.edu (A.A.); b00057412@aus.edu (J.R.); Tel.: +971-5-59517842 (J.R.)

Abstract: Depression is one of the most common mental health disorders, affecting approximately 280 million people worldwide. This condition is defined as emotional dysregulation resulting in persistent feelings of sadness, loss of interest and inability to experience pleasure. Early detection can facilitate timely intervention in the form of psychological therapy and/or medication. With the widespread public adoption of wearable devices such as smartwatches and fitness trackers, it is becoming increasingly possible to gain insights relating the mental states of individuals in an unobtrusive manner within free-living conditions. This work presents a machine learning (ML) approach that utilizes retrospectively collected data-derived consumer-grade wearables for passive detection of depression severity. The experiments conducted in this work reveal that multimodal analysis of physiological signals in terms of their discrete wavelet transform (DWT) features exhibit considerably better performance than unimodal scenarios. Additionally, we conduct experiments to view the impact of severity on emotional valence-arousal detection. We believe that our work has implications towards guiding development in the domain of multimodal wearable-based screening of mental health disorders and necessitates appropriate treatment interventions.

Keywords: affective; depression screening; digital phenotype; emotion; machine learning; passive sensing; wavelet transforms; wearable devices

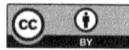

1. Introduction

Depression is one of the prevailing mental health disorders, affecting approximately 280 million people worldwide [1,2]. In the wake of the crippling effects of the pandemic, the global burden of depression continued to worsen, by at least 27.6% on average. This debilitating disorder differs from general mood fluctuations and fleeting emotional reactions along the aspects of intensity, recurrence, and anhedonia [1,2]. Depression often manifests owing to a complex interaction between socioeconomic, psychological and biological factors, and is exacerbated by comorbid physical conditions in an adverse feedback loop. Early screening is critical for timely intervention and the delivery of effective treatment methods such as cognitive behavioral therapy and/or antidepressant medications. However, the social stigma associated with mental health, the scarcity of trained health-care providers, relatively high rates of misdiagnoses and exorbitant service costs discourage individuals from seeking assistance [3].

To improve diagnoses fidelity, it is vital to develop universal screening approaches which reveal useful information without being intrusive or biased, as is the case with the currently adopted surveys [4]. With the proliferation of machine learning (ML) methods in the healthcare domain, where the automatic identification of relevant patterns and relationships among data without specification of a priori hypotheses holds considerable prognostic utility, there is the potential for detecting the presence of elusive disorders such as depression. In parallel, the ubiquity of smartphones and wearable devices such as smartwatches and fitness trackers offer the much sought-after capabilities of long-term unobtrusive monitoring in free-living conditions. Recent studies have employed ML while leveraging passive, non-intrusive modalities such as smartphone call/text logs [4], social media posts [5], gyroscope readings [6] GPS [7] and heart rate [8] for detecting states of depression and mental health distress.

These worthwhile approaches show the potential for depression screening using passive smartphone data while maintaining a fair degree of user privacy. Out of the different parameters measured, those acquired through wearable devices enable continuous and objective monitoring of patients [9]. Moreover, physiological signals, or a combination of them in tandem with ML, can predict symptoms of depression and anxiety [10,11]. This fact, coupled with the increasing ownership of wearables, estimated at 1 billion in 2022, suggest that personalized screening be introduced without revealing any user-specific information as opposed to partial alternatives such as location data or personal message history.

Noticeably, in the most recent literature, the sample population typically consists of depressed and completely healthy participants, and physiological signals are compounded with smartphone-derived biomarkers such as device usage, step count, sleep measures and location. In this work, we aim to quantify the effects of using only unimodal and multimodal signals from wearable sensors in terms of heart rate (HR), galvanic skin response (GSR) and accelerometry (ACC) among a predominantly depressed population.

Another facet of emotional state assessment which can benefit from wearable monitoring is affective experience quantification. As purported by [12], the interplay between the severity of depression and affective emotional activation in terms of valence and arousal can have implications for individual behavior and response to daily stimuli [13]. This manifests a strong influence on processes such as attention, perception, decision-making, learning and mental well-being [14]. Valence captures the extent to which an emotion is positive/negative, while arousal captures the intensity of the experienced emotion. Thus, we also explore this domain as an additional aspect of our central work.

The primary contributions of this work are the following:
- Validating the potential of implementing ML algorithms with retrospectively collected wearable-derived physiological data for classifying between moderately and severely depressed individuals.
- Assessing the quality of low frequency, general signal features extracted using discrete wavelet transforms (DWT) for developing ML algorithms.
- Examining the relative efficacies of heart rate, galvanic skin response and accelerometry readings in distinguishing between depression severity and emotional states.
- Investigating the role of depression severity in emotional valence and arousal detection.

This paper is organized such that Section 2 introduces the dataset and outlines the methodology and Section 3 presents the results and its discussion, with Section 4 concluding the work.

2. Methodology

2.1. Dataset

The DAPPER dataset [15] is an aggregation of ambulatory physiological and psychological data reported over a period of five days by 142 participants. It is segregated into sections as displayed in Table 1.

Table 1. DAPPER Contents.

Physiological Data	Psychological Data
Heart Rate (HR)	ESM (Experience Sampling Method)
Galvanic Skin Response (GSR)	DRM (Daily Reconstruction Method)
ACC Data	-

The volunteers were asked to engage in a pre-test (a data collection procedure preceding the start of the experiment) where they submitted their BDI-II measures amongst other details. During the main experiment, the psychological details were reported by the participants through answering questionnaires on their smartphones. They received six ESM questionnaires per day over 9 a.m.–11 p.m. with a minimum 3-h gap between each questionnaire. The DRM questionnaires were sent at 11 p.m. each day. Nonetheless, our research aimed to utilize the physiological recordings and focus on heart rate, which was collected using photoplethysmography, galvanic skin response, collected using surface electrodes from the wrist, and triaxial accelerometer data to assess depression severity. All the physiological data was recorded using Psychorus, a customized wristband, during Monday–Friday, 9 a.m.–11 p.m. Out of 142 total patients, 87 patients had valid physiological readings. The data was originally recorded with the following sampling rates (HR:20 Hz, GSR:40 Hz, ACC:20 Hz) but later downsampled to 1 Hz by the original authors to reduce complexity for future use by the research community. DAPPER followed the Helsinki standard and all the participants submitted their written permission.

At first, the raw data comprised 2249 signals. However, any signals of duration of less than 30 min were rejected, since the goal was to follow the 30-min ESM event periods. The concluding number of signals were 2034, each over a span of 1800 s for 87 patients. The distinguishing factor of DAPPER is the environment in which the data was collected in. Instead of the more popular laboratory-based controlled experiments, this dataset aimed to provide data gathered during natural day-to-day activities. Furthermore, this approach replicates accurate everyday situations, thus providing a resource with reliable data that can be used in further applications.

The distribution of the BDI-II scores had a mean with standard deviation of 29.73 ± 7.0, with a minimum of 21 and a maximum of 60. Discretizing the data for binary classification, the following four cut-offs are applied to generate four depression severity ranges: minimal severity (≤ 13), mild severity (≥ 14 and ≤ 19), moderate severity (≥ 20 and ≤ 28) and severe severity (≥ 29). Out of the 2034 available data instances, 960 belong to the moderate class and 1074 belong to the severe class. This suggests that all 87 patients in the original study suffered from clinical depression to some degree.

With a pure focus on studying depressed populations, we opt to consider the cases exhibiting minimal depression severity as our experimental control group. In accordance with [16], employing a control group of such close proximity to other experimental cases (in terms of depressive mental state) alleviates the control group's inherent selection bias, and potentially enhances the study's validity.

For binary segregation of arousal and valences, the Likert scale-reported scores of 1 and 2 are treated as low, whereas 3, 4 and 5 are considered as high. For valence, this resulted in 1003 and 1031 for low and high categories, respectively. For arousal, this resulted in 1361 and 673 for low and high categories, respectively. It is observable from Figure 1 that the emotional states stratified across the depressed population congregate towards the higher intensity values.

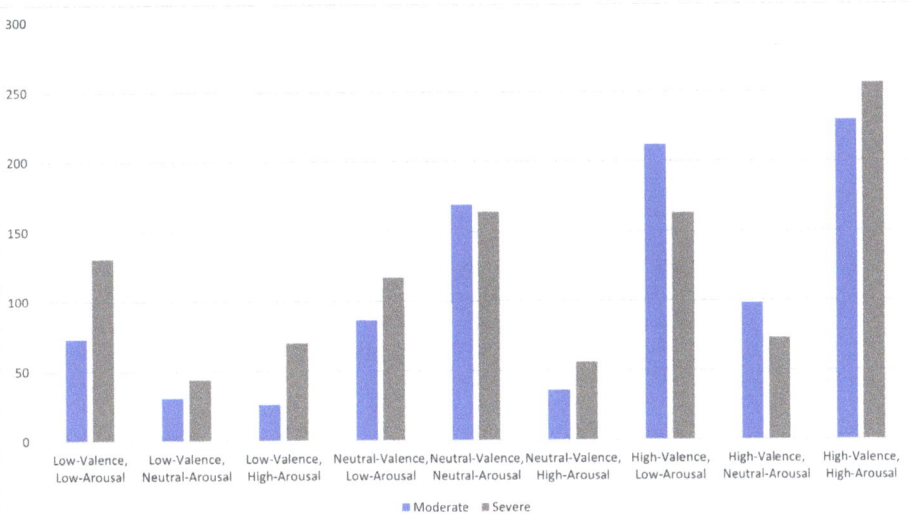

Figure 1. Valence and Arousal frequency grouped by depression severity.

2.2. Feature Extraction

Our complete approach is outlined in Figure 2, consisting of data processing, feature extraction and ML implementation. Discrete wavelet transform (DWT) can be implemented on-devices directly for real-time signal monitoring with relatively lower battery consumption. We derive generic statistical features for all three modalities after DWT analysis with the goals of minimizing computational overhead and preserving the same processing pipeline and introducing a notion of translation invariance to noise or other motion artifacts. Furthermore, a secondary goal is to view the differences in emotional state activation in terms of valence and arousal across the two depressed populations, and the learnable differences with machine learning.

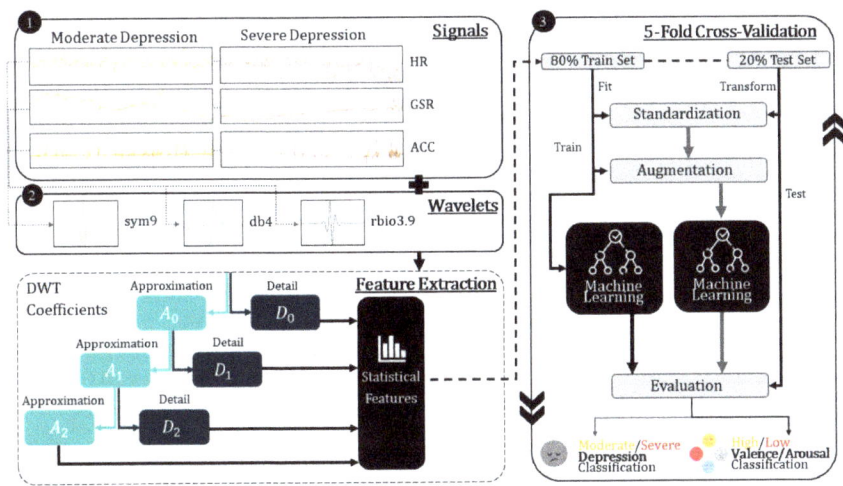

Figure 2. End-to-end model pipeline.

DWT can be considered as the projection of a sum vectored and zero mean signal S into a set of basis functions called wavelets $\phi_{i,k}(n)$ and $\psi_{i,k}(n)$, which localize the time–frequency domain characteristics of the signal. These wavelets $\Psi_{a,b}(t)$ are generated from a single-base wavelet Ψ called the mother wavelet, through a series of dilations and translations of a scaling function as defined in.

$$\begin{aligned}\phi_{i,k}(n) &= 2^{-\frac{i}{2}}\phi\left(2^{-i}n - k\right)\\ \psi_{i,k}(n) &= 2^{-\frac{i}{2}}\psi\left(2^{-i}n - k\right)\end{aligned} \quad (1)$$

In Equation (1), n is the length of the signal S, k is the discrete translations and 2^i are the dyadic dilations.

More specifically, each series is a decomposed time series of coefficients describing the evolution the temporal component within a corresponding frequency band. This is performed using a pair of finite impulse response filters, taken as low-pass and high-pass respectively. With this, the DWT on a signal results in the approximation $A_i(k)$ and detailed coefficients $D_i(k)$ formulated by:

$$\begin{aligned}A_i(k) &= \sum_n S(n)\phi_{i,k}(n)\\ D_i(k) &= \sum_n S(n)\psi_{i,k}(n)\end{aligned} \quad (2)$$

In Equation (2), the approximation coefficients $A_i(k)$ are the low-pass elements, and the detailed coefficients $D_i(k)$ are high-pass elements for a signal S, at a decomposition level i. In the case of multi-level decomposition, numerous stages of decomposition occurs, beginning within the original signal. The former is analyzed further in the same manner to a certain decomposition level, while the latter is not. The decomposition level is determined by the mother wavelet, sampling frequency, and signal length and is generally treated as the optimal decomposition level.

After experimenting with candidate discrete mother wavelets across the families of coiflets, biorthogonal, daubechies, reverse biorthogonal, symlet and haar, the following are selected based on their high performances and accordance with prior physiological signal analysis in literature. For HR, we use the symlet-9 (sym9) which has the properties of near symmetry, orthogonality and biorthogonality. For GSR, we use the daubechies-4 (db4) which has the properties of asymmetry, orthogonality and biorthogonality. For ACC, we use the reverse biorthogonal-3.9 (rbio3.9) which has the properties of symmetry, no orthogonality and biorthogonality. Empirically, we find that the optimal levels of decomposition are 1, 3 and 2 for PPG, GSR and ACC signals, respectively.

The final features pertaining to the coefficients of the signals are Shannon Entropy, Zero Crossing Rate, Mean Crossing Rate, Mean, Standard Deviation, Median, Variance, Root Mean Square, 5th Percentile, 25th Percentile, 75th Percentile, and 95th Percentile values.

2.3. Data Augmentation

While the disparity between the majority and minority classes (0 and 1, no and yes, respectively) were not as extreme, augmentation was applied to observe any quantifiable improvement in overall model performance. Five techniques for augmentation were used, and their breakdown by type is as follows: oversampling: Synthetic Minority Oversampling Technique (SMOTE) and Adaptive Synthetic Sampling (ADASYN), oversampling + undersampling: SMOTE + Tomek links (SMOTEK), SMOTE + Edited Nearest Neighbours (SMOTEEN), and undersampling: Random Under sampling and Edited Nearest Neighbours (ENN).

- SMOTE is an oversampling technique that increases the number of minority samples in the dataset, by generating new samples from existing minority class samples. The approach generates new samples that are not duplicates, but convex combinations of two or more randomly chosen neighboring data samples in the feature space.
- ADASYN is an adaptive data generation method which creates synthetic samples to reduce class imbalances in a dataset. The approach uses weighted distribution for

different minority class samples as per relative difficulty in learning, and generates more samples similar to the harder-to-learn samples. This therefore reduces overall bias present in the dataset, and should improve learning performance of models trained on this data as well.
- SMOTEK and SMOTENN are hybrid techniques that consist of both undersampling and oversampling. Initially, SMOTE performs the over-sampling, then the resulting clusters that overlap on nearby points causing overfitting are removed using Tomek Links, or Nearest Neighbors, respectively, in the methods. The idea here is to clean distributions and lead to a distinct class separation.
- Random under sampling involves randomly discarding samples from the majority class until a balanced class distribution is attained.
- Condensed nearest neighbor undersampling involves the selection of prototypes from the training data, in order to essentially reduce the dataset size for instance-based classification. During this process, the the prototypical instances of the majority class are retained, while likely redundant instances are eliminated from the dataset.

2.4. Machine Learning

We utilized a wide range of standard ML algorithms such as Logistic Regression (LR), Support Vector Classifier (SVC), K-Nearest Neighbors (KNN), Light Gradient Boosting Machines (LGB), and Random Forest (RF) and eXtreme Gradient Boosting (XGB), and CatBoost (CB) to cover both traditional and ensemble techniques. These supervised algorithms span a variety of strategies in learning complexity, and their implementations generally elicit good bias-variance trade-off when data is not particularly voluminous (few hundred to a few thousand unique samples) as shown in [17–19]. Stratified sampling was used to divided 80% training set and 20% testing set through a five-fold cross-validation approach. Random search yielded the final hyperparameters for all algorithms.

3. Results

This section presents the results for (i) depression severity classification, and (ii) valence-arousal detection for each depression category. The performance measures are quantified with the metrics of accuracy, sensitivity, specificity, F1-score and, where pertinent, the Area Under the ROC (receiver operating characteristic) Curve (AUC).

3.1. Detecting Depression Severity

To evaluate the efficacy of the proposed multi-modal inference model, we test a variety of candidate machine learning models and tabulate their performance in Table 2. Despite most of the models scoring similarly (in terms of accuracy, sensitivity, specificity, F1-score, and AUC), we decided on using CatBoost (CB) Classifier in our trails for performing most reliably with an accuracy, sensitivity, and F1-score values of 64 ± 2.0, 68.7 ± 3.0, and 66.8 ± 2.0, respectively. It was observed that data augmentation did not yield any statistically significant increase in performance with this scenario.

Table 2. Quantitative model performance metrics for the multimodal cases.

Model	Accuracy	Sensitivity	Specificity	F1-Score	AUC
LGBM	64.0 ± 3.0	68.2 ± 2.0	59.4 ± 5.0	66.7 ± 2.0	63.8 ± 3.0
RF	64.0 ± 2.0	67.3 ± 2.0	60.2 ± 5.0	66.4 ± 2.0	63.8 ± 2.0
XGB	60.7 ± 2.0	64.8 ± 2.0	56.1 ± 5.0	63.5 ± 1.0	60.5 ± 2.0
CB	64.0 ± 2.0	68.7 ± 3.0	58.8 ± 4.0	66.8 ± 2.0	63.7 ± 2.0
KNN	58.2 ± 2.0	61.0 ± 3.0	55.0 ± 4.0	60.6 ± 2.0	58.0 ± 2.0
SVC	60.2 ± 2.0	63.0 ± 2.0	57.1 ± 5.0	62.6 ± 1.0	60.1 ± 2.0
LR	55.8 ± 2.0	60.2 ± 1.0	50.8 ± 4.0	59.1 ± 1.0	55.5 ± 2.0

In Table 3 we evaluate the performance of uni-modal inference and contrast it against bi- and tri- modal inference to evaluate the added value of multiple-modality and quantify its effectiveness in improving inference quality. Derived from the marginal inference quality increase (in comparison to the tri-modal model) based on the highlighted performance criteria, a holistic score of each permutation's performance is given in the last column of Table 3.

Table 3. Quantitative model performance metrics for exhaustive unimodal and multimodal cases with CB.

Model	Accuracy	Sensitivity	Specificity	F1-Score	AUC	Delta δ_{avg}
PPG	54.0 ± 2.0	62.5 ± 3.0	44.5 ± 2.0	58.9 ± 2.0	53.5 ± 2.0	+9.7
GSR	56.2 ± 1.0	70.7 ± 3.0	40.1 ± 1.0	63.0 ± 2.0	55.4 ± 1.0	+6.8
ACC	59.0 ± 2.0	65.1 ± 6.0	52.3 ± 6.0	62.6 ± 3.0	58.7 ± 2.0	+4.9
PPG + GSR	57.5 ± 2.0	67.9 ± 2.0	45.8 ± 5.0	62.8 ± 1.0	56.9 ± 2.0	+6.2
PPG + ACC	62.1 ± 1.0	65.8 ± 4.0	57.9 ± 4.0	64.7 ± 2.0	61.9 ± 1.0	+1.9
GSR + ACC	62.5 ± 1.0	68.9 ± 2.0	55.4 ± 1.0	66.0 ± 1.0	62.2 ± 1.0	+1.4
PPG + GSR + ACC	64.0 ± 2.0	68.7 ± 3.0	58.8 ± 4.0	66.8 ± 2.0	63.7 ± 2.0	-

For the DAPPER dataset, all possible single-modal models—using either PPG, GSR, or ACC, result in similarly performing models with an average accuracy of 56.4% and average F1-score of 61.5%. When observing combinations of any two modalities, however, we observe an average accuracy and F1-score values of both 60.7% and 64.5%, respectively. Finally, when all three modalities are combined, the resulting model has an accuracy of 64.0% and an F1-score of 66.8%.

Merely looking at the average performance for the learned models of varying number of modalities, we observe a performance increasing trend with each added modality. The move from uni- to bi-modal inference increases accuracy by 7.62%, and F1-score by 4.88%. Analogously, going from bi-modal to tri-modal inference improves the accuracy and F1-score by 5.44% and 3.57%, respectively. This upward trend validates the variability of the proposed multi-modal paradigm for depression severity inference.

3.2. Detecting Emotional Arousal and Valence

Much of performance measures across the metrics range from ~55 to ~60, which belies that only an average level of separability can be obtained between high and low states. In contrast to the depression severity classification case, Tables 4 and 5 exhibit results where one modality fares better than multi-modality. To detect high- and low-valence/arousal states in a moderately depressed population, GSR and ACC proved feasible, with contribution from SMOTE augmentation. The specificity being higher than sensitivity indicates a better recall of the low-valence/arousal states. To detect high- and low-valence/arousal states in the severely depressed population, HR and GSR proved feasible, with contribution from SMOTE and SMOTEEN. The sensitivity for valence is better, while the specificity for arousal is marginally better, indicating that high-valence and low-arousal states are more discernible in the severely depressed population. However, there appears to be no common modality for each kind of emotional state activation, and the results appear to be characteristic of this dataset population with varying degrees of applicability to a general population.

Table 4. Quantitative performance metrics for the moderately depressed population.

State	Modality	Approach	Accuracy	Sensitivity	Specificity	F1-Score
Valence	GSR	SVC + SMOTE	62.9	62.8	66.7	76.6
Arousal	ACC	LR + SMOTE	63.9	48.8	75.9	54.5

Table 5. Quantitative performance metrics for the severely depressed population.

State	Modality	Approach	Accuracy	Sensitivity	Specificity	F1-Score
Valence	HR	KNN + SMOTE	61.2	64.0	53.3	71.0
Arousal	GSR	SVC + SMOTEEN	56.9	56.3	57.8	61.5

4. Discussion

The goal was to separate behaviors of people suffering from depression based on emotional stimuli and possibly identifying affective emotional triggers in response to experienced events. As mentioned previously, there is a prevalence of depression among all surveyed individuals in this dataset who also experience higher-intensity emotional states. This warrants an investigation of the impact of depression in dampening/exacerbating emotional responses to various stimuli or events. As reported by [20], states of depression induce marked dysfunctional regulations of affective experience and affective quality perception. Generally, the neutral arousal/valence state is the most commonly experienced [21], because of the impaired emotional modulation to affective stimuli [22].

The achieved performance measures are in line with a recent study conducted with a similar demographic (race, age and education levels) asserting the potentially useful yet limited predictability of depression severity with wearable devices [23]. It appeared that greater severity of depressive symptoms showed associations with larger variation of night-time heart rate between the hours of 4 a.m. and 6 a.m. Additionally, this led to the findings (adjusted for covariates) that severity was also correlated robustly with weekday circadian activity rhythms. Thereby, our work focusing on individuals during conscious ESM activities serves as a complementary study to the general continuous diurnal and nocturnal biomarkers evaluated in [23].

According to [24], low-arousal states being associated with low-valence fine-grained states such as sadness, lethargy or fatigue is correlated with stronger levels of depression. This is because high arousal occurs when the cortical circuits in the brain are engaged and allocates attention in response to a particular stimuli [25]. However, our results do not agree with these findings, leading to our hypothesis that either the self-reported BDI-II scores were not reflective of the true underlying mental state, or that the self-reported valence and arousal is overly positive by choice of omission. A potential psychological link unifying our results in light of the previous studies is the theory of ambivalence over emotional expression. This is a condition wherein individuals have the propensity to avoid expression of emotions [26], owing to the effects of depression. In [27], it is rationalized that inciting high-arousal states in people with heightened depression thorough memory recalling tests increases help-seeking intentions. It could very well be that the stimuli or events experienced by the participants of the DAPPER dataset creation were involved in positive or familiar environments during the course of study.

Although the heterogeneous nature of different consumer-grade wearables occasionally leads to likely noise saturation, inaccurate values and uncalibrated errors [28], it is rationalized that the characteristic patterns associated with certain mental/physical diseases can indeed be reflected [29]. Additionally, it is not known if the individuals were on prescribed anti-depressants, engaged in psychological counselling or under any treatment which may introduce confounding variables that cannot be adjusted for.

While Deep Learning has demonstrated exemplary results in several fields and recent studies, there are still few limitations and challenges in the biomedical domain pertaining to class imbalance and data complexity, which discouraged its use in our work. As put forward in [30], Deep Learning models tend to capture spurious relations in the training data within clinical studies involving biomedical signals. This occurs, in context of this work, due to the implicit nature of some emotional states such as valence/arousal and depression, which do not manifest across all subjects with the same intensity or magnitude [31]. Thus, it appears that higher volumes of data readings from wearables are necessary to combat the relative sparsity of the wearable measurements, i.e, the ratio of the duration of *normal* physiological behavior to the duration of context-specific instantaneous responses to certain stimuli, and achieve higher performance scores.

Ref. [32] also indicates that with skewed data, the models prioritize the majority group due to higher prior probability. Unlike with summarized measures such as wavelet decomposed features, augmenting continuous raw signals and the rectification of class imbalance requires more complex techniques to account for the profound understanding of the morphology and patterns [33]. We believe the lightweight approaches (DWT + standard ML) are relatively more conducive towards power-efficient deployment on wearable or edge devices, as shown in [34].

We envision this research as an initial baseline for performance benchmarking on the DAPPER dataset, as well as an assessment of the relationship between depression and ephemeral emotional states.

5. Conclusions

In this paper we presented multi-modal depression detection machine learning models while juxtaposing its performance to that of single and double modality models. More specifically, we leverage low-frequency HR, GSR and ACC signals belonging to 87 patients from the Daily Ambulatory Psychological and Physiological recording for Emotional Research (DAPPER) dataset to train multiple ML algorithms to classify between moderate and severe states, as defined by the categorized Beck's Depression Inventory (BDI-II) score. After listing the top performing depression detection models on our dataset's mobile/wearable device-based biomedical signals, we make a case for the introduction of additional modality, with respect to the DAPPER dataset.

In comparison to attempts present in the literature, using a variety of datasets for the detection and prediction of depression trends of individuals using mobile and power-constrained devices, there is a case to be made for the use of multiple-modality devices. One contemporary work [35], describes a smartphone activity monitoring model for the collection of medically relevant metrics and tracking of user activities for the detection of PHQ-9 levels, achieving detection performance metrics of 59.1–60% accuracy, 62.3–72% sensitivity and 47.3–60.8% specificity. In contrast, the metrics of our proposed approach are $64 \pm 2.0\%$ accuracy, $68.7 \pm 3.0\%$ sensitivity and $58.8 \pm 4.0\%$ specificity, which consistently surpass the results in [35]. Therefore, we ultimately conclude that additional modality incorporation could potentially improve the detection accuracy of depression by accounting for different aspects of latent or conscious physiological responses to psychological events.

Author Contributions: Conceptualization, R.A., A.S. and F.A.; data curation, A.A. and S.G.; investigation, J.R., A.A. and S.G.; methodology, J.R.; project administration, R.A. and A.S.; resources, F.A. and A.S.; software, J.R.; supervision, R.A., A.S. and F.A.; validation, J.R., A.A. and S.G.; writing—original draft, J.R., A.A. and S.G.; writing—review and editing, R.A., A.S. and F.A. All authors have read and agreed to the published version of the manuscript.

Funding: This research received no external funding.

Institutional Review Board Statement: Not applicable.

Informed Consent Statement: A consent has been obtained from the patient(s) to use this dataset for research purposes and publishing this paper.

Data Availability Statement: The dataset adopted in this research is openly available in [Synapse] at https://doi.org/10.7303/syn22418021 (accessed on 20 April 2022).

Conflicts of Interest: The authors declare no conflict of interest.

Abbreviations

The following abbreviations are used in this manuscript:

ACC	Accelerometry
BDI-II	Beck's Depression Inventory
CB	CatBoost
DAPPER	Daily Ambulatory Psychological and Physiological recording for Emotional Research
DWT	Discrete Wavelet Transforms
GSR	Galvanic Skin Response
HR	Heart Rate
KNN	K-Nearest Neighbors
LGB	Light Gradient Boosting
ML	Machine Learning
RF	Random Forest
SVC	Support Vector Classifier
XGB	eXtreme Gradient Boosting

References

1. Harris, M.G.; Kazdin, A.E.; Chiu, W.T.; Sampson, N.A.; Aguilar-Gaxiola, S.; Al-Hamzawi, A.; Alonso, J.; Altwaijri, Y.; Andrade, L.H.; Cardoso, G.; et al. Findings from world mental health surveys of the perceived helpfulness of treatment for patients with major depressive disorder. *JAMA Psychiatry* **2020**, *77*, 830–841. [CrossRef] [PubMed]
2. Daly, M.; Robinson, E. Depression and anxiety during COVID-19. *Lancet* **2022**, *399*, 518. [CrossRef]
3. Zhang, F.; Gou, J. Machine Learning Assessment of Risk Factors for Depression in Later Adulthood. *Lancet Reg. Health Eur.* **2022**, *18*, 100399. [CrossRef]
4. Tlachac, M.; Melican, V.; Reisch, M.; Rundensteiner, E. Mobile Depression Screening with Time Series of Text Logs and Call Logs. In Proceedings of the 2021 IEEE EMBS International Conference on Biomedical and Health Informatics (BHI), Athens, Greece, 27–30 July 2021; pp. 1–4. [CrossRef]
5. Zhang, T.; Schoene, A.M.; Ji, S.; Ananiadou, S. Natural Language Processing Applied to Mental Illness Detection: A Narrative Review. *NPJ Digit. Med.* **2022**, *5*, 46. [CrossRef] [PubMed]
6. Choudhary, S.; Thomas, N.; Ellenberger, J.; Srinivasan, G.; Cohen, R. A Machine Learning Approach for Detecting Digital Behavioral Patterns of Depression Using Nonintrusive Smartphone Data (Complementary Path to Patient Health Questionnaire-9 Assessment): Prospective Observational Study. *JMIR Form. Res.* **2022**, *6*, e37736. [CrossRef] [PubMed]
7. Chikersal, P.; Doryab, A.; Tumminia, M.; Villalba, D.K.; Dutcher, J.M.; Liu, X.; Cohen, S.; Creswell, K.G.; Mankoff, J.; Creswell, J.D.; et al. Detecting Depression and Predicting Its Onset Using Longitudinal Symptoms Captured by Passive Sensing: A Machine Learning Approach With Robust Feature Selection. *ACM Trans.-Comput.-Hum. Interact. (TOCHI)* **2021**, *28*, 1–41. [CrossRef]
8. Jacobson, N.C.; Chung, Y.J. Passive Sensing of Prediction of Moment-To-Moment Depressed Mood among Undergraduates with Clinical Levels of Depression Sample Using Smartphones. *Sensors* **2020**, *20*, 3572. [CrossRef]
9. Lee, S.; Kim, H.; Park, M.J.; Jeon, H.J. Current Advances in Wearable Devices and Their Sensors in Patients with Depression. *Front. Psychiatry* **2021**, *12*, 672347. [CrossRef]
10. Long, Y.; Lin, Y.; Zhang, Z.; Jiang, R.; Wang, Z. Objective Assessment of Depression Using Multiple Physiological Signals. In Proceedings of the 2021 14th International Congress on Image and Signal Processing, BioMedical Engineering and Informatics (CISP-BMEI), Online, 23–25 October 2021; pp. 1–6. [CrossRef]
11. Moshe, I.; Terhorst, Y.; Opoku Asare, K.; Sander, L.B.; Ferreira, D.; Baumeister, H.; Mohr, D.C.; Pulkki-Råback, L. Predicting Symptoms of Depression and Anxiety Using Smartphone and Wearable Data. *Front. Psychiatry* **2021**, *12*, 625247. [CrossRef]
12. Xu, M.L.; De Boeck, P.; Strunk, D. An Affective Space View on Depression and Anxiety. *Int. J. Methods Psychiatr. Res.* **2018**, *27*, e1747. [CrossRef]
13. Russell, J.A. Core Affect and the Psychological Construction of Emotion. *Psychol. Rev.* **2003**, *110*, 145–172. [CrossRef] [PubMed]
14. Zitouni, M.S.; Park, C.Y.; Lee, U.; Hadjileontiadis, L.; Khandoker, A. Arousal-Valence Classification from Peripheral Physiological Signals Using Long Short-Term Memory Networks. In Proceedings of the 2021 43rd Annual International Conference of the IEEE Engineering in Medicine & Biology Society (EMBC), Mexico City, Mexico, 1–5 November 2021; pp. 686–689. [CrossRef]
15. Xinyu, S.; Zhang, M.; Li, Z.; Hu, X.; Wang, F.; Zhang, D. A dataset of daily ambulatory psychological and physiological recording for emotion research. *Sci. Data* **2021**, *8*, 161. [CrossRef]
16. Malay, S.; Chung, K.C. The Choice of Controls for Providing Validity and Evidence in Clinical Research. *Plast. Reconstr. Surg.* **2012**, *130*, 959–965. [CrossRef]
17. Pradhan, A.; Prabhu, S.; Chadaga, K.; Sengupta, S.; Nath, G. Supervised Learning Models for the Preliminary Detection of COVID-19 in Patients Using Demographic and Epidemiological Parameters. *Information* **2022**, *13*, 330. [CrossRef]
18. Ramesh, J.; Keeran, N.; Sagahyroon, A.; Aloul, F. Towards Validating the Effectiveness of Obstructive Sleep Apnea Classification from Electronic Health Records Using Machine Learning. *Healthcare* **2021**, *9*, 1450. [CrossRef]

19. Chen, D.; Liu, S.; Kingsbury, P.; Sohn, S.; Storlie, C.B.; Habermann, E.B.; Naessens, J.M.; Larson, D.W.; Liu, H. Deep Learning and Alternative Learning Strategies for Retrospective Real-World Clinical Data. *NPJ Digit. Med.* **2019**, *2*, 43. [CrossRef] [PubMed]
20. Laeger, I.; Dobel, C.; Dannlowski, U.; Kugel, H.; Grotegerd, D.; Kissler, J.; Keuper, K.; Eden, A.; Zwitserlood, P.; Zwanzger, P. Amygdala Responsiveness to Emotional Words Is Modulated by Subclinical Anxiety and Depression. *Behav. Brain Res.* **2012**, *233*, 508–516. [CrossRef]
21. Alskafi, F.A.; Khandoker, A.H.; Jelinek, H.F. A Comparative Study of Arousal and Valence Dimensional Variations for Emotion Recognition Using Peripheral Physiological Signals Acquired from Wearable Sensors. In Proceedings of the 2021 43rd Annual International Conference of the IEEE Engineering in Medicine & Biology Society (EMBC), Mexico City, Mexico, 1–5 November 2021; pp. 1104–1107. [CrossRef]
22. Teismann, H.; Kissler, J.; Berger, K. Investigating the Roles of Age, Sex, Depression, and Anxiety for Valence and Arousal Ratings of Words: A Population-Based Study. *BMC Psychol.* **2020**, *8*, 118. [CrossRef]
23. Rykov, Y.; Thach, T.Q.; Bojic, I.; Christopoulos, G.; Car, J. Digital Biomarkers for Depression Screening with Wearable Devices: Cross-sectional Study with Machine Learning Modeling. *JMIR mHealth uHealth* **2021**, *9*, e24872. [CrossRef] [PubMed]
24. Zhang, L.; Fan, H.; Wang, S.; Li, H. The Effect of Emotional Arousal on Inhibition of Return Among Youth with Depressive Tendency. *Front. Psychol.* **2019**, *10*, 1487. [CrossRef]
25. Moratti, S. Low Emotional Arousal in Depression as Explained by the Motivated Attention Approach. *Escritos-Psicol.-Psychol. Writ.* **2012**, *5*, 20–26. [CrossRef]
26. Brockmeyer, T.; Grosse Holtforth, M.; Krieger, T.; Altenstein, D.; Doerig, N.; Friederich, H.C.; Bents, H. Ambivalence over Emotional Expression in Major Depression. *Personal. Individ. Differ.* **2013**, *54*, 862–864. [CrossRef]
27. Straszewski, T.; Siegel, J.T. Differential Effects of High- and Low-Arousal Positive Emotions on Help-Seeking for Depression. *Appl. Psychol. Health Well-Being* **2020**, *12*, 887–906. [CrossRef] [PubMed]
28. Hickey, B.A.; Chalmers, T.; Newton, P.; Lin, C.T.; Sibbritt, D.; McLachlan, C.S.; Clifton-Bligh, R.; Morley, J.; Lal, S. Smart Devices and Wearable Technologies to Detect and Monitor Mental Health Conditions and Stress: A Systematic Review. *Sensors* **2021**, *21*, 3461. [CrossRef] [PubMed]
29. De Angel, V.; Lewis, S.; White, K.; Oetzmann, C.; Leightley, D.; Oprea, E.; Lavelle, G.; Matcham, F.; Pace, A.; Mohr, D.C.; et al. Digital Health Tools for the Passive Monitoring of Depression: A Systematic Review of Methods. *NPJ Digit. Med.* **2022**, *5*, 1–14. [CrossRef] [PubMed]
30. Dinsdale, N.K.; Bluemke, E.; Sundaresan, V.; Jenkinson, M.; Smith, S.; Namburete, A.I. Challenges for machine learning in clinical translation of big data imaging studies. *arXiv* **2021**, arXiv:2107.05630. [CrossRef]
31. Christensen, M.C.; Wong, C.M.J.; Baune, B.T. Symptoms of Major Depressive Disorder and Their Impact on Psychosocial Functioning in the Different Phases of the Disease: Do the Perspectives of Patients and Healthcare Providers Differ? *Front. Psychiatry* **2020**, *11*, 280. [CrossRef]
32. Johnson, J.M.; Khoshgoftaar, T.M. Survey on deep learning with class imbalance. *J. Big Data* **2019**, *6*, 27. [CrossRef]
33. Zhang, K.; Xu, G.; Han, Z.; Ma, K.; Zheng, X.; Chen, L.; Duan, N.; Zhang, S. Data Augmentation for Motor Imagery Signal Classification Based on a Hybrid Neural Network. *Sensors* **2020**, *20*, 4485. [CrossRef]
34. Pope, G.C.; Halter, R.J. Design and Implementation of an Ultra-Low Resource Electrodermal Activity Sensor for Wearable Applications. *Sensors* **2019**, *19*, 2450. [CrossRef]
35. Wahle, F.; Kowatsch, T.; Fleisch, E.; Rufer, M.; Weidt, S. Mobile Sensing and Support for People with Depression: A Pilot Trial in the Wild. *JMIR mHealth uHealth* **2016**, *4*, e111. [CrossRef] [PubMed]

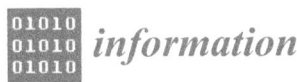

Article

Predicting Emergency Department Utilization among Older Hong Kong Population in Hot Season: A Machine Learning Approach

Huiquan Zhou [1], Hao Luo [1], Kevin Ka-Lun Lau [2], Xingxing Qian [3], Chao Ren [4] and Puihing Chau [3],*

[1] Department of Social Work and Social Administration, Faculty of Social Sciences, The University of Hong Kong, Hong Kong SAR, China
[2] Department of Civil, Environmental and Natural Resources Engineering, Luleå University of Technology, SE-97187 Luleå, Sweden
[3] School of Nursing, Li Ka Shing Faculty of Medicine, The University of Hong Kong, Hong Kong SAR, China
[4] Department of Architecture, Faculty of Architecture, The University of Hong Kong, Hong Kong SAR, China
* Correspondence: phchau@graduate.hku.hk; Tel.: +852-3917-6626; Fax: +852-2872-6079

Abstract: Previous evidence suggests that temperature is associated with the number of emergency department (ED) visits. A predictive system for ED visits, which takes local temperature into account, is therefore needed. This study aimed to compare the predictive performance of various machine learning methods with traditional statistical methods based on temperature variables and develop a daily ED attendance rate predictive model for Hong Kong. We analyzed ED utilization among Hong Kong older adults in May to September from 2000 to 2016. A total of 103 potential predictors were derived from 1- to 14-day lag of ED attendance rate and meteorological and air quality indicators and 0-day lag of holiday indicator and month and day of week indicators. LASSO regression was used to identify the most predictive temperature variables. Decision tree regressor, support vector machine (SVM) regressor, and random forest regressor were trained on the selected optimal predictor combination. Deep neural network (DNN) and gated recurrent unit (GRU) models were performed on the extended predictor combination for the previous 14-day horizon. Maximum ambient temperature was identified as a better predictor in its own value than as an indicator defined by the cutoff. GRU achieved the best predictive accuracy. Deep learning methods, especially the GRU model, outperformed conventional machine learning methods and traditional statistical methods.

Keywords: emergency department; machine learning; temperature; older adult; Hong Kong

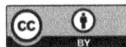

1. Introduction

Global warming is becoming an increasingly important concern worldwide. The global surface temperature rose by 1.09 °C in 2011–2020 as compared to 1850–1900 and the continuous rise was projected to exceed 2 °C during this century [1]. In metropolitan areas, the air temperature, especially at nighttime, is amplified by urban heat island (UHI) effect [2]. The older population is vulnerable to extreme heat due to their impaired physiological ability to regulate heat [3]. Previous studies have demonstrated the association between heat exposure and increased Emergency Department (ED) attendance risk. A United Kingdom (UK) study demonstrated a 0.6% increase in daily ED attendance risk in people aged 65–74 with 1 °C increase in mean ambient temperature [4]. In Asia, increased risk of ED visits due to cardiovascular diseases and respiratory diseases among older adults was also shown to be associated with high indoor temperatures (such as 31 °C lasting over one hour) during the hot season in Taiwan [5,6]. While temperature had been used as predictor for ED visits in many studies, its prediction performance varied. A previous study found that meteorological information, including daily mean temperature, improved the predictive performance of a hierarchical Bayesian model on daily ED visits [7]. In contrast, there were evidence showed that incorporating climatic factors (including mean, maximum, and minimum ambient temperature) did not improve the predictive performance [8,9]. A recent study using linear regression reported association between ED visits and heat stress defined by Universal Thermal Climate Index, which incorporated ambient temperature, humidity, wind speed, and radiant temperature into an index [10].

Globally, EDs face increasing emergency care demand, especially with an aging population. Older adults are reported as frequent users of EDs [11,12]. In the United States (US), the ED usage of older people aged 65 or over increased by 25% from 2001 to 2009 [13]. The growing demand accompanied by the shortage of healthcare resources might increase the workload of healthcare providers and adversely affect care quality, which may in turn decrease patients' satisfaction and prognosis outcomes, or even increase the mortality rate [13]. Service providers have taken actions to address those issues by adopting strategies on regulating patient flow and improving the capacity of EDs. However, the effectiveness of these strategies relies heavily on reliable forecasts of ED visits and an early warning of the peaks of future patient flow. Therefore, there is a need to have an accurate prediction of healthcare utilization to help healthcare providers facilitate medical resources in advance, in case of summer surges.

Most previous studies have used conventional statistical models, such as time series models or regression models, to predict ED demand based on records of previous ED visits. Autoregressive integrated moving average (ARIMA) and its variations were a class of widely applied time-series data prediction models. The model eliminated the non-stationarity of data by initial differencing and made the prediction based on the history of time-series data. However, it was difficult to incorporate covariates and unstable to changes in observations and model specification [14]. Generalized linear models (GLMs) were simpler to implement compared to ARIMA. Previous studies demonstrated that GLMs outperformed ARIMA in predicting ED visits [8,15]. However, GLM were usually inefficient for big data volumes and prone to noise and overfitting. While conventional statistical models are more useful in inferring associations between variables, machine learning methods are superior in predictive tasks with capability of handling non-stationary data and robustness to outliers [16].

Machine learning methods have been applied to healthcare utilization prediction tasks since the last decade. For example, a previous study predicted hospital bed demand in ED attendances by support vector machine (SVM) and demonstrated 80% accuracy, which was comparable with experienced physicians [17]. Besides, ensemble learning methods, such as random forest (RF) and gradient boosting classifier (GBC), were also demonstrated as effective models for ED prediction [18]. Artificial neural network (ANN) was the most popular machine learning method used to predict ED visits. A US study applied an ANN classifier to forecast the peaks of ED demand due to respiratory diseases and achieved high classification accuracy [19]. A study from Hong Kong identified that ANN was superior to regression models in modelling the association between contributing predictors and daily non-critical patient arrivals at a local emergency department [20]. The ARIMA-ANN hybrid model, a variation of ANN, was demonstrated to outperform both linear regression and ARIMA in predicting the ED demand [21]. Advanced deep learning methods, such as deep neural network (DNN) and recurrent neural network (RNN), have been increasingly used to model massive electronic health records (EHRs). However, their application in prediction of healthcare utilization is scarce. Initial evidence showed that convolutional neural network (CNN), an advanced ANN with convolutional cells, and long short-term memory (LSTM), an efficient recurrent unit based on RNN architecture achieved better predictive performance than conventional machine learning models [16].

Over the past decade, there has been a significant increase in ED service demand accompanied by population growth and aging in Hong Kong. Meanwhile, global warming has taken its toll in the subtropical city Hong Kong. There was an average rise of 0.13 °C per decade from 1885 to 2021, with an accelerated growing trend reaching 0.31 °C per decade from 1992 to 2021 [22]. In addition, the urban heat island effect is prominent in Hong Kong, resulting from the high-density compact urban setting. The frequency, magnitude, and duration of extreme hot weather have been estimated to keep increasing during this century [23]. The extreme weather conditions have a noticeable negative effect on the residents' health. Literature demonstrated that females and members of the older population were the most affected populations in Hong Kong during extremely hot weather [23]. Prior evidence also suggested that the help-seeking behavior of the older Hong Kong population significantly increased when they were exposed to hot weather, and females were even more sensitive to elevated temperature [24]. The public-funded healthcare providers in Hong Kong also encountered summer surges in recent years in addition to winter surges. It was reported that hospitalizations increased by 4.5% for every 1 °C increase in mean daily temperature above 29 °C [25]. There were always long queues in EDs of Hong Kong; the average waiting time ranged from 1 h to over 8 h. A reliable prediction model of ED attendance in Hong Kong remains lacking. Existing predictive models developed from other populations are specifically trained to serve the forecast needs in countries with different physical environments from Hong Kong and thus cannot be directly applied to Hong Kong. Hence, it is essential to develop a local model for application purpose in Hong Kong. Even though temperature was demonstrated to be associated with ED visits, its predictive ability and relative importance in the predictive model remains ambiguous. Besides, the choice of predictors is still a challenge in training predictive models especially when there are various measures of temperature. For instance, the predictor can be the daily minimum, maximum, or mean temperature at their own values, while the other option is to transfer these variables into indicators by a threshold. For own values, it is direct, but a possible U-shape may occur if the choice of the period under study is not starting with the tip of the U-shape. For the use of indicators, it can reduce the redundancy with the categorization, but the determination of the threshold is critical, and the information entropy decreases.

This study aimed to: (i) comprehensively compare the predictive performance of traditional statistical method, conventional machine learning approach, and advanced deep learning approach in predicting ED attendance rate; and (ii) identify the optimal predictive model that can be applied to Hong Kong. The findings of this study were of practical value. First, researchers around the world could repeat the algorithm with their local data and develop prediction models for their own settings. Second, service providers in Hong Kong could apply the prediction algorithm to better plan for ED resources. Third, the public could also be alerted with the high-risk period and initiate preventive measures.

2. Materials and Methods

2.1. Data Sources

Daily healthcare utilization data of ED admission for older people aged 65 and above from 1 January 2000 to 31 December 2016 were obtained from the Hong Kong Hospital Authority. Since the Hong Kong Hospital Authority manages all Accident and Emergency Departments under the public hospitals in Hong Kong, these data reflect all Hong Kong ED utilization at public hospitals. Population statistics were obtained from the Census and Statistics Department of Hong Kong. Daily maximum/mean/minimum ambient temperature data from the Hong Kong Observatory (HKO) Headquarter station were extracted from the HKO. Air quality data in terms of general Air Quality Health Index (AQHI) were obtained from the Environmental Protection Department of Hong Kong government [26].

2.2. Outcomes

The primary outcome of this study was the gender-specific daily ED attendance rate, which was measured as the daily ED attendance per 100,000 population.

2.3. Predictors

Previous works in the literature have reported predictors of ED utilization, including maximum, mean, and minimum ambient temperature [25,27,28]. We included the maximum, mean, and minimum ambient temperature from 1 to 14 days lag, resulting in 42 continuous variables. The lag of 1 to 14 days was chosen since the maximum number of lag studied in the literature was 13 [29], although shorter lags were considered elsewhere [23]. According to the HKO's extreme hot weather warning system, Very Hot Day (VHD) was defined as daily maximum ambient temperature $\geq 33\,°C$ and Hot Nights (HN) was defined as daily minimum ambient temperature $\geq 28\,°C$). We further included VHD and HN from 1 to 14 days lag, resulting in 28 binary indicators of extreme hot weather.

Apart from ambient temperature, we have a base variable set comprising 33 variables. We included ED attendance rates of lags 1 to 14 days, as there was evidence about autoregressive nature of the ED attendance [30]. AQHI was also included, since previous literature suggested that air pollution (ozone, nitrogen dioxide, sulfur dioxide, and particulate matter) was associated with short-term health risk, which may lead to hospital admissions [26]. We included lags 1 to 14 days of the daily general AQHI. A binary variable indicating whether the day was a holiday (including Sunday) was included to control the holiday effect. Finally, we exploited four sine- and cosine-transformed variables, two in a pair, to describe the cyclical patterns of month and day in the week across years [31]. An example of sine- and cosine-transformed month variables is visualized in Figure S1.

A total of 103 potential predictors, including the base set (33 variables), the ambient temperature set (42 variables), and the extreme hot weather indicator set (28 variables) were included (Table S1).

2.4. Statistical Analysis

We excluded data in 2003 to avoid the impact of the SARS outbreak in Hong Kong. A training data set comprising 10-years' data (2000 to 2010, excluding 2003) was used to develop the models. A validation data set comprising three-years' data (2011 to 2013) was used to select the optimal model. A testing data set comprising three-years' data (2014 to 2016) was used to evaluate the performance of the model. Since the ED data is time-series data, we split the data in this way instead of random splitting.

We adopted typical models covering all of the three classes of predictive models (i.e., traditional statistics models, conventional machine learning models, advanced deep learning models). We applied linear regression (i.e., GLM with Gaussian distribution assumption) from traditional statistical models; decision tree, SVM and random forest from conventional machine learning models, and DNN and GRU from advanced deep learning models, based on their relative superior performance from literatures [16,17,32]. A detailed process of the analysis is presented in Figure 1.

We applied the least absolute shrinkage and selection operator (LASSO) regression to select significant predictors from the candidate ambient temperature variable set and the candidate extreme hot weather indicator set separately to identify the significant predictors within each set. In each gender subgroup, we applied 10-fold cross validation on the standardized data to find the optimal hyperparameter and substituted it back to the regression formula to shrink the scale of candidate variables. We removed variables with zero coefficient and kept the rest as selected variables. We then fit a linear regression model (Model 1) by including the base variable set (i.e., ED attendance rates and general AHQI at lags 1–14, the current holiday indicator, and paired month and week indicating variables). Then, Model 2 was built on Model 1 plus the selected ambient temperature variables; and Model 3 was built on Model 1 plus the selected extreme hot weather indicators. We applied linear regression to evaluate the performance of the three models on the test data set in terms of evaluation metrics (see Formula (2) and (3)). The model with the best performance was named as the baseline model. The variables in the baseline model were chosen to be used in the machine learning algorithm. Based on the variables in the baseline model, we applied 10-fold cross validation to decide the hyperparameters of conventional machine learning models: decision tree, support vector machine (SVM), and random forest. Then, we tested the predictive ability of each model from conventional machine learning and the baseline model from linear regression. This would inform us if conventional machine learning could have better prediction performance than the linear regression given the same set of predictors. On the other hand, deep learning methods could do the feature selection automatically without the need to go through the feature selection step, although the shortcoming is that the selected feature was not visualized. We tested the performance of deep learning models based on two methods, namely deep neural network (DNN) and gated recurrent unit (GRU), and compared with those from conventional machine learning models. For deep learning, an extended feature set had to be used as all of the features had to be on the same 14-day horizon (1–14 lags).

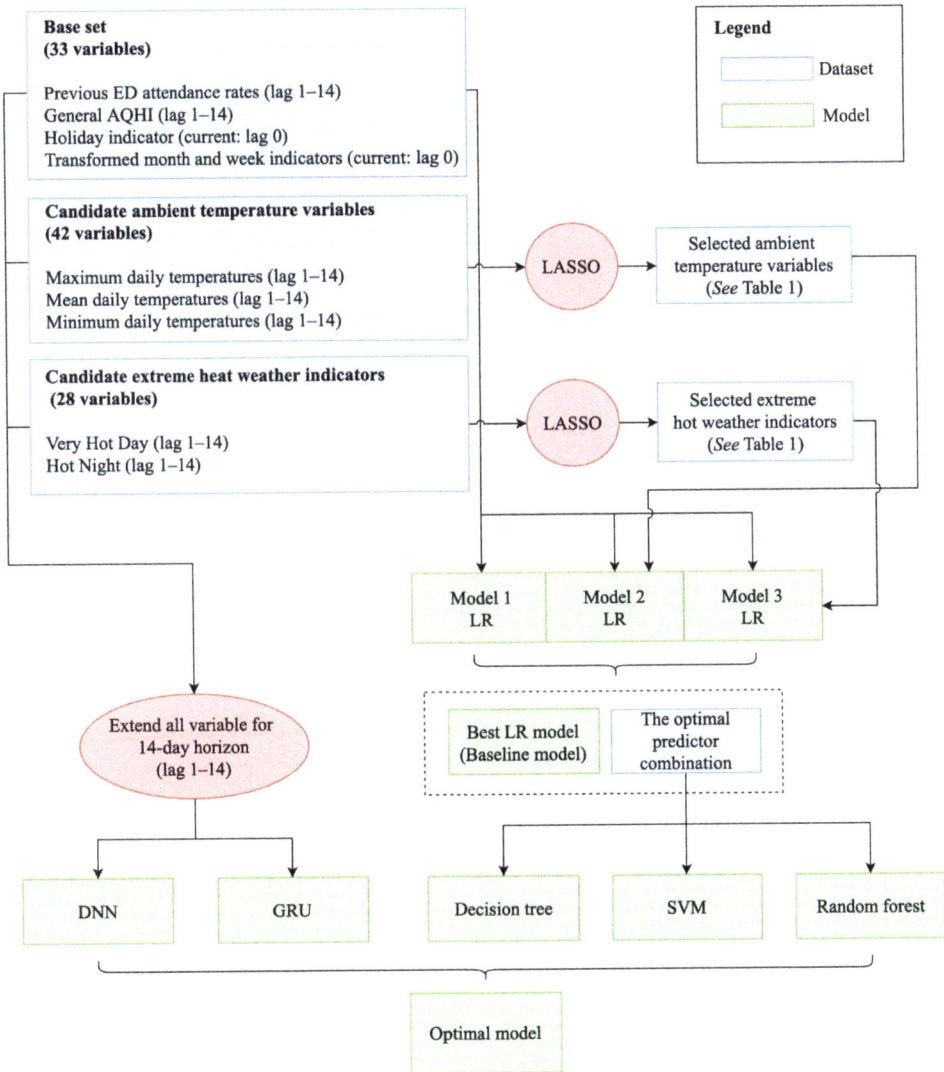

Figure 1. Process of the statistical analysis. Note: LASSO denotes least absolute shrinkage and selection operator, LR denotes linear regression, SVM denotes support vector machine, DNN denotes deep neural network, and GRU denotes gated recurrent unit.

Decision trees and SVM are two conventional machine learning methods in regression and classification tasks. The decision tree generates the optimal tree structure by deciding the feature and the split at each node [33]. In contrast, SVM aims at optimizing a maximum-margin hyperplane to achieve the best prediction performance [33]. Compared with the ordinary least squares (OLS) method, decision trees and SVM support non-linear solutions. Random forest is an efficient ensemble learning method that operates by constructing many base learners (decision tree). It follows the bagging method and bootstrap sampling and is less prone to overfitting than the decision tree and gives a more generalized solution [34]. A deep neural network (DNN) is an extension of artificial neural network (ANN) with a minimum of three stacked hidden layers followed by a non-linear activation function [35]. Figure 2 describes the structure of DNN in our study. The blue circles denote the input vector containing previous 14-day ED attendance rate, general AQHI, calendar information (i.e., holiday, month, and week indicators), and extended chosen ambient temperature variables and extreme hot weather indicators from Model 1–3 comparison. Each orange circle is a neuron within the hidden layers (layers between the input layer and the output layer), which assigns weights to inputs and passes on the values through an activation function as outputs. We used a rectified liner unit (ReLU) activation function [36]. We fine-tuned the hyperparameters (including the hidden layer structure, learning rate, and batch size) based on the predictive performance on the validation data set. The red circle is the output where we generate the predicted ED attendance rate in our study.

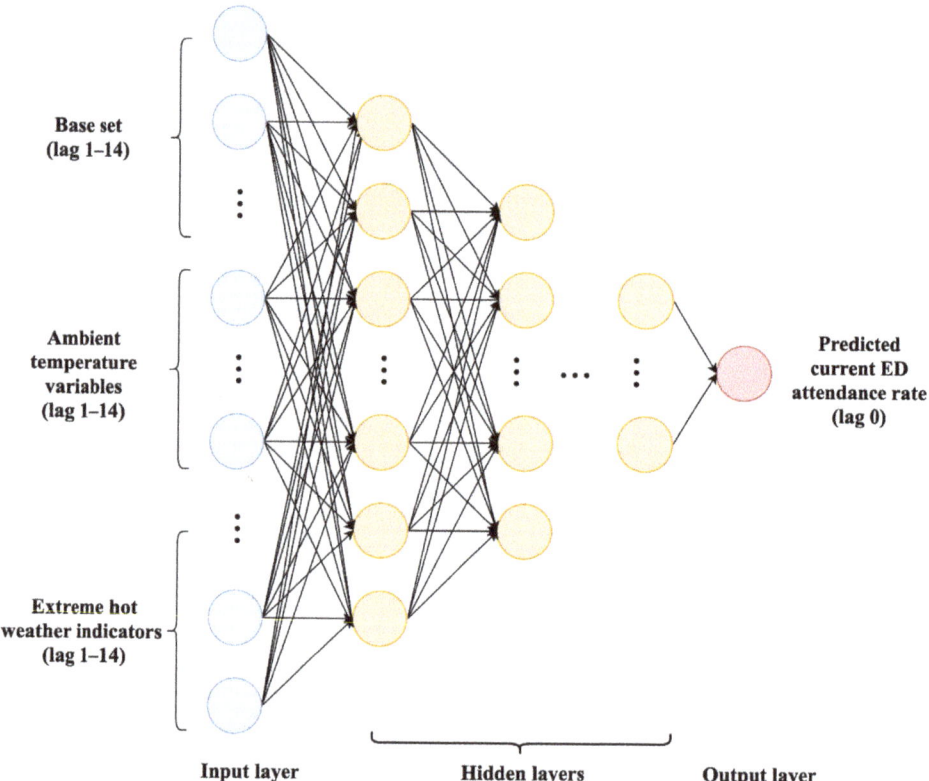

Figure 2. Proposed DNN structure.

A GRU model is a transformed recurrent neural network (RNN) with a gating mechanism. Figure 3 shows the inner implementation of GRU, which is constructed by a reset gate (r_t), an update gate (z_t), and a candidate status ($\overline{h}_t$) to decide what information can be passed to the output [37]. x_t denotes the input vector, which was composed by ED attendance rate, general AQHI, calendar information, ambient temperature variables, and extreme hot weather indicators at time t. h_t is the output vector of current unit and it passes the kept information to another stacked GRU. The orange bricks denote a fully connected layer with activation function. The formula is presented as follows.

$$\begin{aligned} z_t &= \sigma(W_{xz}x_t + W_{hz}h_{t-1} + b_z) \\ r_t &= \sigma(W_{xr}x_t + W_{hr}h_{t-1} + b_r) \\ \overline{h_t} &= tanh(W_{xh}x_t + r_t \odot h_{t-1} + b_h) \\ h_t &= (1 - z_t) \odot h_{t-1} + z_t \odot \overline{h_t} \end{aligned} \quad (1)$$

where W denotes weight parameters, $\odot$ denotes elementwise product (Hadamard product) operator.

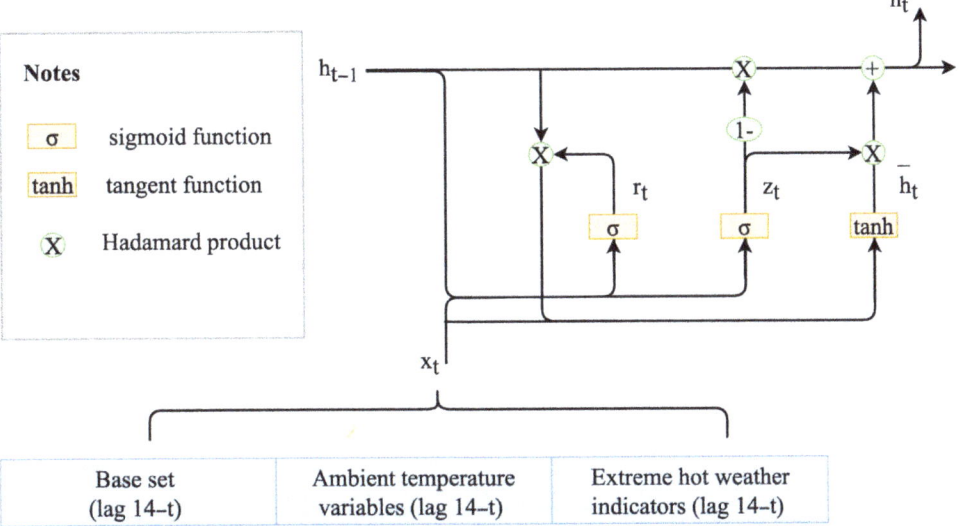

Figure 3. Proposed GRU structure.

For model evaluations, we adopted two widely adopted evaluation metrics to compare the predictive performance of each model: root mean square error (*RMSE*) and normalized root mean square error (*NMSE*). The corresponding formulae are

$$RMSE = \sqrt{\frac{\sum_{i=1}^{n}(y_i - \hat{y}_i)^2}{n}} \quad (2)$$

and

$$NRMSE = \frac{RMSE}{y_{max} - y_{min}} \quad (3)$$

where y_i and $\hat{y}_i$ denote the observed and predicted current ED attendance rate in the test set, respectively; n denotes the number of observations; y_{max} and y_{min} denote the maximum and minimum values of observations separately.

The optimal value of *RMSE* is zero, with lower values indicating better predictive performance. *NRMSE* normalizes *RMSE* by the scale of observation and makes the result comparable across datasets and scales. It also indicates better fitting with minor value. In the public health area, a predictive model with a *NRMSE* less than 30% is regarded as an effective model [38].

All analyses were conducted in Python version 3.8.5 [39]. Linear regression, decision tree, SVM, random forest, and DNN were implemented using the *Sklearn* package [40]. GRU was developed using the *PyTorch* package [41].

3. Results

3.1. Data Descriptions

From May to September 2000 to 2016 (except 2003), the daily ED attendance rate varied, in general, between 140 to 200 per 100,000 population. A higher attendance rate was consistently observed in males (Figure 4).

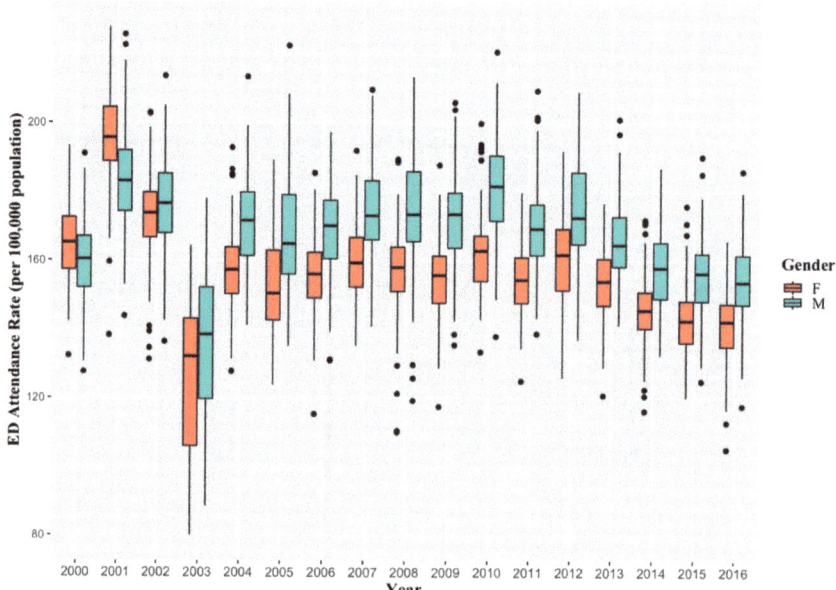

Figure 4. Distribution of daily ED attendance rate across year. Distributions are presented in form of box plots.

In the hot seasons, the mean temperature generally varied between 25 °C and 35 °C. Substantially higher frequencies of VHD and HN were observed in 2009 and the most recent three years (2014–2016) than in previous years (see Figure S1). Hong Kong remained a low level of air pollution with the health risk straying moderate and lower (AQHI $\leq$ 6) most of the years (see Figure S2). After 2009, few days with very high health risk of air pollution (AQHI > 8) were observed (see Figure S3).

3.2. Selection of Predictors by LASSO

After LASSO selection, we identified 11 out of 42 ambient temperature variables (previous 14-day maximum/mean/minimum daily temperature) and 19 out of 28 extreme hot weather indicators (previous 14-day VHD and HN) for the female group. The numbers of selected ambient temperature variables and extreme hot weather indicators for the male group were 10 and 17, respectively. These selected variables are presented in Table 1. Among the ambient temperature variables, maximum daily temperature was most commonly selected. Among the extreme hot weather indicators, VHD was slightly more commonly selected than HN.

In Model 1 (ED attendance on previous 14-day ED attendance and general AQHI, with current calendar information), the predictive performance for the female group (*RMSE*: 8.53×10^{-5}, *NRMSE*: 12.05%) and the male group (*RMSE*: 9.04×10^{-5}, *NRMSE*: 12.47%) were both good. Model 2 (ED attendance on the same predictors as Model 1 plus those LASSO-selected ambient temperature variables) achieved better performance than Model 1 for both female (*RMSE*: 8.44×10^{-5}, *NRMSE*: 11.93%) and male groups (*RMSE*: 8.87×10^{-5}, *NRMSE*: 12.23%). Model 3 (ED attendance on the same predictors as Model 1 plus those LASSO-selected extreme hot weather indicators) had the worst performance among the three models for both female (*RMSE*: 8.68 × 10^{-5}, *NRMSE*: 12.27%) and male groups (*RMSE*: 9.20 × 10^{-5}, *NRMSE*: 12.69%). Detailed information is listed in Table 2. Hence, Model 2 was chosen as the baseline model, with the optimal variables composed by previous 14-day ED attendance and general AQHI, current calendar information, and the LASSO-selected ambient temperature variables presented in Table 1.

Table 1. LASSO selected ambient temperature variables for each group.

	Female		Male	
	Ambient Temperature Variables	Extreme Hot Weather Indicators	Ambient Temperature Variables	Extreme Hot Weather Indicators
	Max 2	VHD 1	Max 1	VHD 1
	Max 8	VHD 2	Max 4	VHD 3
	Max 10	VHD 3	Max 6	VHD 4
	Max 11	VHD 4	Max 7	VHD 5
	Max 12	VHD 5	Max 9	VHD 6
	Max 13	VHD 6	Mean 2	VHD 7
	Max 14	VHD 7	Min 6	VHD 9
	Mean 6	VHD 9	Min 7	VHD 11
	Min 1	VHD 12	Min 10	VHD 13
	Min 12	VHD 13	Min 12	HN 3
	Min 13	VHD 14		HN 4
		HN 1		HN 5
		HN 2		HN 6
		HN 3		HN 7
		HN 6		HN 8
		HN 7		HN 12
		HN 11		HN 14
		HN 13		
		HN 14		
Count	11	19	10	17

Note. Max denotes maximum temperature; Mean denotes mean temperature; Min denotes minimum. Temperature; VHD denotes very hot day; HN denotes hot night, and the numbers denote lags.

Table 2. Predictive performance of three linear regression models with different predictor combinations.

		Methods		
Groups	Metric	Model 1	Model 2	Model 3
Female	*RMSE* (10^{-5})	8.53	8.44	8.68
	NRMSE	12.05%	11.93%	12.27%
Male	*RMSE* (10^{-5})	9.04	8.87	9.20
	NRMSE	12.47%	12.23%	12.69%

Note. Model 1 denotes base set; Model 2 denotes base set plus candidate ambient temperature variables; Model 3 denotes base set plus candidate extreme hot weather indicators. *RMSE* denotes root mean square error and NMSE denotes normalized root mean square error.

3.3. Predictive Performance of Machine Learning Methods

On the optimal variable combination, the performance of the conventional machine learning methods were tested on the same test dataset. The results show that random forest (Female: *RMSE*: 9.18 × 10^{-5}, *NRMSE*: 12.97%; Male: *RMSE*: 10.23 × 10^{-5}, *NRMSE*: 14.10%) achieved better performance than decision tree (Female: *RMSE*: 11.24 × 10^{-5}, *NRMSE*: 15.88%; Male: *RMSE*: 11.66 × 10^{-5}, *NRMSE*: 16.01%) and SVM (Female: *RMSE*: 21.62 × 10^{-5}, *NRMSE*: 30.5%; Male: *RMSE*: 20.41 × 10^{-5}, *NRMSE*: 28.15%) for both sexes (Table 3). However, none of these methods improved the predictive accuracy of the baseline model on this task. Then, deep learning methods DNN and GRU models were tested on the extended variable combination. The GRU model achieved the best performance in both female (*RMSE*: 7.98 × 10^{-5}, *NRMSE*: 11.28%) and male (*RMSE*: 8.52 × 10^{-5}, *NRMSE*: 11.75%) groups. DNN (Female: *RMSE*: 8.30 × 10^{-5}, *NRMSE*: 11.73%; Male: *RMSE*: 8.75 × 10^{-5}, *NRMSE*: 12.08%) also obtained slightly improved predictive accuracy than baseline but not better than the GRU model. (Table 3). The ground-truth observations, the linear regression (baseline), and the GRU predictions are shown in Figure 5. Compared with the baseline model, GRU showed a better ability in capturing the peaks.

Table 3. Predictive performance of model comparison among baseline model, conventional machine learning methods and deep learning methods.

Groups	Metric	Methods					
		Linear Regression (Baseline)	Decision Tree	Random Forest	SVM	DNN	GRU
Female	RMSE (10^{-5})	8.44	11.24	9.18	21.62	8.30	7.98
	NRMSE	11.93%	15.88%	12.97%	30.5%	11.73%	11.28%
Male	RMSE (10^{-5})	8.87	11.66	10.23	20.41	8.75	8.52
	NRMSE	12.23%	16.01%	14.10%	28.15%	12.08%	11.75%

Note. *RMSE* denotes root mean square error and NMSE denotes normalized root mean square error.

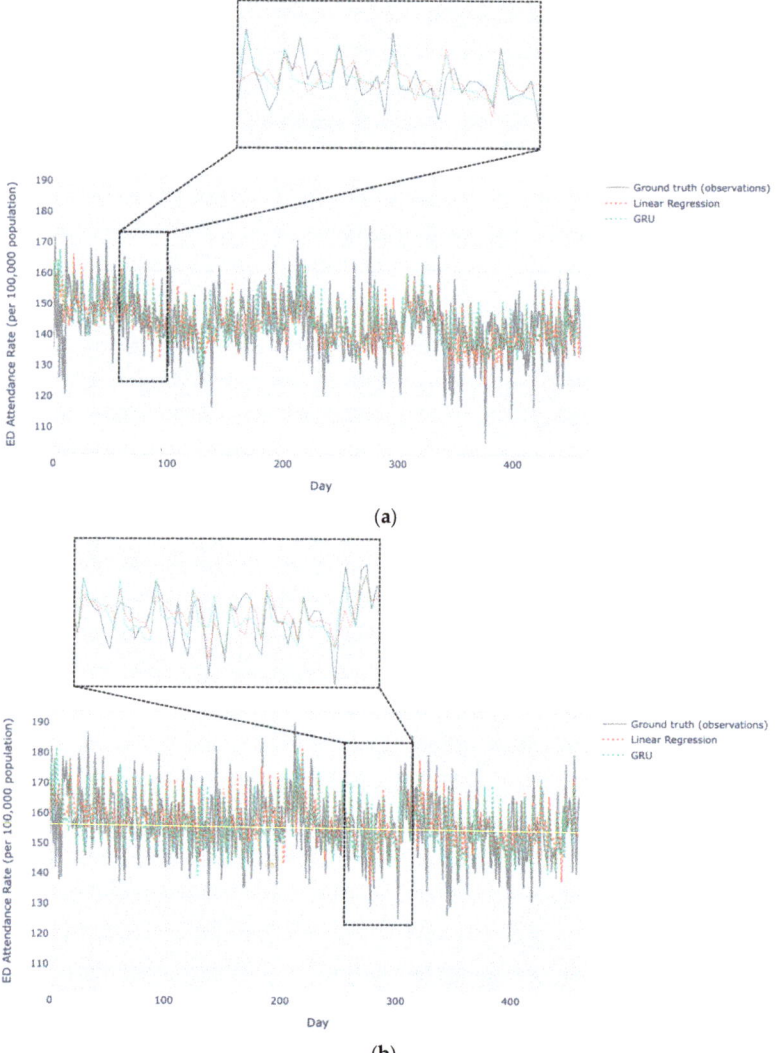

(a)

(b)

Figure 5. Visualization of ground truth and predictions from linear regression model (baseline) and GRU. (**a**) Female group; (**b**) male group.

4. Discussion

With the development of machine learning methods, many advanced methods have been developed and have achieved better performance than previous methods. This study compared the predictive performance of ambient temperature variables at their own value and those using these variables as indicators, as well as the predictive power among various models, including traditional statistical method (i.e., linear regression), three typical conventional machine learning approaches (i.e., decision tree, SVM, and RF), and two widely-adopted deep learning approaches (i.e., DNN and GRU) in predicting daily ED attendance rate, using Hong Kong as an example. Also, we were the first to compare the ability and shrink the candidate pool to a reasonable size by use of LASSO. We also applied state-of-the art deep learning methods in the ED prediction task and suggested how to apply the model in practice. It was found that ambient temperatures at their own values had better predictive power than those indicators defined by cutoffs, and the advanced deep learning approaches had better predictive performance than traditional statistical models and conventional machine learning with acceptable computational complexity.

Literature using ambient temperature at its own value or as an indicator defined by thresholds for prediction purpose were mixed. Some researchers reported that heat waves defined by VHD and HN were associated with excess mortality [42]. On the other hand, some researchers reported hospital admissions as a function of ambient temperature [25]. Another local study used thresholds of various meteorological variables to define extreme weather in the prediction of mortality among older adults [43]. In a local study using time series approach to study suicide death among older adults in summer, it was reported that minimum temperature at its own value had the best predictive power for violent method suicides, but maximum ambient temperature exceeding a threshold of 32.7°C was better at predicting non-violent method suicides [44]. In clinical studies, categorization of continuous variables is common and it also helps simplify analyses and leads to more interpretable results [45]. Moreover, binarization potentially conceals any non-linearity between the variable and the outcome [45]. However, dichotomizing a variable leads to excessive information loss, thus reducing its statistical power. The considerable within-group variability after categorization may be suppressed. Our results supported these conclusions with evidence that temperature variables at their own values had better predictive performance than extreme hot weather indicators. This implies that temperature variables at their own values are more effective predictors, as they contain essential information in predicting ED attendance rates. The data-driven predictor selection approach also showed that daily maximum ambient temperatures were more important than mean and minimum ambient temperatures in predicting ED attendance rates, which might be due to their ability to reflect the more extreme hot weather.

Most previous studies were limited to application of one kind of machine learning model and had mixed conclusions when comparing the predictive performance among different models [20,32]. Our study included state-of-the-art machine learning models, including base learner (i.e., decision tree and SVM), ensemble learning model (i.e., random forest) and deep learning models (i.e., DNN and GRU). We found that random forest outperformed decision tree and SVM with a maximum of 2.91% and 14.62% improvement regarding *NRMSE*, which was consistent with the previous literature that ensemble learning methods had better performance than base learners and supported the effectiveness of the dragging mechanism and the bootstrap sampling [34]. However, these three conventional machine learning methods did not outperform the linear regression model with a minimum of 1.04% lower regarding *NRMSE*. This is in agreement with a previous study [32], which also found that simple methods such as penalized linear regression models were better or at least comparable with ensemble learning methods such as GBC and random forest to predict ED demand in England. Decision tree, SVM and random forest were conventional machine learning models that were not designed for time-series predictive tasks, which did not fit well for the increasing or decreasing trends of time-series data. Besides, the increased algorithm complexity might decrease the performance when the number of variables was prominent, and when the data size was relatively small. A review also indicated that machine learning models were more suitable to pioneering fields with large data volume, such as radio diagnostics, precision medicine and omics [46]. Meanwhile, deep machine learning approaches, namely DNN and GRU, outperformed linear regression and conventional machine learning models studied in both female and male groups. Up to date, GRU is one of the state-of-the-art machine learning algorithms, in the way that the gating mechanism effectively handles data with timestamps by repeatedly updating gates and resetting gates to keep important information and remove irrelevant information [47]. LSTM has been applied to ED predictive tasks in a previous study and achieved better predictive accuracy for moderate-term prediction compared to CNN and random forest, with a 1.49% improvement of current day prediction than CNN and 2.06% improvement than random forest regarding mean absolute percentage error (MAPE) [16]. While the mechanism of LSTM indicates it can remember longer sequences theoretically, GRU usually had better performance than LSTM with faster training speed and lower memory cost on low complexity sequences in practice [48]. Still the application of GRU in predicting ED visits is in the nascent stage. Our study showed GRU achieved the best performance among all models with 0.71%, 1.69%, and 4.3% improvement over linear regression, random forest, and decision tree separately regarding $NRMSE$ in the female group and similar results in the male group, supporting GRU as a suitable method for predicting ED visits regardless of gender. Even though the performance improvement of GRU was not considerable in value, its ability in capturing the peaks of ED visits revealed its potential application as an early signal of ED unit utilization.

As older people are vulnerable to hot weather, it is essential to develop a targeted predictive model for the older Hong Kong population. Although there are both winter and summer surges in ED visits, the summer surge was not given enough attention. Hence, our study filled a knowledge gap by focusing on the prediction of ED visits by older adults in the hot season in Hong Kong. As GRU showed the optimal prediction power, we attempt to apply GRU to build an ED visit forecast system, so that the healthcare providers can rely on the sequential predictions to allocate resources for the coming period. We first pre-train a GRU model, store it in a reliable server, and build portal links from the web or mobile devices. The healthcare providers can get access to the precise prediction of ED attendance rates in the coming period through the website, mobile app, or messages, and thus be able to plan for the potential surge. Although the prediction for the coming day is validated, based on the feature of GRU that the predictive period is extensible, we can also provide longer-term predictions (say, for one to two weeks in advance) for the healthcare providers. Although 9-day weather forecasts are available in Hong Kong, the sequential prediction does not require such input since the GRU can internally model the temperature pattern based on the data with 1–14 days lag and predict future ED visits. Thus, no extra information is needed to do the prolonged sequential prediction compared to traditional methods. Nevertheless, it is admitted that the predictive performance will decline as the prediction period gets longer and longer. Meanwhile, this study is a proof-of-concept study to demonstrate the feasibility of real-time predictions. Firstly, the dataset we used for training and testing spans more than a decade, whereas the predictive accuracy is still demonstrated competitive on the testing dataset. Thus, our model will likely be applicable for the future data. Secondly, the variables we selected are strictly based on previous literatures and robust selection algorithms, which are practical for real-time predictions. Lastly, the deep learning method, GRU we used to build our model, is of superior generalization ability, which extracts effective features and identifying patterns adaptively by approximating complex non-linear functions, and thus is robust for unobserved data over the time. Nevertheless, the COVID pandemic might affect the current pattern of ED admission. However, our model is convenient to adapt to the changes by retraining at low memory cost and fast speed. Therefore, for future studies, we may retrain the prediction rule regularly using the most updated data. Other variables such as the hospitalization of COVID confirmed cases and the trend of COVID need to be included in future model. A real time training and prediction model should also be explored to enhance the timeliness and thus the usefulness of the predictions. With the advancement in the machine learning techniques, more advanced models may perform more accurate predictions. Researchers should keep on investigating better models.

Apart from the ED healthcare providers, the general public and other health and social services providers should also get access to the forecast system and be informed of the sequential prediction results. A high predicted ED visit rate implies a higher health risk. Although we cannot claim causation with an observational study, the population, particularly the older adults, would still be well-advised to take preventive measures, such as staying in cool places and maintaining adequate fluid intake, to ameliorate adverse health risk from extreme hot weather. Future studies with more vigorous experimental designs should be conducted to facilitate health and social services providers to develop heat action plans to protect vulnerable populations.

The strength of our study includes the long-time data series used. We used a 10-year data for training and three-year data for validation and testing, respectively, which significantly increased the reliability of our predictive model. Although we achieved high predictive performance of ED attendance rate prediction, there was limitation related to the lack of the cause-specific or hospital-specific ED attendance information, limiting more efficient application to Eds. Further works are needed to develop cause-specific and hospital-specific prediction models for more targeted warnings. Secondly, we did not decide the optimal lag time, although we covered a moderate interval to balance the short-term and long-term effect. Prolonged lag effect or dynamic lag effect will be assessed in future studies. Further work will also include more meteorological variables such as relative humidity, wind speed, and sunshine duration as potential predictors. The data used in this study were only collected up to 2016. Future studies are needed to revisit the situation using the most updated, or even real time data. In this study, we only compared the machine learning methods with one type of traditional statistical methods, namely linear regression. Moreover, not all available machine learning methods were attempted in this study. Comparisons with other traditional statistical methods and other machine learning methods should be performed in future studies in order to complete the comparisons.

5. Conclusions

To our knowledge, this was the first study to comprehensively compare the predictive ability of linear regression, conventional machine learning methods, and advanced deep learning methods, with prediction of the ED attendance rates in Hong Kong as illustration. We found that deep learning methods, especially the GRU model, outperformed conventional machine learning methods and traditional statistical methods. Future robust predictive system for ED attendance could be developed based on GRU model with ambient temperatures at their own values as predictors. Such predictions could provide healthcare providers and the older Hong Kong population timely ED crowding forecasts.

Supplementary Materials: The following supporting information can be downloaded at: https://www.mdpi.com/article/10.3390/info13090410/s1, Figure S1: Visualization of sine and cosine transform of Month; Figure S2. Frequency of VHD and HN in hot season from 2000 to 2016; Figure S3. Frequency of general AQHI in hot season from 2000 to 2016. Table S1: A summary of potential predictors used in developing the prediction models.

Author Contributions: Conceptualization: P.C., K.K.-L.L., C.R. and H.L.; data curation: X.Q., K.K.-L.L. and C.R.; methodology and formal analysis: H.Z., H.L., P.C., K.K.-L.L. and C.R.; resources: K.K.-L.L., C.R. and P.C.; software: H.Z. and H.L.; writing—original draft preparation: H.Z. and P.C.; writing—review and editing: K.K.-L.L., X.Q., H.L. and C.R. All authors have read and agreed to the published version of the manuscript.

Funding: This work was supported by The University of Hong Kong [Project No. 201811159222].

Institutional Review Board Statement: The study was conducted in accordance with the Declaration of Helsinki and approved by the Institutional Review Board the University of Hong Kong/Hospital Authority, Hong Kong West Cluster (reference number UW19-388 and date of approval 28 May 2019).

Informed Consent Statement: Not applicable.

Data Availability Statement: Not applicable.

Conflicts of Interest: The authors declare that they have no known competing financial interest or personal relationships that could have appeared to influence the work reported in this paper.

References

1. Masson-Delmotte, V.; Zhai, P.; Pirani, A.; Connors, S.L.; Péan, C.; Berger, S.; Caud, N.; Chen, Y.; Goldfarb, L.; Gomis, M.I.; et al. *Climate Change 2021: The Physical Science Basis. Contribution of Working Group I to the Sixth Assessment Report of the Intergovernmental Panel on Climate Change*; Cambridge University Press: Cambridge, UK, 2021.
2. Houghton, J.T.; Ding, Y.; Griggs, D.J.; Noguer, M.; van der Linden, P.J.; Dai, X.; Maskell, K.; Johnson, C.A. *Climate Change 2001: The Scientific Basis: Contribution of Working Group I to the Third Assessment Report of the Intergovernmental Panel on Climate Change*; Cambridge University Press: Cambridge, UK, 2001.
3. Balmain, B.N.; Sabapathy, S.; Louis, M.; Morris, N.R. Aging and thermoregulatory control: The clinical implications of exercising under heat stress in older individuals. *BioMed Res. Int.* **2018**, *2018*, 8306154. [CrossRef] [PubMed]
4. Corcuera Hotz, I.; Hajat, S. The effects of temperature on accident and emergency department attendances in London: A time-series regression analysis. *Int. J. Environ. Res. Public Health* **2020**, *17*, 1957. [CrossRef] [PubMed]
5. Jung, C.C.; Hsia, Y.F.; Hsu, N.Y.; Wang, Y.C.; Su, H.J. Cumulative effect of indoor temperature on cardiovascular disease-related emergency department visits among older adults in Taiwan. *Sci. Total Environ.* **2020**, *731*, 138958. [CrossRef]
6. Jung, C.C.; Chen, N.T.; Hsia, Y.F.; Hsu, N.Y.; Su, H.J. Influence of Indoor Temperature Exposure on Emergency Department Visits Due to Infectious and Non-Infectious Respiratory Diseases for Older People. *Int. J. Environ. Res. Public Health* **2021**, *18*, 5273. [CrossRef]
7. Sahu, S.K.; Baffour, B.; Harper, P.R.; Minty, J.H.; Sarran, C. A hierarchical Bayesian model for improving short-term forecasting of hospital demand by including meteorological information. *J. R. Stat. Soc. Ser. A Stat. Soc.* **2014**, *177*, 39–61. [CrossRef]
8. Marcilio, I.; Hajat, S.; Gouveia, N. Forecasting daily emergency department visits using calendar variables and ambient temperature readings. *Acad. Emerg. Med.* **2013**, *20*, 769–777. [CrossRef]
9. Calegari, R.; Fogliatto, F.S.; Lucini, F.R.; Neyeloff, J.; Kuchenbecker, R.S.; Schaan, B.D. Forecasting daily volume and acuity of patients in the emergency department. *Comput. Math. Methods Med.* **2016**, *2016*, 3863268. [CrossRef]
10. Chau, P.H.; Lau, K.K.; Qian, X.X.; Luo, H.; Woo, J. Visits to the accident and emergency department in hot season of a city with subtropical climate: Association with heat stress and related meteorological variables. *Int. J. Biometeorol.* **2022**, *2022*, 1–17. [CrossRef]
11. Moe, J.; O'Sullivan, F.; McGregor, M.J.; Schull, M.J.; Dong, K.; Holroyd, B.R.; Grafstein, E.; Hohl, C.M.; Trimble, J.; McGrail, K.M. Identifying subgroups and risk among frequent emergency department users in British Columbia. *J. Am. Coll. Emerg. Physicians Open* **2021**, *2*, e12346. [CrossRef]
12. Soril, L.J.; Leggett, L.E.; Lorenzetti, D.L.; Noseworthy, T.W.; Clement, F.M. Characteristics of frequent users of the emergency department in the general adult population: A systematic review of international healthcare systems. *Health Policy* **2016**, *120*, 452–461. [CrossRef]
13. Berchet, C. *Emergency Care Services: Trends, Drivers and Interventions to Manage the Demand*; OECD Health Working Papers; OECD Publishing: Paris, France, 2015.
14. Chen, G.; Xie, J.; Li, W.; Li, X.; Hay Chung, L.C.; Ren, C.; Liu, X. Future "local climate zone" spatial change simulation in Greater Bay Area under the shared socioeconomic pathways and ecological control line. *Build. Environ.* **2021**, *203*, 108077. [CrossRef]
15. Hertzum, M. Forecasting hourly patient visits in the emergency department to counteract crowding. *Ergon. Open J.* **2017**, *10*, 1–13. [CrossRef]
16. Sudarshan, V.K.; Brabrand, M.; Range, T.M.; Wiil, U.K. Performance evaluation emergency department patient arrivals forecasting models by including meteorological and calendar information: A comparative study. *Comput. Biol. Med.* **2021**, *135*, 104541. [CrossRef]
17. Lucini, F.R.; Dos Reis, M.A.; Da Silveira, G.J.C.; Fogliatto, F.S.; Anzanello, M.J.; Andrioli, G.G.; Nicolaidis, R.; Beltrame, R.C.F.; Neyeloff, J.L.; Schaan, B.D. Man vs. machine: Predicting hospital bed demand from an emergency department. *PLoS ONE* **2020**, *15*, e0237937. [CrossRef]
18. Rahimian, F.; Salimi-Khorshidi, G.; Payberah, A.H.; Tran, J.; Ayala Solares, R.; Raimondi, F.; Nazarzadeh, M.; Canoy, D.; Rahimi, K. Predicting the risk of emergency admission with machine learning: Development and validation using linked electronic health records. *PLoS Med.* **2018**, *15*, e1002695. [CrossRef]
19. Khatri, K.L.; Tamil, L.S. Early detection of peak demand days of chronic respiratory diseases emergency department visits using artificial neural networks. *IEEE J. Biomed. Health Inform.* **2017**, *22*, 285–290. [CrossRef] [PubMed]

20. Xu, M.; Wong, T.C.; Chin, K.S. Modeling daily patient arrivals at emergency epartment and quantifying the relative importance of contributing variables using artificial neural network. *Decis. Support Syst.* **2013**, *54*, 1488–1498. [CrossRef]
21. Yucesan, M.; Gul, M.; Celik, E. A multi-method patient arrival forecasting outline for hospital emergency departments. *Int. J. Healthc. Manag.* **2020**, *13*, 283–295. [CrossRef]
22. Hong Kong Observatory. Climate Change in Hong Kong. Available online: https://www.hko.gov.hk/en/climate_change/obs_hk_temp.htm (accessed on 12 August 2022).
23. Wang, D.; Lau, K.K.L.; Ren, C.; Goggins, W.B.I.; Shi, Y.; Ho, H.C.; Lee, T.-C.; Lee, L.-S.; Woo, J.; Ng, E. The impact of extremely hot weather events on all-cause mortality in a highly urbanized and densely populated subtropical city: A 10-year time-series study (2006–2015). *Sci. Total Environ.* **2019**, *690*, 923–931. [CrossRef]
24. Chan, E.Y.Y.; Goggins, W.B.; Kim, J.J.; Griffiths, S.; Ma, T.K. Help-seeking behavior during elevated temperature in Chinese population. *J. Urban Health* **2011**, *88*, 637–650. [CrossRef]
25. Chan, E.Y.; Goggins, W.B.; Yue, J.S.; Lee, P. Hospital admissions as a function of temperature, other weather phenomena and pollution levels in an urban setting in China. *Bull. World Health Organ.* **2013**, *91*, 576–584. [CrossRef] [PubMed]
26. Wong, T.W.; Tam, W.W.S.; Yu, I.T.S.; Lau, A.K.H.; Pang, S.W.; Wong, A.H. Developing a risk-based air quality health index. *Atmos. Environ.* **2013**, *76*, 52–58. [CrossRef]
27. Van Loenhout, J.A.F.; Delbiso, T.D.; Kiriliouk, A.; Rodriguez-Llanes, J.M.; Segers, J.; Guha-Sapir, D. Heat and emergency room admissions in the Netherlands. *BMC Public Health* **2018**, *18*, 108. [CrossRef] [PubMed]
28. Thomas, N.; Ebelt, S.T.; Newman, A.J.; Scovronick, N.; D'Souza, R.R.; Moss, S.E.; Warren, J.L.; Strickland, M.J.; Darrow, L.A.; Chang, H.H. Time-series analysis of daily ambient temperature and emergency department visits in five US cities with a comparison of exposure metrics derived from 1-km meteorology products. *Environ. Health* **2021**, *20*, 55. [CrossRef]
29. Luo, Y.; Zhang, Y.; Liu, T.; Rutherford, S.; Xu, Y.; Xu, X.; Wu, W.; Xiao, J.; Zeng, W.; Chu, C.; et al. Lagged effect of diurnal temperature range on mortality in a subtropical megacity of China. *PLoS ONE* **2013**, *8*, e55280.
30. Sun, Y.; Heng, B.H.; Seow, Y.T.; Seow, E. Forecasting daily attendances at an emergency department to aid resource planning. *BMC Emerg. Med.* **2009**, *9*, 1–9. [CrossRef]
31. Adams, A.; Vamplew, P. Encoding and decoding cyclic data. *South Pac. J. Nat. Sci.* **1998**, *16*, 54–58.
32. Vollmer, M.A.; Glampson, B.; Mellan, T.; Mishra, S.; Mercuri, L.; Costello, C.; Klaber, R.; Cooke, G.; Flaxman, S.; Bhatt, S. A unified machine learning approach to time series forecasting applied to demand at emergency departments. *BMC Emerg. Med.* **2021**, *21*, 1–14. [CrossRef]
33. Wu, X.; Kumar, V.; Quinlan, J.R.; Ghosh, J.; Yang, Q.; Motoda, H.; McLachlan, G.J.; Ng, A.; Liu, B.; Yu, P.S.; et al. Top 10 algorithms in data mining. *Knowl. Inf. Syst.* **2008**, *14*, 1–37. [CrossRef]
34. Ali, J.; Khan, R.; Ahmad, N.; Maqsood, I. Random forests and decision trees. *Int. J. Comput. Sci. Issues* **2012**, *9*, 272.
35. Liu, W.; Wang, Z.; Liu, X.; Zeng, N.; Liu, Y.; Alsaadi, F.E. A survey of deep neural network architectures and their applications. *Neurocomputing* **2017**, *234*, 11–26. [CrossRef]
36. Xu, B.; Wang, N.; Chen, T.; Li, M. Empirical evaluation of rectified activations in convolutional network. *arXiv* **2015**, arXiv:1505.00853.
37. Chung, J.; Gulcehre, C.; Cho, K.; Bengio, Y. Empirical evaluation of gated recurrent neural networks on sequence modeling. *arXiv* **2014**, arXiv:1412.3555.
38. Chai, Y.; Luo, H.; Zhang, Q.; Cheng, Q.; Lui, C.S.; Yip, P.S. Developing an early warning system of suicide using Google Trends and media reporting. *J. Affect. Disord.* **2019**, *255*, 41–49. [CrossRef] [PubMed]
39. Van Rossum, G.; Drake, F.L. *The Python Language Reference Manual*; Network Theory Ltd.: Godalming, UK, 2011.
40. Pedregosa, F.; Varoquaux, G.; Gramfort, A.; Michel, V.; Thirion, B.; Grisel, O.; Blondel, M.; Prettenhofer, P.; Weiss, R.; Dubourg, V.; et al. Scikit-learn: Machine learning in Python. *J. Mach. Learn. Res.* **2011**, *12*, 2825–2830.
41. Paszke, A.; Gross, S.; Massa, F.; Lerer, A.; Bradbury, J.; Chanan, G.; Killeen, T.; Lin, Z.; Gimelshein, N.; Antiga, L.; et al. Pytorch: An imperative style, high-performance deep learning library. *Adv. Neural Inf. Processing Syst.* **2019**, *32*, 8026–8037.
42. Ho, H.C.; Lau, K.K.; Ren, C.; Ng, E. Characterizing prolonged heat effects on mortality in a sub-tropical high-density city, Hong Kong. *Int. J. Biometeorol.* **2017**, *61*, 1935–1944. [CrossRef]
43. Chau, P.H.; Woo, J. The trends in excess mortality in winter vs. summer in a sub-tropical city and its association with extreme climate conditions. *PLoS ONE* **2015**, *10*, e0126774.
44. Chau, P.H.; Yip, P.S.F.; Lau, E.H.Y.; Ip, Y.T.; Law, F.Y.W.; Ho, R.T.H.; Leung, A.Y.M.; Wong, J.Y.H.; Woo, J. Hot weather and suicide deaths among older adults in Hong Kong, 1976–2014: A retrospective study. *Int. J. Environ. Res. Public Health* **2020**, *17*, 3449. [CrossRef]
45. Altman, D.G.; Royston, P. The cost of dichotomising continuous variables. *BMJ* **2006**, *332*, 1080. [CrossRef]
46. Rajula, H.S.R.; Verlato, G.; Manchia, M.; Antonucci, N.; Fanos, V. Comparison of conventional statistical methods with machine learning in medicine: Diagnosis, drug development, and treatment. *Medicina* **2020**, *56*, 455. [CrossRef] [PubMed]
47. Cho, K.; Van Merriënboer, B.; Gulcehre, C.; Bahdanau, D.; Bougares, F.; Schwenk, H.; Bengio, Y. Learning phrase representations using RNN encoder-decoder for statistical machine translation. *arXiv* **2014**, arXiv:1406.1078.
48. Cahuantzi, R.; Chen, X.; Güttel, S. A comparison of LSTM and GRU networks for learning symbolic sequences. *arXiv* **2021**, arXiv:2107.02248.

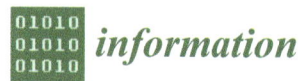

Article

A Fuzzy Knowledge Graph Pairs-Based Application for Classification in Decision Making: Case Study of Preeclampsia Signs

Hai Van Pham [1,*], Cu Kim Long [1,2,*], Phan Hung Khanh [1] and Ha Quoc Trung [2]

1 School of Information Communication Technology, Hanoi University of Science and Technology (HUST), Hanoi 100000, Vietnam
2 Information Technology Center, Ministry of Science and Technology (MOST), Hanoi 100000, Vietnam
* Correspondence: haipv@soict.hust.edu.vn (H.V.P.); longck.2006@gmail.com (C.K.L.)

Abstract: Problems of preeclampsia sign diagnosis are mostly based on symptom data with the characteristics of data collected periodically in uncertain, ambiguous, and obstetrician opinions. To reduce the effects of preeclampsia, many studies have investigated the disease, prevention, and complication. Conventional fuzzy inference techniques can solve several diagnosis problems in health such as fuzzy inference systems (FIS), and Mamdani complex fuzzy inference systems with rule reduction (M-CFIS-R), however, the computation time is quite high. Recently, the research direction of approximate inference based on fuzzy knowledge graph (FKG) has been proposed in the M-CFIS-FKG model with the combination of regimens in traditional medicine and subclinical data gathered from medical records. The paper has presented a proposed model of FKG-Pairs3 to support patients' disease diagnosis, together with doctors' preferences in decision-making. The proposed model has been implemented in real-world applications for disease diagnosis in traditional medicine based on input data sets with vague information, quantified by doctor's preferences. To validate the proposed model, it has been tested in a real-world case study of preeclampsia signs in a hospital for disease diagnosis with the traditional medicine approach. Experimental results show that the proposed model has demonstrated the model's effectiveness in the decision-making of preeclampsia signs.

Keywords: fuzzy knowledge graph; FKG-Pairs; disease diagnosis; preeclampsia; decision making

1. Introduction

Recently, preeclampsia signs have several typical clinical symptoms such as high blood pressure, proteinuria, and edema. Severe cases may be accompanied by convulsions and narcotisms [1–3]. Preeclampsia is a sort of multi-organ dysfunction related to pregnancy, accounting for about 2–10% during the entire pregnancy [1,3,4]. Over the past two decades, the preeclampsia rate has increased by about 25%, especially in the early preeclampsia group. In Asia, a statistic from 2001 to 2014 shows that preeclampsia increased quickly, from 0.5% to 0.8% during the entire pregnancy [1]. In Viet Nam, the preeclampsia rate before 34 weeks is 0.43%, the preeclampsia rate from 34 to 37 weeks is 0.7%, and the preeclampsia rate after 37 weeks is 1.68% compared to the entire pregnancy. A series of studies from 2012 to 2016 in Hue showed the preeclampsia rate is about 2.8–5.5% [2]. In applied AI healthcare applications, many studies of preeclampsia pathology in recent years have focused on the field of disease occurrence prediction, disease progression prediction, and pregnancy outcomes diagnosis as well as preeclampsia prophylaxis.

Preeclampsia is a pathology with multi-variable evidence for both mother and fetus. This causes of death maternal and perinatal mortality worldwide. Maternal mortality associated with hypertension in general pregnancy and preeclampsia accounts for about 14%. Death rate maternal mortality is associated with an increase in hypertension during

Citation: Pham, H.V.; Long, C.K.; Khanh, P.H.; Trung, H.Q. A Fuzzy Knowledge Graph Pairs-Based Application for Classification in Decision Making: Case Study of Preeclampsia Signs. *Information* 2023, 14, 104. https://doi.org/10.3390/info14020104

Academic Editors: Shlomo Berkovsky, Sidong Liu and Cristián Castillo Olea

Received: 16 December 2022
Revised: 1 February 2023
Accepted: 2 February 2023
Published: 7 February 2023

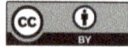

Copyright: © 2023 by the authors. Licensee MDPI, Basel, Switzerland. This article is an open access article distributed under the terms and conditions of the Creative Commons Attribution (CC BY) license (https://creativecommons.org/licenses/by/4.0/).

pregnancy in the range of 12.9–16.1% [1,4]. Besides, the effects of preeclampsia are given after birth, in relation to subsequent births, and are a risk factor for later cardiovascular diseases [5]. Despite efforts in the management of the prenatal phase, preeclampsia is still one of the disease burdens in maternal and child healthcare. To reduce the effects of preeclampsia, many investigations have been given to aim disease forecasting and prophylaxis, optimally export prophylaxis presents the disease, prevents severe progression, and prevents complications. Since 2011, WHO has issued recommendations for forecasting and prophylaxis of preeclampsia pathology [1]. Many organizations (Federation Obstetrics and Gynecology International (FIGO), American Society of Obstetricians and Gynecologists (ACOG), Healthcare Institute British National and Clinical Health (NICE), Canadian Society of Obstetricians and Gynecologists (SOGC)) and other specialized associations have also provided guidance on forecasting and redundancy preeclampsia [6–9]. With the motivation to apply information technology in early disease diagnosis, the authors have endeavored to deploy an application based on regimes in traditional medicine to solve the problem of preeclampsia sign diagnosis in pregnant women.

To handle problems in disease diagnosis, a knowledge graph-based approach is considered to support doctors in disease diagnosis [10–12]. KG is considered a powerful technique to support decision support systems, predictive analysis systems, and recommendation systems. It can be combined with other techniques to find the output labels of new samples. However, knowledge graphs face difficulties in representing knowledge and making approximate inferences based on input data sets with unclear information (such as subclinical symptom data with amplitude factor in the medical sector).

To solve the limitations of the knowledge graph, several techniques based on fuzzy inference systems are applied to build real-world applications. It has received much attention from many researchers all over the world, such as fuzzy inference systems (FIS) [13–18], complex fuzzy inference systems (CFIS) [19–21], and Mamdani-type complex fuzzy inference systems (M-CFIS) [22], M-CFIS-R [23]. These techniques cannot generate the output labels when new samples are not in the fuzzy rule base. Furthermore, these techniques can also show that the computation time is still quite high. Nevertheless, the M-CFIS-FKG still has low accuracy with incomplete information input data sets. Recently, the research direction of approximate inference based on fuzzy knowledge graph (FKG) has been proposed in the M-CFIS-FKG model [24] with the combination of regimens in traditional medicine and subclinical data gathered from electric medical records. This helps FKG to overcome the previous works' drawbacks.

From the above limitations of the M-CFIS-FKG, a new model (so-called FKG-Pairs) was proposed in [25]. It is considered an extension of FKG in the M-CFIS-FKG model [24]. It improved the single-pairs FKG (FKG-Pairs1) by using combinations of attribute pairs to compute the weights and inference of the output label (e.g., double-pairs FKG (FKG-Pairs2), triple-pairs FKG (FKG-Pairs3), quadruple-pairs FKG (FKG-Pairs4), and quintuple-pairs FKG (FKG-Pairs5)). These methods have been applied to improve the inference performance of decision-making systems in terms of accuracy. In related works [26–28], the investigations have proposed Decision Support System to apply ontology-based for diabetic patients [26], Fuzzy Knowledge applied to give decision-making in diagnosis Decision Support System [27]. Further investigations have focused on human hearing abilities classification [28], applied U-Net with Deep Learning of glaucoma [29], and multiple Machine Learning techniques for decision making of chronic kidney disease [30], Prediction and analysis using dynamic neural network, genetic algorithm [31], and medical system has been applied to use deep learning techniques for clinic diagnosis [32]. In clinical decision support systems, knowledge reasoning and linguistics can be used in decision-making [33], multi-attribute decision-making [34,35], and group decision-making [36] for significant contributions to medical diagnosis. As mentioned in the related works, with incomplete information input data sets, conventional methods or fuzzy inference techniques have not been considered fully effective solutions. Studying to deploy easy and convenient FKG-Pairs-based applications is to meet the requirements for real-world problems.

The paper has presented a proposed model of FKG-Pairs3 to support patients' disease diagnosis, together with doctors' preferences in decision-making. The proposed model has been tested in a real-world case study of preeclampsia signs in a hospital for disease diagnosis with the traditional medicine approach. The **main contributions** of this study are as follows:

- Proposing the FKG-Pairs3-based preeclampsia sign diagnosis model. This proposed model is used to quantify incomplete and vague information input data sets including qualitative and quantitative factors, quantified from doctor's preferences.
- Applying FKG-Pairs3 for consideration of patient's symptom pairs to approximate reasoning to find the output labels of new samples, matched with the class of classification in decision-making problems with incomplete information input data sets.
- Implementing the proposed model for the development of real-world applications using datasets collected from medical records in accordance with the preferences of doctors through a case study of preeclampsia sign diagnosis for support of traditional medicine inpatient medical records.

The rest of this paper is organized as follows. Part 2 presents the background knowledge of the research process. Part 3 describes the detailed proposed model in medical diagnosis including the problem statement and the process of building and applying the FKG-Pairs to solve the problem. Experimental results and performance evaluation of the application are shown in Part 4. The final part is to give conclusions and future investigations.

2. Research Background

2.1. Fuzzy Sets

Fuzzy sets were first introduced by Zadeh in 1965 [37], introduced as a new mathematical tool for solving problems with ambiguous, uncertain information. Unlike normal sets, which evaluate the membership of the set according to the binary logic "an element belongs or not to the set", fuzzy logic [38,39] evaluates the membership of a part element through a membership function $\mu \to [0, 1]$, which represents the membership of an element to a set.

2.2. Fuzzy Inference System

A fuzzy inference system (FIS) is a popular computational framework based on the concept of fuzzy set theory, often applied when building decision support systems in case the input information is not clear [16]. The general framework of the FIS as shown in Figure 1 can be summarized with three main parts: fuzzification, knowledge base, and defuzzification. The FIS has the basic structure as follows:

- Fuzzification: It is responsible for converting input values into language values.
- The knowledge base consists of two parts: The database (definition of fuzzy set membership functions used in fuzzy rules) and the set of rules (including IF-THEN structural fuzzy rules).
- Engine: Perform inference operations in the fuzzy rule base.

Defuzzification: It is responsible for converting the fuzzy result values of the fuzzy inference system into clear values.

Fuzzy inference is the process of finding a conclusion for a set of input values, based on the synthesized fuzzy rule system. Fuzzy inference methods are regularly referred to as FIS, CFIS, and M-CFIS. These inference systems, also known as classical inference methods, have been widely used in automatic control systems and decision support systems. The FKG [24] is known as a new, efficient, and more accurate inference method than previous fuzzy inference methods. Fuzzy inference systems are classified into three main methods: Mamdani fuzzy inference systems, Takagi-Sugeno fuzzy inference systems, and Tsukamoto fuzzy inference systems.

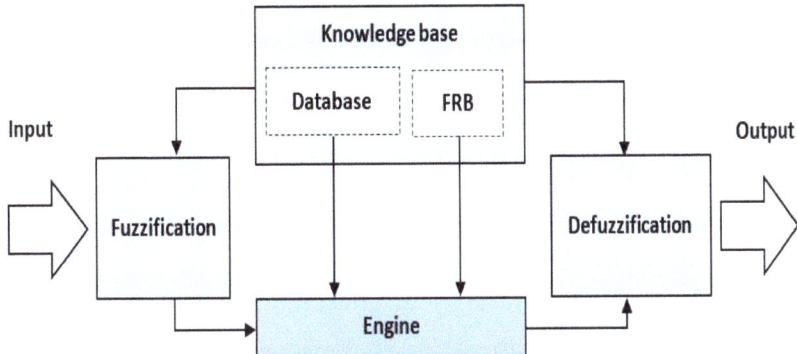

Figure 1. The general framework of the FIS.

2.3. Knowledge Graph

Knowledge graph (KG) was first introduced by Google in 2012 [40]. The main purpose of KG is to analyze to maximize the value of knowledge, detect and avoid errors, and to be able to infer new conclusions from existing data. The selection of new entity representations and their relationships through the KG model can gain a lot of useful information and can be more supportive for practical applications. It is for this reason that KG is researched, proposed, and applied by the community of researchers in many practical problems, especially in models with approximate reasoning. It is considered a powerful technique to support decision support systems, predictive analysis systems, and recommendation systems [41–43].

2.4. Fuzzy Knowledge Graph

The FKG was first proposed in 2020 [24] to solve the limitations of KG in representing knowledge and making approximate inferences based on input data sets with unclear or incomplete information by using linguistic labels for the attributes in the training set connected to the output labels. It represents inference through natural law where the impact of language labels is capable of generating corresponding output labels. By accumulating single events (or single pairs in the FKG), it can determine the final output of a new sample. The FKG has two main phases including representation and approximate reasoning.

In the representation phase, the weights of edges are calculated and are briefly summarized as follows. Firstly, for edges connecting among vertices or input attributes' labels on FKG, the weight A_{ij}^t of these edges is calculated by using Equation (1):

$$A_{ij}^t = \frac{|X_i \text{ is related to } X_j \text{ in rule } t|}{|R|} \quad (1)$$

where: X_i, X_j are input attribute vertices, $1 \leq i \leq j \leq m$, R_t is the tth rule, $t = \overline{1,k}$.

Secondly, for edges connecting the input attribute label and the output label on FKG, the weight B_{il}^t of these edges is calculated by using Equation (2):

$$B_{il}^t = \left(\sum A_{ij}^t\right) \times \frac{|X_i \text{ is related to the label } l \text{ in rule } t|}{|R|} \quad (2)$$

where: X_i is input attribute vertex, $1 \leq i < j < m$, R_t is the tth rule, $t = \overline{1,k}$, l is output label vertex and $l = \overline{1,C}$.

The results of the two sets of weights are stored in an adjacency matrix, which can be used in the FISA algorithm in the next phase.

In the approximate reasoning phase, the FISA algorithm [24] is applied to approximate reasoning and find the output labels of the new records.

2.5. Approximate Reasoning and Decision Making

Approximate reasoning is defined as a tool for inferences from propositions of unspecified meaning through fuzzy logic [43]. Usually, the approximate inference method has a lower accuracy than the conventional inference techniques based on clear data, but the advantage of approximation reasoning unclear data with language variables. In [24], it is applied in the FISA algorithm to find the output labels of the new records.

Decision-making is considered the core of decision-support systems. It supports leaders and managers make accurate, timely, and effective decisions. It is applied in many sectors in the real world, such as healthcare, finance, stock, transportation, environment, agriculture, business, and other studies [31,42–46].

3. The Proposed Model for Preeclampsia Sign Diagnosis in Decision Making

This section describes the preeclampsia sign diagnosis proposed model in detail. The main contents are presented in this section including the problem statement, the proposed model, and a numerical example to elucidate the solving problem.

3.1. Problem Statement

Input: Suppose that we have an original database after extracting from pregnancy patients' medical records. By supporting of doctors and obstetricians, the subclinical features are selected to construct the FKG-Pairs (*such as Blood Pressure, HGB, PLT, Urea, Creatinine, Acid Uric, ALT, AST, Total Protein, Albumin, LDH, Proteinuria and so on*). The training and testing data sets, with splitting 70% and 30% respectively, are obtained after applying the data preprocessing method and the rule-generated mechanism.

A fuzzy rule base of the training data set is described in detail in Table 1. It includes n rules $(P_1, P_2, P_3, \ldots, P_{n-1}, P_n)$ representing patients' medical records, m input features $(S_1, S_2, S_3, \ldots, S_{m-1}, S_m)$ representing the symptoms of the preeclampsia, and C output labels $(1, 2, 3, \ldots, C)$ representing the doctor's diagnosis results.

In addition, the testing data set includes samples after applying the rule-generated mechanism with the IF-THEN structure similar to the rules in Table 1. For instance:

IF S_1 is "L_1" and S_2 is "L_2" and S_3 is "H_2" and S_4 is "VH_4" and ... and S_{m-1} is "H_{m-1}" and S_m is "L_m" THEN Output label = 3.

Table 1. The fuzzy rule bases.

P_i \ S_j	S_1	S_2	...	S_{m-1}	S_m	Output Labels
P_1	H_1	H_2	...	VH_{m-1}	H_m	2
P_2	M_1	M_2	...	M_{m-1}	L_m	1
...	...	...	...	...	...	...
P_{n-1}	M_1	M_2	...	M_{m-1}	M_m	1
P_n	L_1	M_2	...	L_{m-1}	L_m	3
Patients' symptoms	$\{H_1, M_1, L_1\}$	$\{H_2, M_2\}$	...	$\{VH_{m-1}, H_{m-1}, M_{m-1}, L_{m-1}\}$	$\{H_m, M_m, L_m\}$	$\{1, 2, 3, \ldots, C\}$

Output: Find the output label of the new records with subclinical data inputted by doctors or patients based on the preeclampsia sign diagnosis module.

3.2. Proposed Model

In this subsection, we have presented the main contents related to the construction of triple-pairs FKG (FKG-Pairs3) for the problem of disease diagnosis based on symptom data, namely: Giving a model for the problem of preeclampsia sign diagnosis in gestational women; Describing steps to follow the proposed model; and give numerical examples to illustrate the proposed model.

3.2.1. The Preeclampsia Sign Diagnosis Proposed Model

The preeclampsia sign diagnosis proposed model consists of two phases (preparation phase; diagnosis phase) as shown in Figure 2. In the problem statement, assuming we have a fuzzy rule base of the preeclampsia sign diagnosis problem after applying several steps (including the pre-processing, the rule-generated mechanism, and the training). Then, the preeclampsia sign diagnosis module (based on FKG-Pairs3) is constructed by using the training data set and is validated by using the testing data set. Finally, obstetricians and gestational women can use this module to check the preeclampsia signs by inputting the subclinical data.

3.2.2. The Steps to Implement the Application

To implement the preeclampsia sign diagnosis application based on FKG-Pairs3, several steps are obligated strictly as follows:

Step 1. Gather data sets to establish the original database.

From the medical records of the patients, the features related to the preeclampsia signs are extracted. Then, the clinical and subclinical signs data are gathered with the doctor's support. The data are stored in a database (considered the original database).

Step 2. Prepare the fuzzy rule base.

In this step, we conduct some tasks before constructing the FKG-Pairs3 as follows:

- Conducting the data preprocessing.
- Applying the rule-generated mechanism (herein FIS or M-CFIS).
- Applying the cluster sampling method and splitting the dataset into two parts including the training set and testing set with rates of 70% and 30% respectively.

Step 3. Construct the FKG-Pairs3 based on the training data set.

This step is considered the most important step to implement the preeclampsia sign diagnosis application in the proposed model as shown in Figure 2. There are three main tasks in this step as follows:

Firstly, for the edges connecting among vertices (input features' labels) on FKG, the weight $\widetilde{A}^t_{ijhk}$ of these edges is calculated by using Equation (3):

$$\widetilde{A}^t_{ijhk} = \frac{|S_i \to S_j \to S_h \to S_k \text{ in rule } t|}{|R|} \qquad (3)$$

in which $t = \overline{1,n}, 1 \leq i \leq j < h < k < m-1$, $|R|$ is the number of rules in the training data set.

Secondly, for edges connecting the input feature label and the output label on FKG, the weight $\widetilde{B}^t_{ijhl}$ of these edges is calculated by using Equation (4):

$$\widetilde{B}^t_{ijhl} = \left(\sum \widetilde{A}^t_{ijhk}\right) \times \text{MIN}\left(\frac{|S_i \to l \text{ in rule } t|}{|R|}, \frac{|S_j \to l \text{ in rule } t|}{|R|}, \frac{|S_h \to l \text{ in rule } t|}{|R|}\right) \qquad (4)$$

in which $t = \overline{1,n}$; $1 \leq i < j < h \leq m$; $l = \overline{1,C}$, $|R|$ is the number of rules in the training data set.

Finally, the FKG-Pairs algorithm in [37] (with $k = 3$ or FKG-Pairs3) is applied to approximate reasoning and find the output labels of the new records. The algorithm is described briefly below.

Calculating the sum of the weights of the edges $\left(\widetilde{C}\right)$ connecting from the super-nodes (i.e., each node is the combination among three features' labels) is given to the output label by using Equation (5).

$$\widetilde{C}_{ijhl} = \sum_t \widetilde{B}^t_{ijhl} \qquad (5)$$

in which $t = \overline{1,n}$; $1 \leq i < j < h \leq m$; $l = \overline{1,C}$.

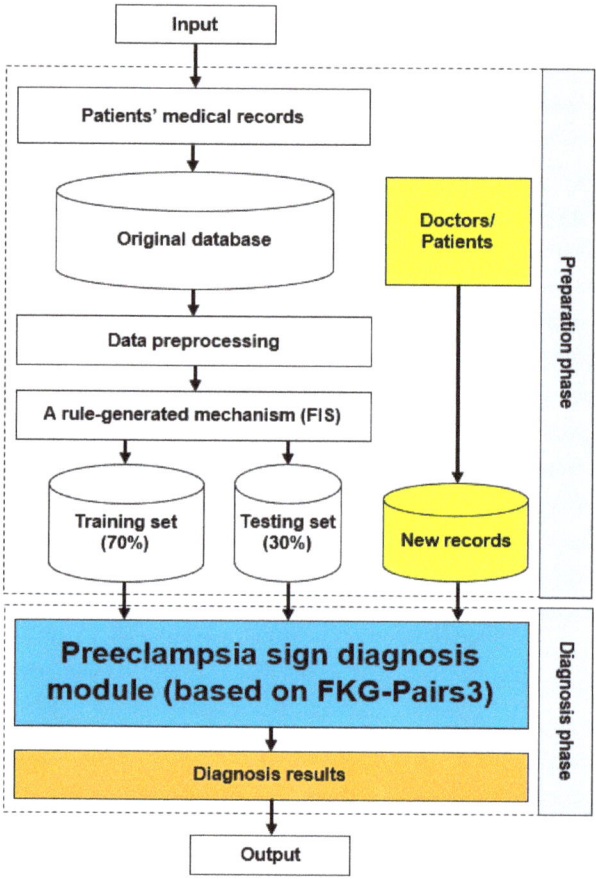

Figure 2. The proposed model of preeclampsia sign diagnosis.

Calculating the membership value ($\widetilde{D}_l$) by using the $Max - Min$ operator, given by Equation (6).

$$\widetilde{D}_l = Max_{1 \leq i < j < h \leq m}\left(\widetilde{C}_{ijhl}\right) + Min_{1 \leq i < j < h \leq m}\left(\widetilde{C}_{ijhl}\right) \quad (6)$$

in which $t = \overline{1,n}$; $1 \leq i < j < h \leq m$; $l = \overline{1,C}$.

Finding the labels of the new records by using the Max operator, given by Equation (7).

$$Label = p \; if \; \widetilde{D}_p = Max_{l=\overline{1,C}}\left(\widetilde{D}_l\right) \quad (7)$$

Step 4. Validate the testing data set.

Before applying the preeclampsia sign diagnosis module for new records validated on the testing data set, which supports the application becoming more reliable. In case, the confidence of the diagnosis module cannot meet the doctors' requirements, we have to return to step 1 to get more data from new medical records to enrich the fuzzy rule base.

Step 5. Input the subclinical data of a gestational woman.

This step permits the patients (or users) to input the subclinical data to check the preeclampsia signs. Note that the data entered into the program has to meet the system's requirements (i.e., in the valued range).

Step 6. Get the diagnosis results.

After processing and approximate reasoning based on the subclinical data entered by patients or users, the application calculates and finds the output label corresponding to the diagnosis result (users can recheck it from obstetricians if possible).

3.2.3. A numerical Example to Illustrate the Proposed Model

To deeply understand the proposed model, a numerical example is given in this subsection.

Input: Suppose that we have six rules $\{R_1, R_2, R_3, R_4, R_5, R_6\}$ representing six gestational women. Each gestational woman has five features $\{S_1, S_2, S_3, S_4, S_5\}$ representing the preeclampsia signs test results. The above cases of gestational women were examined and diagnosed based on the test results by the doctor. The output labels are 0, 1, and 2 corresponding to the doctor's diagnosis conclusions "*Normal*", "*Preeclampsia*" and "*Severe Preeclampsia*" respectively. After going through the data preprocessing step as well as applying the fuzzification of the input value by using the linguistic variables, a fuzzy rule base system is obtained as shown in Table 2.

Table 2. The fuzzy rule base assumes that the medical examination results of six gestational women have been concluded to be diagnosed by doctors.

	S_1	S_2	S_3	S_4	S_5	S_6	Output Label
R_1	H_1	M_2	M_3	M_4	H_5	H_6	2
R_2	H_1	M_2	M_3	M_4	M_5	M_6	1
R_3	VH_1	M_2	M_3	M_4	H_5	H_6	2
R_4	M_1	M_2	M_3	M_4	M_5	M_6	0
R_5	H_1	M_2	M_3	M_4	M_5	M_6	1
R_6	VH_1	L_2	L_3	M_4	M_5	M_6	2

In addition, we have also a new gestational woman after applying the rule-generated mechanism with the IF-THEN structure similar to the rules in Table 2. For instance: **IF** S_1 is "H_1" and S_2 is "H_2" and S_3 is "M_3" and S_4 is "M_4" and S_5 is "H_5" and S_6 is "H_6" **THEN** the output label = ?

Output: Find the output label of several new gestational women based on the fuzzy rule base in Table 2.

To solve the requirements given in the output, two steps are performed as follows:

Step 1: Constructing the FKG-Pairs3 based on the fuzzy rule base as shown in Table 2.

Firstly, we calculate the set of weights $\widetilde{A}^t_{ijhk}$ by applying Equation (3). With the rule R_1, we have:

$$\widetilde{A}^1_{1234} = \frac{|H_1 \to M_2 \to M_3 \to M_4|}{|R|} = \frac{1}{6} = 0.17, \quad \widetilde{A}^1_{1235} = \frac{|H_1 \to M_2 \to M_3 \to H_5|}{|R|} = \frac{1}{6} = 0.17,$$

$$\widetilde{A}^1_{1236} = \frac{|H_1 \to M_2 \to M_3 \to H_6|}{|R|} = \frac{1}{6} = 0.17, \quad \widetilde{A}^1_{1245} = \frac{|H_1 \to M_2 \to M_4 \to H_5|}{|R|} = \frac{1}{6} = 0.17,$$

$$\widetilde{A}^1_{1246} = \frac{|H_1 \to M_2 \to M_4 \to H_6|}{|R|} = \frac{1}{6} = 0.17, \quad \widetilde{A}^1_{1256} = \frac{|H_1 \to M_2 \to H_5 \to H_6|}{|R|} = \frac{1}{6} = 0.17,$$

$$\widetilde{A}^1_{1345} = \frac{|H_1 \to M_3 \to M_4 \to H_5|}{|R|} = \frac{1}{6} = 0.17, \quad \widetilde{A}^1_{1346} = \frac{|H_1 \to M_3 \to M_4 \to H_6|}{|R|} = \frac{1}{6} = 0.17,$$

$$\widetilde{A}^1_{1356} = \frac{|H_1 \to M_3 \to H_5 \to H_6|}{|R|} = \frac{1}{6} = 0.17, \quad \widetilde{A}^1_{1456} = \frac{|H_1 \to M_4 \to H_5 \to H_6|}{|R|} = \frac{1}{6} = 0.17,$$

$$\widetilde{A}^1_{2345} = \frac{|M_2 \to M_3 \to M_4 \to H_5|}{|R|} = \frac{1}{3} = 0.33, \quad \widetilde{A}^1_{2346} = \frac{|M_2 \to M_3 \to M_4 \to H_6|}{|R|} = \frac{1}{3} = 0.33,$$

$$\widetilde{A}^1_{2356} = \frac{|M_2 \to M_3 \to H_5 \to H_6|}{|R|} = \frac{1}{3} = 0.33, \quad \widetilde{A}^1_{2456} = \frac{|M_2 \to M_4 \to H_5 \to H_6|}{|R|} = \frac{1}{3} = 0.33,$$

$$\widetilde{A}^1_{3456} = \frac{|M_3 \to M_4 \to H_5 \to H_6|}{|R|} = \frac{1}{3} = 0.33$$

By the same calculation, we obtain the weights $\widetilde{A}^t_{ijhk}$ for six rules in Table 3 as follows.

Table 3. Results of weight matrix calculation $\widetilde{A}$.

$\widetilde{A}$	R_1	R_2	R_3	R_4	R_5	R_6
$\widetilde{A}^t_{1234}$	0.17	0.33	0.17	0.17	0.33	0.17
$\widetilde{A}^t_{1235}$	0.17	0.33	0.17	0.17	0.33	0.17
$\widetilde{A}^t_{1236}$	0.17	0.33	0.17	0.17	0.33	0.17
$\widetilde{A}^t_{1245}$	0.17	0.33	0.17	0.17	0.33	0.17
$\widetilde{A}^t_{1246}$	0.17	0.33	0.17	0.17	0.33	0.17
$\widetilde{A}^t_{1256}$	0.17	0.33	0.17	0.17	0.33	0.17
$\widetilde{A}^t_{1345}$	0.17	0.33	0.17	0.17	0.33	0.17
$\widetilde{A}^t_{1346}$	0.17	0.33	0.17	0.17	0.33	0.17
$\widetilde{A}^t_{1356}$	0.17	0.33	0.17	0.17	0.33	0.17
$\widetilde{A}^t_{1456}$	0.17	0.33	0.17	0.17	0.33	0.17
$\widetilde{A}^t_{2345}$	0.33	0.33	0.33	0.17	0.33	0.17
$\widetilde{A}^t_{2346}$	0.33	0.33	0.33	0.17	0.33	0.17
$\widetilde{A}^t_{2356}$	0.33	0.33	0.33	0.17	0.33	0.17
$\widetilde{A}^t_{2456}$	0.33	0.33	0.33	0.17	0.33	0.17
$\widetilde{A}^t_{3456}$	0.33	0.33	0.33	0.17	0.33	0.17

Secondly, after calculating the set of weights $\widetilde{A}^t_{ijhk}$, we calculate the set of weights $\widetilde{B}^t_{ijhl}$ by applying the Equation (4). With the rule R_1, it is expressed by:

$$\widetilde{B}^1_{1231} = \left(\widetilde{A}^1_{1234} + \widetilde{A}^1_{1235} + \widetilde{A}^1_{1236} + \widetilde{A}^1_{1245} + \widetilde{A}^1_{1246} + \widetilde{A}^1_{1256} + \widetilde{A}^1_{1345} + \widetilde{A}^1_{1346} + \widetilde{A}^1_{1356}\right.$$
$$\left. + \widetilde{A}^1_{1456} + \widetilde{A}^1_{2345} + \widetilde{A}^1_{2346} + \widetilde{A}^1_{2356} + \widetilde{A}^1_{2456} + \widetilde{A}^1_{3456}\right)$$
$$\times MIN\left(\frac{|H_1 \to 1|}{|R|}, \frac{|M_2 \to 1|}{|R|}, \frac{|M_3 \to 1|}{|R|}\right) = 3.33 \times MIN\left(\frac{1}{3}, \frac{1}{3}, \frac{1}{3}\right)$$
$$= 3.33 \times \frac{1}{3} = 1.11$$

By similar calculation, we find $\widetilde{B}^1_{1241} = \widetilde{B}^1_{1251} = \widetilde{B}^1_{1261} = \widetilde{B}^1_{1341} = \widetilde{B}^1_{1351} = \widetilde{B}^1_{1361} = \widetilde{B}^1_{1451} = \widetilde{B}^1_{1461} = \widetilde{B}^1_{1561} = \widetilde{B}^1_{2341} = \widetilde{B}^1_{2351} = \widetilde{B}^1_{2361} = \widetilde{B}^1_{2451} = \widetilde{B}^1_{2461} = \widetilde{B}^1_{3451} = \widetilde{B}^1_{3461} = \widetilde{B}^1_{3561} = \widetilde{B}^1_{4561} = 1.11$.

After applying Equation (4) for six rules, we obtain results of the entire weighted matrix $\widetilde{B}^t_{ijhl}$, given in Table 4.

Table 4. Results of weight matrix calculation $\widetilde{B}$.

$\widetilde{B}$	R_1	R_2	R_3	R_4	R_5	R_6
$\widetilde{B}_{1231}$	1.11	1.67	0.56	0.42	1.67	0.42
$\widetilde{B}_{1241}$	1.11	1.67	0.56	0.42	1.67	0.42
$\widetilde{B}_{1251}$	1.11	1.67	0.56	0.42	1.67	0.42
$\widetilde{B}_{1261}$	1.11	1.67	0.56	0.42	1.67	0.42
$\widetilde{B}_{1341}$	1.11	1.67	0.56	0.42	1.67	0.42
$\widetilde{B}_{1351}$	1.11	1.67	0.56	0.42	1.67	0.42
$\widetilde{B}_{1361}$	1.11	1.67	0.56	0.42	1.67	0.42

Table 4. *Cont.*

$\widetilde{B}$	R_1	R_2	R_3	R_4	R_5	R_6
$\widetilde{B}_{145l}$	1.11	1.67	0.56	0.42	1.67	0.42
$\widetilde{B}_{146l}$	1.11	1.67	0.56	0.42	1.67	0.42
$\widetilde{B}_{156l}$	1.11	1.67	0.56	0.42	1.67	0.42
$\widetilde{B}_{234l}$	1.11	1.67	1.11	0.42	1.67	0.42
$\widetilde{B}_{235l}$	1.11	1.67	1.11	0.42	1.67	0.42
$\widetilde{B}_{236l}$	1.11	1.67	1.11	0.42	1.67	0.42
$\widetilde{B}_{245l}$	1.11	1.67	1.11	0.42	1.67	0.42
$\widetilde{B}_{246l}$	1.11	1.67	1.11	0.42	1.67	0.42
$\widetilde{B}_{256l}$	1.11	1.67	1.11	0.42	1.67	0.42
$\widetilde{B}_{345l}$	1.11	1.67	1.11	0.42	1.67	0.42
$\widetilde{B}_{346l}$	1.11	1.67	1.11	0.42	1.67	0.42
$\widetilde{B}_{356l}$	1.11	1.67	1.11	0.42	1.67	0.42
$\widetilde{B}_{456l}$	1.11	1.67	1.11	0.42	1.67	0.42

Finally, the FKG-Pairs3 module is built by applying the FKG-Pairs algorithm in [37] (with $k = 3$ or FKG-Pairs3) to approximate reasoning and find the output labels.

After calculating the weights $\widetilde{A}_{ijhk}^t$ and $\widetilde{B}_{ijhl}^t$ for six rules in the fuzzy rule base, we calculate the sum of the weights of the edges $\left(\widetilde{C}\right)$ connecting from the super-nodes (i.e., each node is the combination among three feature labels) to the output label by using Equation (5). Let's consider the rule R_1:

- With label $l = 0$, we have:

$$\widetilde{C}_{1230} = \widetilde{C}_{1240} = \widetilde{C}_{1250} = \widetilde{C}_{1260} = \widetilde{C}_{1340} = \widetilde{C}_{1350} = \widetilde{C}_{1360} = \widetilde{C}_{1450} = \widetilde{C}_{1460} = \widetilde{C}_{1560} = \widetilde{C}_{2340}$$
$$= \widetilde{C}_{2350} = \widetilde{C}_{2360} = \widetilde{C}_{2450} = \widetilde{C}_{2460} = \widetilde{C}_{2560} = \widetilde{C}_{3450} = \widetilde{C}_{3460} = \widetilde{C}_{3560}$$
$$= \widetilde{C}_{4560} = 0$$

- With label $l = 1$, we have:

$$\widetilde{C}_{1231} = \widetilde{C}_{1241} = \widetilde{C}_{1251} = \widetilde{C}_{1261} = \widetilde{C}_{1341} = \widetilde{C}_{1351} = \widetilde{C}_{1361} = \widetilde{C}_{1451} = \widetilde{C}_{1461} = \widetilde{C}_{1561} = \widetilde{C}_{2341}$$
$$= \widetilde{C}_{2351} = \widetilde{C}_{2361} = \widetilde{C}_{2450} = \widetilde{C}_{2461} = \widetilde{C}_{2561} = \widetilde{C}_{3451} = \widetilde{C}_{3461} = \widetilde{C}_{3561}$$
$$= \widetilde{C}_{4561} = 0$$

- With label $l = 2$, we have:

$$\widetilde{C}_{1232} = \widetilde{C}_{1252} = \widetilde{C}_{1262} = \widetilde{C}_{1342} = \widetilde{C}_{1352} = \widetilde{C}_{1362} = \widetilde{C}_{1452} = \widetilde{C}_{1462} = \widetilde{C}_{1562} = \widetilde{C}_{2352} = \widetilde{C}_{2362}$$
$$= \widetilde{C}_{2452} = \widetilde{C}_{2462} = \widetilde{C}_{2562} = \widetilde{C}_{3450} = \widetilde{C}_{3452} = \widetilde{C}_{3462} = \widetilde{C}_{3562} = \widetilde{C}_{4562}$$
$$= \widetilde{B}_{1232}(Rule\ R_1) = 1.11$$

$$\widetilde{C}_{2342} = \widetilde{B}_{2342}(Rule\ R_1) + \widetilde{B}_{2342}(Rule\ R_3) = 2.22$$

By the same calculation with the rules R_2, R_3, R_4, R_5, R_6, we obtain results of the set of weights $\left(\widetilde{C}\right)$, given in Table 5.

From the values $(\widetilde{C}_{ijhl})$ in Table 5, we continue to compute the membership value $(\widetilde{D}_l)$ for each label ($l = 0, 1, 2$) by using the $Max - Min$ operator, given by Equation (6). For instance, in rule R_1 we have:

$$\tilde{D}_0 = Max(\tilde{C}_{1230}, \tilde{C}_{1240}, \tilde{C}_{1250}, \tilde{C}_{1260}, \tilde{C}_{1340}, \tilde{C}_{1350}, \tilde{C}_{1360}, \tilde{C}_{1450}, \tilde{C}_{1460}, \tilde{C}_{1560}, \tilde{C}_{2340},$$
$$\tilde{C}_{2350}, \tilde{C}_{2360}, \tilde{C}_{2450}, \tilde{C}_{2460}, \tilde{C}_{2560}, \tilde{C}_{3450}, \tilde{C}_{3460}, \tilde{C}_{3560}, \tilde{C}_{4560}) + Min(\tilde{C}_{1230}, \tilde{C}_{1240},$$
$$\tilde{C}_{1250}, \tilde{C}_{1260}, \tilde{C}_{1340}, \tilde{C}_{1350}, \tilde{C}_{1360}, \tilde{C}_{1450}, \tilde{C}_{1460}, \tilde{C}_{1560}, \tilde{C}_{2340}, \tilde{C}_{2350}, \tilde{C}_{2360}, \tilde{C}_{2450}, \tilde{C}_{2460},$$
$$\tilde{C}_{2560}, \tilde{C}_{3450}, \tilde{C}_{3460}, \tilde{C}_{3560}, \tilde{C}_{4560}) = 0$$

$$\tilde{D}_1 = Max(\tilde{C}_{1231}, \tilde{C}_{1241}, \tilde{C}_{1251}, \tilde{C}_{1261}, \tilde{C}_{1341}, \tilde{C}_{1351}, \tilde{C}_{1361}, \tilde{C}_{1451}, \tilde{C}_{1461}, \tilde{C}_{1561}, \tilde{C}_{2341},$$
$$\tilde{C}_{2351}, \tilde{C}_{2361}, \tilde{C}_{2451}, \tilde{C}_{2461}, \tilde{C}_{2561}, \tilde{C}_{3451}, \tilde{C}_{3461}, \tilde{C}_{3561}, \tilde{C}_{4561}) + Min(\tilde{C}_{1231}, \tilde{C}_{1241},$$
$$\tilde{C}_{1251}, \tilde{C}_{1261}, \tilde{C}_{1341}, \tilde{C}_{1351}, \tilde{C}_{1361}, \tilde{C}_{1451}, \tilde{C}_{1461}, \tilde{C}_{1561}, \tilde{C}_{2341}, \tilde{C}_{2351}, \tilde{C}_{2361}, \tilde{C}_{2451}, \tilde{C}_{2461},$$
$$\tilde{C}_{2561}, \tilde{C}_{3451}, \tilde{C}_{3461}, \tilde{C}_{3561}, \tilde{C}_{4561}) = 0$$

$$\tilde{D}_2 = Max(\tilde{C}_{1232}, \tilde{C}_{1242}, \tilde{C}_{1252}, \tilde{C}_{1262}, \tilde{C}_{1342}, \tilde{C}_{1352}, \tilde{C}_{1362}, \tilde{C}_{1452}, \tilde{C}_{1462}, \tilde{C}_{1562}, \tilde{C}_{2342},$$
$$\tilde{C}_{2352}, \tilde{C}_{2362}, \tilde{C}_{2452}, \tilde{C}_{2462}, \tilde{C}_{2562}, \tilde{C}_{3452}, \tilde{C}_{3462}, \tilde{C}_{3562}, \tilde{C}_{4562}) + Min(\tilde{C}_{1232}, \tilde{C}_{1242},$$
$$\tilde{C}_{1252}, \tilde{C}_{1262}, \tilde{C}_{1342}, \tilde{C}_{1352}, \tilde{C}_{1362}, \tilde{C}_{1452}, \tilde{C}_{1462}, \tilde{C}_{1562}, \tilde{C}_{2342}, \tilde{C}_{2352}, \tilde{C}_{2362}, \tilde{C}_{2452}, \tilde{C}_{2462},$$
$$\tilde{C}_{2562}, \tilde{C}_{3452}, \tilde{C}_{3462}, \tilde{C}_{3562}, \tilde{C}_{4562}) = 2.22 + 1.11 = 3.33$$

Table 5. Results of calculating the set of weights $\tilde{C}$.

	$\tilde{C}$	R_1	R_2	R_3	R_4	R_5	R_6
Label 0	$\tilde{C}_{1230}$	0.00	0.00	0.00	0.42	0.00	0.00
	$\tilde{C}_{1240}$	0.00	0.00	0.00	0.42	0.00	0.00
	$\tilde{C}_{1250}$	0.00	0.00	0.00	0.42	0.00	0.00
	$\tilde{C}_{1260}$	0.00	0.00	0.00	0.42	0.00	0.00
	$\tilde{C}_{1340}$	0.00	0.00	0.00	0.42	0.00	0.00
	$\tilde{C}_{1350}$	0.00	0.00	0.00	0.42	0.00	0.00
	$\tilde{C}_{1360}$	0.00	0.00	0.00	0.42	0.00	0.00
	$\tilde{C}_{1450}$	0.00	0.00	0.00	0.42	0.00	0.00
	$\tilde{C}_{1460}$	0.00	0.00	0.00	0.42	0.00	0.00
	$\tilde{C}_{1560}$	0.00	0.00	0.00	0.42	0.00	0.00
	$\tilde{C}_{2340}$	0.00	0.00	0.00	0.42	0.00	0.00
	$\tilde{C}_{2350}$	0.00	0.00	0.00	0.42	0.00	0.00
	$\tilde{C}_{2360}$	0.00	0.00	0.00	0.42	0.00	0.00
	$\tilde{C}_{2450}$	0.00	0.00	0.00	0.42	0.00	0.00
	$\tilde{C}_{2460}$	0.00	0.00	0.00	0.42	0.00	0.00
	$\tilde{C}_{2560}$	0.00	0.00	0.00	0.42	0.00	0.00
	$\tilde{C}_{3450}$	0.00	0.00	0.00	0.42	0.00	0.00
	$\tilde{C}_{3460}$	0.00	0.00	0.00	0.42	0.00	0.00
	$\tilde{C}_{3560}$	0.00	0.00	0.00	0.42	0.00	0.00
	$\tilde{C}_{4560}$	0.00	0.00	0.00	0.42	0.00	0.00
	$\tilde{C}_{1231}$	0.00	3.33	0.00	0.00	3.33	0.00
	$\tilde{C}_{1241}$	0.00	3.33	0.00	0.00	3.33	0.00
	$\tilde{C}_{1251}$	0.00	3.33	0.00	0.00	3.33	0.00

Table 5. Cont.

	$\tilde{C}$	R_1	R_2	R_3	R_4	R_5	R_6
Label 1	$\tilde{C}_{1261}$	0.00	3.33	0.00	0.00	3.33	0.00
	$\tilde{C}_{1341}$	0.00	3.33	0.00	0.00	3.33	0.00
	$\tilde{C}_{1351}$	0.00	3.33	0.00	0.00	3.33	0.00
	$\tilde{C}_{1361}$	0.00	3.33	0.00	0.00	3.33	0.00
	$\tilde{C}_{1451}$	0.00	3.33	0.00	0.00	3.33	0.00
	$\tilde{C}_{1461}$	0.00	3.33	0.00	0.00	3.33	0.00
	$\tilde{C}_{1561}$	0.00	3.33	0.00	0.00	3.33	0.00
	$\tilde{C}_{2341}$	0.00	3.33	0.00	0.00	3.33	0.00
	$\tilde{C}_{2351}$	0.00	3.33	0.00	0.00	3.33	0.00
	$\tilde{C}_{2361}$	0.00	3.33	0.00	0.00	3.33	0.00
	$\tilde{C}_{2451}$	0.00	3.33	0.00	0.00	3.33	0.00
	$\tilde{C}_{2461}$	0.00	3.33	0.00	0.00	3.33	0.00
	$\tilde{C}_{2561}$	0.00	3.33	0.00	0.00	3.33	0.00
	$\tilde{C}_{3451}$	0.00	3.33	0.00	0.00	3.33	0.00
	$\tilde{C}_{3461}$	0.00	3.33	0.00	0.00	3.33	0.00
	$\tilde{C}_{3561}$	0.00	3.33	0.00	0.00	3.33	0.00
	$\tilde{C}_{4561}$	0.00	3.33	0.00	0.00	3.33	0.00
Label 2	$\tilde{C}_{1232}$	1.11	0.00	0.56	0.00	0.00	0.42
	$\tilde{C}_{1242}$	1.11	0.00	0.56	0.00	0.00	0.42
	$\tilde{C}_{1252}$	1.11	0.00	0.56	0.00	0.00	0.42
	$\tilde{C}_{1262}$	1.11	0.00	0.56	0.00	0.00	0.42
	$\tilde{C}_{1342}$	1.11	0.00	0.56	0.00	0.00	0.42
	$\tilde{C}_{1352}$	1.11	0.00	0.56	0.00	0.00	0.42
	$\tilde{C}_{1362}$	1.11	0.00	0.56	0.00	0.00	0.42
	$\tilde{C}_{1452}$	1.11	0.00	0.56	0.00	0.00	0.42
	$\tilde{C}_{1462}$	1.11	0.00	0.56	0.00	0.00	0.42
	$\tilde{C}_{1562}$	1.11	0.00	0.56	0.00	0.00	0.42
	$\tilde{C}_{2342}$	2.22	0.00	2.22	0.00	0.00	0.42
	$\tilde{C}_{2352}$	1.11	0.00	1.11	0.00	0.00	0.42
	$\tilde{C}_{2362}$	1.11	0.00	1.11	0.00	0.00	0.42
	$\tilde{C}_{2452}$	1.11	0.00	1.11	0.00	0.00	0.42
	$\tilde{C}_{2462}$	1.11	0.00	1.11	0.00	0.00	0.42
	$\tilde{C}_{2562}$	1.11	0.00	1.11	0.00	0.00	0.42
	$\tilde{C}_{3452}$	1.11	0.00	1.11	0.00	0.00	0.42
	$\tilde{C}_{3462}$	1.11	0.00	1.11	0.00	0.00	0.42
	$\tilde{C}_{3562}$	1.11	0.00	1.11	0.00	0.00	0.42
	$\tilde{C}_{4562}$	1.11	0.00	1.11	0.00	0.00	0.42

By using the *Max* operator, given by Equation (7), the label of rule R_1 is **2** because of $\tilde{D}_2 = Max\left(\tilde{D}_0, \tilde{D}_1, \tilde{D}_2\right)$. Similarly, we obtain the labels of rules R_2, R_3, R_4, R_5, R_6 being **1, 2, 0, 1, 2** respectively.

Step 2: Validating with the new records.

Case 1: The new record is in the fuzzy rule base system in Table 1, the output label is the same as the result of one of the six rules.

Case 2: The new record is not in the fuzzy rule base system in Table 1. For instance, **IF** S_1 is "H_1" and S_2 is "H_2" and S_3 is "M_3" and S_4 is "M_4" and S_5 is "H_5" and S_6 is "H_6" **THEN** the output label = ?. The output label of this new record is found by applying Equations (5)–(7). We have:

- With label $l = 0$,

$$\tilde{C}_{1230} = \tilde{C}_{1240} = \tilde{C}_{1250} = \tilde{C}_{1260} = \tilde{C}_{1340} = \tilde{C}_{1350} = \tilde{C}_{1360} = \tilde{C}_{1450} = \tilde{C}_{1460} = \tilde{C}_{1560} = \tilde{C}_{2340}$$
$$= \tilde{C}_{2350} = \tilde{C}_{2360} = \tilde{C}_{2450} = \tilde{C}_{2460} = \tilde{C}_{2560} = \tilde{C}_{3450} = \tilde{C}_{3460} = \tilde{C}_{3560}$$
$$= \tilde{C}_{4560} = 0$$

- With label $l = 1$,

$$\tilde{C}_{1231} = \tilde{C}_{1241} = \tilde{C}_{1251} = \tilde{C}_{1261} = \tilde{C}_{1341} = \tilde{C}_{1351} = \tilde{C}_{1361} = \tilde{C}_{1451} = \tilde{C}_{1461} = \tilde{C}_{1561} = \tilde{C}_{2341}$$
$$= \tilde{C}_{2351} = \tilde{C}_{2361} = \tilde{C}_{2450} = \tilde{C}_{2461} = \tilde{C}_{2561} = \tilde{C}_{3451} = \tilde{C}_{3461} = \tilde{C}_{3561}$$
$$= \tilde{C}_{4561} = 0$$

- With label $l = 2$,

$$\tilde{C}_{1232} = \tilde{C}_{1252} = \tilde{C}_{1262} = \tilde{C}_{2342} = \tilde{C}_{2352} = \tilde{C}_{2362} = \tilde{C}_{2452} = \tilde{C}_{2462} = \tilde{C}_{2562} = \tilde{C}_{3450} = 0$$
$$\tilde{C}_{1342} = \tilde{C}_{1352} = \tilde{C}_{1362} = \tilde{C}_{1452} = \tilde{C}_{1462} = \tilde{C}_{1562} = 0.56$$
$$\tilde{C}_{3452} = \tilde{C}_{3462} = \tilde{C}_{3562} = \tilde{C}_{4562} = 1.11$$

Therefore, $\tilde{D}_0 = \tilde{D}_1 = 0$, $\tilde{D}_2 = 1.11$. The result of the new record: **IF** S_1 is "H_1" and S_2 is "H_2" and S_3 is "M_3" and S_4 is "M_4" and S_5 is "H_5" and S_6 is "H_6" **THEN** the output label = **2**. The output label is 2 corresponding to the doctor's diagnosis conclusion "*Severe Preeclampsia*".

4. Experimental Results

4.1. Experiments

To simulate the proposed model in real-world applications, the data set was gathered from pregnant women who came for regular check-ups to monitor the fetus at the National Hospital of Obstetrics and Gynecology in Vietnam. After receiving expert comments from the obstetrician, the preeclampsia data set includes 210 samples with 19 test parameters, such as Blood Pressure, Hemoglobin (HGB), Platelet Count (PLT), Urea, Creatinine, Acid Uric, Alanine Aminotransferase (ALT), Aspartate Aminotransferase (AST), Total Protein, Albumin, Lactate Dehydrogenase (LDH), Proteinuria and so on (in detail given in Table 6). In this data set, according to the diagnostic conclusion (in which 118 women with signs of normal pregnancy, 60 preeclampsia women, and 32 severe preeclampsia women).

Table 6. List of features in the preeclampsia dataset.

No.	Feature's Name	Domain
1	Pregnant Woman's Age	18–66 years old
2	Fetus's Age	15–40 weeks
3	Occupation	Officer, Teacher, Doctor, Worker, Farmer, Freelancer, and so on.
4	Number of Pregnancies	0–9 times
5	Pregnant Woman's Height	1.40–1.90 m

Table 6. Cont.

No.	Feature's Name	Domain
6	Pregnant Woman's Weight	45–95 kg
7	Upper Blood Pressure	90–129 mmHg
8	Lower Blood Pressure	60–84 mmHg
9	Hemoglobin (HGB)	120–160 g/L
10	Platelet Count (PLT)	150–450 g/L
11	Urea	2.5–6.7 mmol/L
12	Creatinine	50.4–98.1 µmol/L
13	Acid Uric	150–350 µmol/L
14	Alanine Aminotransferase (ALT)	<31/37 Ul/L
15	Aspartate Aminotransferase (AST)	<31/37 Ul/L
16	Total Protein	64–83 g/L
17	Albumin	35–52 g/L
18	Lactate Dehydrogenase (LDH)	<247 U/L
19	Proteinuria	0.1–0.25 g/L
Output	Output labels (Diagnostic results)	0: Normal 1: Preeclampsia 2: Severe preeclampsia

The preeclampsia application is built using Python 3.10 language installed on a laptop (ASUS Intel(R) Core (TM) i5-8300H CPU @ 2.30 GHz).

4.2. Evaluation Method

To evaluate the proposed model-based system's performance, the parameters are used including the accuracy and calculation time, specifically as follows:

Accuracy is evaluated by the ratio of the number of correctly classified samples over the total number of performed samples, estimated by Formula (8).

$$Accuracy = \frac{TP + TN}{TP + FP + TN + FN} \quad (8)$$

where:

- *TP*: True Positive
- *TN*: True Negative
- *FP*: False Positive
- *FN*: False Negative

Time is estimated by the total execution time of the classification system (unit: seconds).

4.3. Test Results in Simulations

After implementing the application based on the above data set, the authors established three different scenarios, namely:

- Scenario 1: the systematic random sampling method and the splitting method with training set (70%) and testing set (30%).
- Scenario 2: the systematic random sampling method and the splitting method with training set (10%) and testing set (90%).
- Scenario 3: the systematic random sampling method and the splitting method with training set (5%) and testing set (95%).

The comparison criteria include accuracy and computation time as given in Section 4.2. The experimental results are shown in Figures 3 and 4.

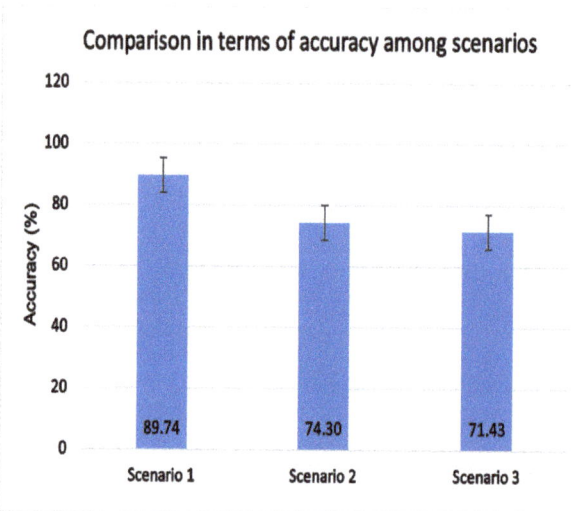

Figure 3. Comparison in terms of accuracy among scenarios.

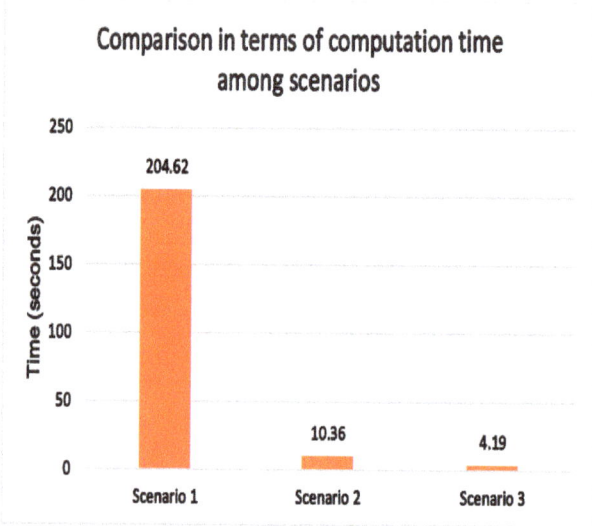

Figure 4. Comparison in terms of computation time among scenarios.

As shown in the results of Figure 3, it is clear to see that the accuracy of scenario 1 is significantly higher than that of the other two scenarios. For example, the accuracy of scenario 1 is **15.44%** higher than scenario 2 and **18.31%** higher than scenario 3. It proves that the accuracy depends on the number of samples in the training data set.

However, the data in Figure 4 shows that the computation time of scenario 1 is also much higher than that of the other scenarios. Specifically, the computation time of scenario 1 is approximately **20 times** higher than that of scenario 2, and nearly **50 times** that of scenario 3. This demonstrated that the data set splitting method contributed significantly to improving the application's performance in terms of time consumption.

After building and evaluating the model's confidence, the authors proceed to build a simple application to diagnose the preeclampsia signs of the built model. Several illustrated images of the preeclampsia sign diagnosis application have been shown in Figures 5–8.

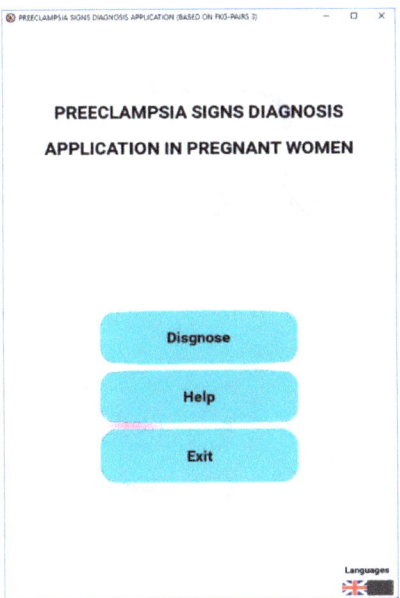

Figure 5. The main screen of the application.

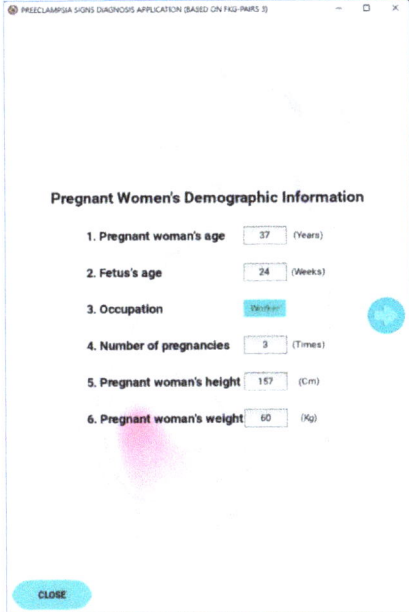

Figure 6. Screen for entering demographic information.

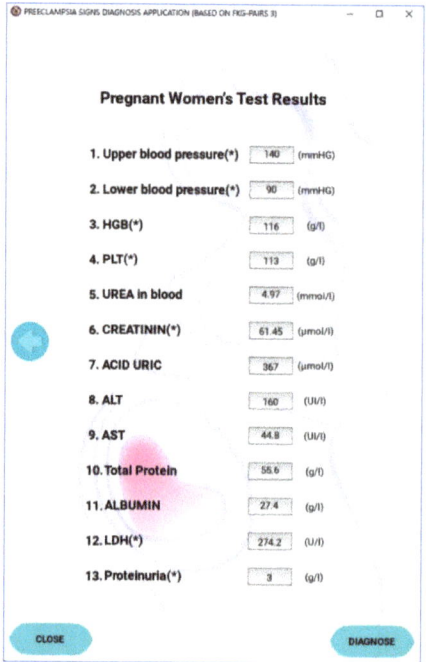

Figure 7. Screen for entering subclinical test results.

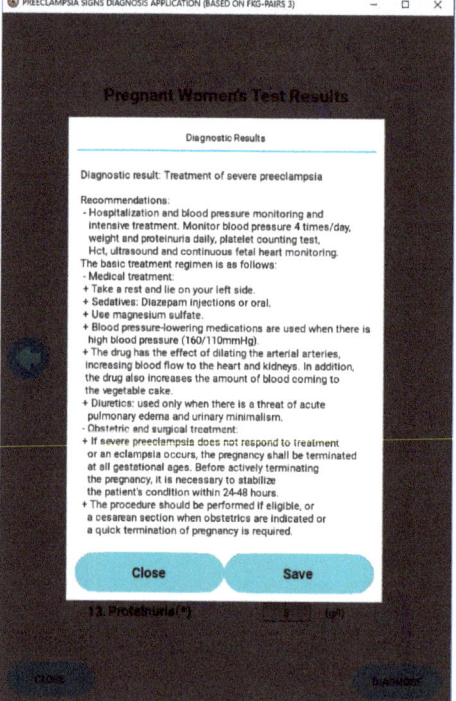

Figure 8. Diagnostic results screen and recommendations.

5. Conclusions

This paper has proposed the FKG-Pairs3-based preeclampsia signs in the diagnosis by combining regimens in traditional medicine and the information in medical records. The proposed model has been performed as a case study on the diagnosis of preeclampsia signs in gestational women based on the clinical and subclinical data collected from pregnant women attending routine antenatal care. The proposed model has been tested for an accuracy performance of **89.74%** with the implementation designed scenario, in which the systematic random sampling method and the splitting method with training set (70%) and testing set (30%).

With complete information input data sets, the accuracy of the preeclampsia sign diagnosis system will continue to improve. However, the limitation of the proposed model is identified with two drawbacks in extreme cases as follows:

- Firstly, with large input data sets, the computation time is high based on the traditional data set splitting method (e.g., in scenario 1).
- Secondly, with too-small training data sets, the accuracy is low (e.g., in scenario 2 and scenario 3).

To expand this research work, the investigation will continue to study the approach of using the FKG-Pairs3 proposed model combined with Q-learning techniques in reinforcement learning to improve the accuracy of a system in extreme cases in which the training data set is much smaller than the testing data set (e.g., in cases scenarios 2 and 3 where the training sets only 10% and 5%, respectively).

6. Patents

This section is not mandatory but may be added if there are patents resulting from the work reported in this manuscript.

Author Contributions: Conceptualization, methodology, C.K.L. and H.V.P.; software, P.H.K. and C.K.L.; validation, H.V.P., C.K.L. and H.Q.T.; formal analysis, C.K.L. and H.Q.T.; investigation, C.K.L. and P.H.K.; data curation, P.H.K.; writing—original draft preparation, C.K.L. and P.H.K.; writing—review and editing, H.V.P. and H.Q.T.; project administration, H.V.P.; All authors have read and agreed to the published version of the manuscript.

Funding: This research is funded by Vietnam National Foundation for Science and Technology Development (NAFOSTED) under grant number 102.05-2019.316.

Data Availability Statement: The dataset and source codes of this paper can be downloaded at: https://github.com/FKGHUST/Preeclampsia.git (accessed on 15 December 2022).

Conflicts of Interest: The authors declare no conflict of interest. This research does not involve any human or animal participation. All authors have checked and agreed with the submission.

References

1. World Health Organization. *WHO Recommendations for Prevention and Treatment of Pre-Eclampsia and Eclampsia*; World Health Organization: Geneva, Switzerland, 2011.
2. Nguyen, T.H.; Bui, T.C.; Vo, T.M.; Tran, Q.M.; Luu, L.T.; Nguyen, T.D. Predictive value of the sFlt-1 and PlGF in women at risk for preeclampsia in the south of Vietnam. *Pregnancy Hypertens* **2018**, *14*, 37–42. [CrossRef] [PubMed]
3. Masini, G.; Foo, L.F.; Tay, J.; Wilkinson, I.B.; Valensise, H.; Gyselaers, W.; Lees, C.C. Preeclampsia has two phenotypes which require different treatment strategies. *Am. J. Obstet. Gynecol.* **2021**, *226*, S1006–S1018. [CrossRef] [PubMed]
4. American College of Obstetricians and Gynecologists. Hypertension in Pregnancy: Executive Summary. *Obstet. Gynecol.* **2013**, *122*, 1122–1131. [CrossRef] [PubMed]
5. Wright, D.; Syngelaki, A.; Akolekar, R.; Poon, L.C.; Nicolaides, K.H. Competing risks model in screening for preeclampsia by maternal characteristics and medical history. *Am. J. Obstet. Gynecol.* **2015**, *213*, 62.e1–62.e10. [CrossRef]
6. American College of Obstetricians and Gynecologists. ACOG Practice Bulletin No. 202: Gestational Hypertension and Preeclampsia. *Obstet. Gynecol.* **2019**, *133*, e1–e25.
7. SOGC guideline, Diagnosis, Evaluation, and Management of the Hypertensive Disoder of Pregnancy: Executive Summary. *J. Obstet. Gynaecol. Can.* **2014**, *36*, 416–438. [CrossRef]

8. NICE. Hypertension in pregnancy: The management of hypertensive disorders during pregnancy. *NICE Clin. Guidel* **2019**. No. 107.
9. Poon, L.C.; Shennan, A.; Hyett, J.A.; Kapur, A.; Hadar, E.; Divakar, H.; McAuliffe, F.; da Silva Costa, F.; von Dadelszen, P.; McIntyre, H.D.; et al. The International Federation of Gynecology and Obstetrics initiative on pre-eclampsia: A pragmatic guide for first-trimester screening and prevention. *Int. J. Gynecol. Obstet.* **2019**, *145*, 1–33. [CrossRef]
10. Yu, T.; Li, J.; Yu, Q.; Tian, Y.; Shun, X.; Xu, L.; Zhu, L.; Gao, H. Knowledge graph for TCM health preservation: Design, construction, and applications. *Artif. Intell. Med.* **2017**, *77*, 48–52. [CrossRef]
11. Gyrard, A.; Gaur, M.; Shekarpour, S.; Thirunarayan, K.; Sheth, A. Personalized health knowledge graph. In *CEUR Workshop Proceedings*; NIH Public Access: Bethesda, MD, USA, 2018; Volume 2317.
12. Chai, X. Diagnosis Method of thyroid disease combining knowledge graph and deep learning. *IEEE Access* **2020**, *8*, 149787–149795. [CrossRef]
13. Troussas, C.; Chrysafiadi, K.; Virvou, M. An intelligent adaptive fuzzy-based inference system for computer-assisted language learning. *Expert Syst. Appl.* **2019**, *127*, 85–96. [CrossRef]
14. Bakhshipour, A.; Zareiforoush, H.; Bagheri, I. Application of decision trees and fuzzy inference system for quality classification and modeling of black and green tea based on visual features. *J. Food Meas. Charact.* **2020**, *14*, 1402–1416. [CrossRef]
15. Tiwari, L.; Raja, R.; Sharma, V.; Miri, R. Fuzzy Inference System for Efficient Lung Cancer Detection. In *Computer Vision and Machine Intelligence in Medical Image Analysis, Advances in Intelligent Systems and Computing*; Springer: Singapore, 2020; Volume 992. [CrossRef]
16. Ortega, L.C.; Otero, L.D.; Otero, C. Fuzzy Inference System Framework to Prioritize the Deployment of Resources in Low Visibility Traffic Conditions. *IEEE Access* **2019**, *7*, 174368–174379. [CrossRef]
17. Johann, G.; dos Santos, C.S.; Montanher, P.F.; de Oliveira, R.A.P.; Carniel, A.C. Fuzzy inference systems for predicting the mass yield in extractions of chia cake extract. *Softw. Impacts* **2021**, *10*, 100145. [CrossRef]
18. Saini, J.; Dutta, M.; Marques, G. Fuzzy Inference System Tree with Particle Swarm Optimization and Genetic Algorithm: A novel approach for PM10 forecasting. *Expert Syst. Appl.* **2021**, *183*, 115376. [CrossRef]
19. Man, J.Y.; Chen, Z.; Dick, S. Towards inductive learning of complex fuzzy inference systems. In Proceedings of the NAFIPS 2007: 2007 Annual Meeting of the North American Fuzzy Information Processing Society, San Diego, CA, USA, 24–27 June 2007; pp. 415–420. [CrossRef]
20. Tu, C.H.; Li, C. Multiple Function Approximation-A New Approach Using Complex Fuzzy Inference System. In *Intelligent Information and Database Systems. ACIIDS 2018. Lecture Notes in Computer Science*; Springer: Cham, Switzerland, 2018; Volume 10751.
21. Ngan, T.T.; Lan, L.T.H.; Tuan, T.M.; Son, L.H.; Tuan, L.M.; Minh, N.H. Colorectal Cancer Diagnosis with Complex Fuzzy Inference System. In *Frontiers in Intelligent Computing: Theory and Applications. Advances in Intelligent Systems and Computing*; Springer: Singapore, 2019; Volume 2013. [CrossRef]
22. Selvachandran, G.; Quek, S.G.; Lan, L.T.H.; Son, L.H.; Giang, N.L.; Ding, W.; Abdel-Basset, M.; de Albuquerque, V.H.C. A New Design of Mamdani Complex Fuzzy Inference System for Multiattribute Decision Making Problems. *IEEE Trans. Fuzzy Syst.* **2019**, *29*, 716–730. [CrossRef]
23. Tuan, T.M.; Lan, L.T.H.; Chou, S.-Y.; Ngan, T.T.; Son, L.H.; Giang, N.L.; Ali, M. M-CFIS-R: Mamdani complex fuzzy inference system with rule reduction using complex fuzzy measures in granular computing. *Mathematics* **2020**, *8*, 707. [CrossRef]
24. Lan, L.T.H.; Tuan, T.M.; Ngan, T.T.; Son, L.H.; Giang, N.L.; Ngoc, V.T.N.; Van Hai, P. A New Complex Fuzzy Inference System With Fuzzy Knowledge Graph and Extensions in Decision Making. *IEEE Access* **2020**, *8*, 164899–164921. [CrossRef]
25. Long, C.K.; Van Hai, P.; Tuan, T.M.; Lan, L.T.H.; Chuan, P.M.; Son, L.H. A Novel Fuzzy Knowledge Graph Pairs Approach in Decision Making. *Multimedia Tools Appl.* **2022**, *81*, 26505–26534. [CrossRef]
26. Sherimon, P.C.; Krishnan, R. OntoDiabetic: An Ontology-Based Clinical Decision Support System for Diabetic Patients. *Arab. J. Sci. Eng.* **2015**, *41*, 1145–1160. [CrossRef]
27. Sweidan, S.; El-Sappagh, S.; El-Bakry, H.; Sabbeh, S.; Badria, F.A.; Kwak, K.-S. A Fibrosis Diagnosis Clinical Decision Support System Using Fuzzy Knowledge. *Arab. J. Sci. Eng.* **2018**, *44*, 3781–3800. [CrossRef]
28. Ibrahim, I.A.; Ting, H.-N.; Moghavvemi, M. Formulation of a Novel Classification Indices for Classification of Human Hearing Abilities According to Cortical Auditory Event Potential signals. *Arab. J. Sci. Eng.* **2019**, *44*, 7133–7147. [CrossRef]
29. Sudhan, M.; Sinthuja, M.; Raja, S.P.; Amutharaj, J.; Latha, G.C.P.; Rachel, S.S.; Anitha, T.; Rajendran, T.; Waji, Y.A. Segmentation and Classification of Glaucoma Using U-Net with Deep Learning Model. *J. Healthc. Eng.* **2022**, *2022*, 1601354. [CrossRef]
30. Jhou, M.-J.; Chen, M.-S.; Lee, T.-S.; Yang, C.-T.; Chiu, Y.-L.; Lu, C.-J. A Hybrid Risk Factor Evaluation Scheme for Metabolic Syndrome and Stage 3 Chronic Kidney Disease Based on Multiple Machine Learning Techniques. *Healthcare* **2022**, *10*, 2496. [CrossRef]
31. Son, L.H.; Ciaramella, A.; Huyen, D.T.T.; Staiano, A.; Tuan, T.M.; Van Hai, P. Predictive reliability and validity of hospital cost analysis with dynamic neural network and genetic algorithm. *Neural Comput. Appl.* **2020**, *32*, 15237–15248. [CrossRef]
32. Ngoc, V.T.N.; Viet, D.H.; Tuan, T.M.; Van Hai, P.; Thang, N.P.; Tuyen, D.N.; Son, L.H. VNU-diagnosis: A novel medical system based on deep learning for diagnosis of periapical inflammation from X-Rays images. *J. Intell. Fuzzy Syst.* **2022**, *43*, 1417–1427. [CrossRef]
33. Van Pham, H.; Moore, P.; Cuong, B.C. Applied picture fuzzy sets with knowledge reasoning and linguistics in clinical decision support system. *Neurosci. Inform.* **2022**, *2*, 100109. [CrossRef]

34. Garg, H.; Ahmad, A.; Ullah, K.; Mahmood, T.; Ali, Z. Algorithm for multi-attribute decision-making using T-spherical fuzzy Maclaurin symmetric mean operator. *Iran. J. Fuzzy Syst.* **2022**, *19*, 111–124.
35. Garg, H.; Deng, Y.; Ali, Z.; Mahmood, T. Decision-making strategy based on Archimedean Bonferroni mean operators under complex Pythagorean fuzzy information. *Comput. Appl. Math.* **2022**, *41*, 152. [CrossRef]
36. Van Pham, H.; Khoa, N.D.; Bui, T.T.; Giang, N.T.; Moore, P. Applied Picture Fuzzy Sets for Group Decision-Support in the Evaluation of Pedagogic Systems. *Int. J. Math. Eng. Manag. Sci.* **2022**, *7*, 243–257.
37. Zadeh, L. Fuzzy sets. *Inf. Control.* **1965**, *8*, 338–353. [CrossRef]
38. Chen, X.; Hu, Z.; Sun, Y. Fuzzy Logic Based Logical Query Answering on Knowledge Graphs. *Proc. Conf. AAAI Artif. Intell.* **2022**, *36*, 3939–3948. [CrossRef]
39. Zadeh, L.A. Approximate reasoning based on fuzzy logic. In Proceedings of the 6th International Joint Conference on Artificial Intelligence, Tokyo, Japan, 20–23 August 1979; Volume 2, pp. 1004–1010.
40. Singhal, A. "Introducing the Knowledge Graph: Things, Not Strings", Official Google Blog. Available online: https://blog.google/products/search/introducing-knowledge-graph-things-not/ (accessed on 22 June 2022).
41. Paulheim, H. Knowledge graph refinement: A survey of approaches and evaluation methods. *Semantic Web* **2016**, *8*, 489–508. [CrossRef]
42. Tian, L.; Zhou, X.; Wu, Y.-P.; Zhou, W.-T.; Zhang, J.-H.; Zhang, T.-S. Knowledge graph and knowledge reasoning: A systematic review. *J. Electron. Sci. Technol.* **2022**, *20*, 100159. [CrossRef]
43. Moussa, S.; Kacem, S.B.H. Symbolic approximate reasoning with fuzzy and multi-valued knowledge. *Procedia Comput. Sci.* **2017**, *112*, 800–810. [CrossRef]
44. Rajabi, E.; Kafaie, S. Knowledge Graphs and Explainable AI in Healthcare. *Information* **2022**, *13*, 459. [CrossRef]
45. Sachdeva, S.; Bhalla, S. Using Knowledge Graph Structures for Semantic Interoperability in Electronic Health Records Data Exchanges. *Information* **2022**, *13*, 52. [CrossRef]
46. Long, C.K.; Van Hai, P.; Tuan, T.M.; Lan, L.T.H.; Ngan, T.T.; Chuan, P.M.; Son, L.H. A novel Q-learning-based FKG-Pairs approach for extreme cases in decision making. *Eng. Appl. Artif. Intell.* **2023**, *120*, 105920. [CrossRef]

Disclaimer/Publisher's Note: The statements, opinions and data contained in all publications are solely those of the individual author(s) and contributor(s) and not of MDPI and/or the editor(s). MDPI and/or the editor(s) disclaim responsibility for any injury to people or property resulting from any ideas, methods, instructions or products referred to in the content.

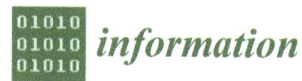

Article

NUMSnet: Nested-U Multi-Class Segmentation Network for 3D Medical Image Stacks

Sohini Roychowdhury [1,2]

[1] AI Engineering, Accenture LLP, Palo Alto, CA 94304, USA; sohini.roychowdhury@accenture.com
[2] Adjunct Faculty, Computer Engineering, Santa Clara University, Santa Clara, CA 95053, USA

Abstract: The semantic segmentation of 3D medical image stacks enables accurate volumetric reconstructions, computer-aided diagnostics and follow-up treatment planning. In this work, we present a novel variant of the Unet model, called the *NUMSnet*, that transmits pixel neighborhood features across scans through nested layers to achieve accurate multi-class semantic segmentation with minimal training data. We analyzed the semantic segmentation performance of the NUMSnet model in comparison with several Unet model variants in the segmentation of 3–7 regions of interest using only 5–10% of images for training per Lung-CT and Heart-CT volumetric image stack. The proposed NUMSnet model achieves up to 20% improvement in segmentation recall, with 2–9% improvement in *Dice* scores for Lung-CT stacks and 2.5–16% improvement in *Dice* scores for Heart-CT stacks when compared to the Unet++ model. The NUMSnet model needs to be trained with ordered images around the central scan of each volumetric stack. The propagation of image feature information from the six nested layers of the Unet++ model are found to have better computation and segmentation performance than the propagation of fewer hidden layers or all ten up-sampling layers in a Unet++ model. The NUMSnet model achieves comparable segmentation performance to previous works while being trained on as few as 5–10% of the images from 3D stacks. In addition, transfer learning allows faster convergence of the NUMSnet model for multi-class semantic segmentation from pathology in Lung-CT images to cardiac segmentation in Heart-CT stacks. Thus, the proposed model can standardize multi-class semantic segmentation for a variety of volumetric image stacks with a minimal training dataset. This can significantly reduce the cost, time and inter-observer variability associated with computer-aided detection and treatment.

Keywords: semantic segmentation; multi-class; 3D image stacks; region of interest; Dice score; Unet; CT images; overfitting

Citation: Roychowdhury, S. NUMSnet: Nested-U Multi-Class Segmentation Network for 3D Medical Image Stacks. *Information* 2023, *14*, 333. https://doi.org/10.3390/info14060333

Academic Editors: Sidong Liu, Cristián Castillo Olea and Shlomo Berkovsky

Received: 2 April 2023
Revised: 30 May 2023
Accepted: 9 June 2023
Published: 13 June 2023

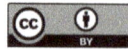

Copyright: © 2023 by the author. Licensee MDPI, Basel, Switzerland. This article is an open access article distributed under the terms and conditions of the Creative Commons Attribution (CC BY) license (https://creativecommons.org/licenses/by/4.0/).

1. Introduction

Deep learning approaches for vision-based detection have seen significant breakthroughs over the past five years [1]. From autonomous driving to virtual reality and from facial detection for phone unlocking to home security camera systems, several deep-learning-based object detection and segmentation models have been developed to date to keep up with speed, precision and hardware requirements [2]. For semantic segmentation tasks, where objects or regions of interest (ROIs) are enclosed within a closed polygon, the Unet model [3] and its variants have been a widely preferred method owing to the relatively low computational complexity and high adaptability across use cases due to short- and long-range skip connections. This allows the Unet and variant models to be well trained from only a few hundred images, as opposed to requiring thousands of annotated images for deep learning models with dense connections, which are preferred in the real-time use cases of autonomous driving and augmented reality [4,5]. However, segmenting multiple ROIs with varying sizes and shapes in continuous image stacks or videos can be challenging due to the biases introduced by foreground regions with varying sizes and can result in jittery detection across subsequent frames. In this work, we present a novel

Unet model variant, called the NUMSnet, that is capable of accurately segmenting multiple shapes and sizes of ROIs and transferring information across subsequent images in a stack to provide superior segmentation performance while training with only a fraction of the training images when compared to state-of-the art approaches.

Deep learning approaches for medical imaging use cases have a unique requirement to maintain high recall for pathological detection: i.e., the over-detection of pathology is acceptable since a specialist will always look at the report and confirm, but detection failures must be minimized. To enhance the *quality of detection* and enable explainability, semantic segmentation and explainable classification models are preferred across medical domain use cases to identify pathology in patients and also localize the pathological sites. For example, the recent work in [6] demonstrated the significance of segmentation for detecting Leukemia using bloodstream images. A review of several deep learning approaches/models developed to detect pathology is presented in [7] for the use case of detecting monkeypox from RGB images. Another work in [8] reviewed recent advances in deep learning models for chest disease detection using X-ray images. Unet and its variant models continue to be the preferred method in the medical imaging domain owing to the fewer parameters involved when compared to dense-connection models. The Unet and variant models have thus far been applied to a variety of medical imaging use cases, from dental segmentation in [9] and human skin classification in [10] to polyp segmentation tasks in colonoscopy images in [11]. This demonstrates the versatility of the Unet and variant models in the medical imaging domain, thereby necessitating the development of advanced Unet model versions.

The medical imaging domain often requires the semantic segmentation of multiple ROIs, also known as multi-class segmentation, from 3D medical image stacks of CT or MRI images for diagnostics and pre-procedural planning tasks. Performing such segmentation manually can be both costly and time-intensive [12]. Additionally, the manual segmentation process suffers from inter-observer variability, where two medical practitioners may disagree on the exact locations of the ROIs [12]. The challenge associated with training deep learning models using annotated images isolated across patient stacks is that 3D medical image stacks often have variable pixel resolutions and vary in additive image noise owing to imaging and storage conditions. This can impede the scalability of automated deep learning solutions to other patient image stacks acquired under different imaging settings [13]. Several previous works on medical image semantic segmentation performed binary segmentation for each image [3,14] or two-stage multi-class segmentation for image stacks [15] to overcome such image-level variations. In this work, we present a novel single-stage variant of the Unet model, as shown in Figure 1, that propagates image features across scans, which results in faster network convergence with few training images for volumetric medical image stacks. The proposed NUMSnet model requires training images to be in order, but not necessarily subsequent images in a sequence. The training set is shown in Figure 1 for the image stack $[T_0$ to $T_n]$. Once trained, the test set of images can be ordered or randomized per stack, as represented by sets S_m and $S_{m'}$ in Figure 1.

The novel multi-class semantic segmentation NUMSnet model presented in this paper achieves multi-class semantic segmentation with only 10% of frames per 3D image stack. It is noteworthy that the proposed model has significantly less computational complexity than the 3D Unet model and its variants that perform 3D convolutions across image stacks but has a comparable volumetric segmentation performance [16]. We investigated three main analytical questions regarding the multi-class semantic segmentation of 3D medical image stacks. (1) Does the transmission of image features from some of the layers of a Unet variant model enhance the semantic segmentation performance for multi-class segmentation tasks? (2) Is the order of training and test frames significant to segmentation tasks for 3D volumes? (3) How many layers should be optimally propagated to ensure model optimality while working with sparse training data? The key contributions of this work are as follows:

1. A novel multi-scan semantic segmentation model that propagates feature-level information from a few nested layers across ordered scans to enable feature learning from as few as 10% of annotated images per 3D medical image stack.
2. The transfer learning performance analysis of the proposed model compared to existing Unet variants on multiple CT image stacks from Lung-CT (thoracic region) scans to Heart-CT regions. The NUMSnet model achieves up to 20% improvement in segmentation recall and 2–16% improvement in *Dice* scores for multi-class semantic segmentation across image stacks.
3. The identification of a minimal number of optimally located training images per volumetric stack for multi-class semantic segmentation.
4. The identification of the optimal number of layers that can be transmitted across scans to prevent model over- or underfitting for the segmentation of up to seven ROIs with variables shapes and sizes.

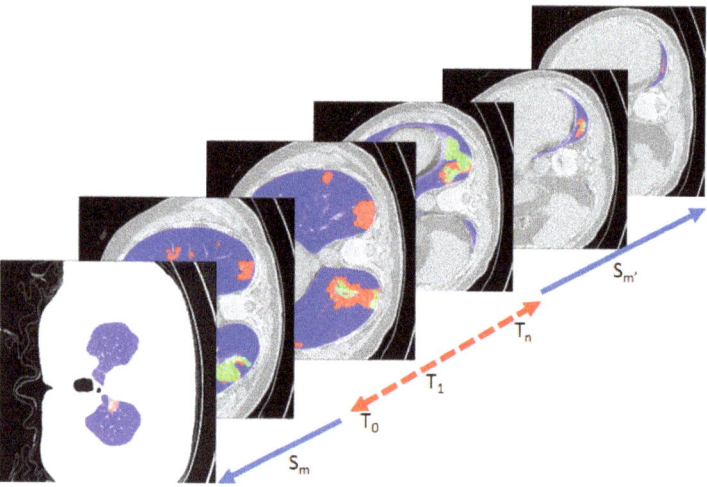

Figure 1. An example of the proposed NUMSnet system on a Lung-CT image stack. The training images (T) are selected in order or in sequence, while test images (S) can be random or in sequence.

This paper is organized as follows. The existing literature and related works are reviewed in Section 2. The datasets under analysis and the NUMSnet model are explained in Section 3. The experiments and results are shown in Section 4. A discussion regarding the limiting conditions is presented in Section 5, and the final conclusions are presented in Section 6.

2. Related Work

Deep learning models have been highly popular for computer-aided detection in the past decade and preferred over the signal processing methods in [17,18]. This is primarily due to the ability of deep learning models to automatically learn features that are indicative of an ROI if a significant volume of annotated data is provided. Signal processing models, on the other hand, rely on hand-generated features that may lead to faulty detections due to the high variability across imaging modalities and storage and transmission formats. The prior work in [19] demonstrates a two-path CNN model that can take filtered Lung-CT images followed by fuzzy c-means clustering to segment the opacity in each Lung-CT image. While such feature-based works have low data dependence, the models often do not scale across datasets.

Unet models with the default 2D architecture have been used extensively for medical image segmentation applications since 2015 [3]. While other deep learning models, such as MaskRCNN [20] and fully convolutional neural networks (FCNs) [21], are more popular in non-medical domains, Unet and its variants have continued to be the preferred deep learning model for medical image segmentation tasks. The 2D Unet model and its variants apply long and short skip connections that ensure that the number of trainable parameters is low, thereby leading to quicker training with fewer images. Over the last few years, several Unet model variants have been applied for dense volumetric scan segmentation. In instances where high volumes of annotated data are readily available, such as anatomical regions in Heart-CT scans in [15], multi-stage Unet variants have been introduced. The works in [15,22] trained two separate Unet models with separate loss functions, with the objective of zooming into the foreground regions in the first network, followed by separating the foreground into various ROIs. Other variants of multi-2D-Unet models, such as the work in [23], implement trained Unet models at different resolutions, i.e., one Unet model trained on images with dimensions of [256 × 256], another trained at a resolution of [512 × 512] and so on for lung segmentation. However, these methods require significantly high volumes of annotated data to train multiple Unet models.

Other recent works in [13,24] applied variations to the 2D Unet model to achieve the segmentation of opacity and lung regions in chest CT scans to aid in COVID-19 detection. Additionally, in [25], Inf-net and Semi-Inf net models are presented that can perform binary segmentation for lung opacity detection with *Dice* scores in the range of 0.74–0.76. Most of these existing methods require several hundred annotated training images across scans and patients and can efficiently be trained for binary semantic segmentation tasks.

Some of the well-known 2D Unet model variants used in the medical imaging domain are the wide Unet (wU-net) and Nested Unet (Unet++) [14]. While a typical Unet model with a depth of 5 will have filter kernel widths of [32, 64, 128, 256, 512] at model depths of 1 through 5, the wUnet model has filter kernel widths of [35, 70, 140, 280, 560] at model depths of 1 through 5. Thus, wUnet has more parameters and thus can enhance segmentation performance when compared to Unet. The Unet++ model, on the other hand, generates dense connections with nested up-sampling layers to further enhance the performance of semantic segmentation, as presented in [26,27]. In this work, we propose an enhanced Unet++ architecture called the NUMSnet, where the features from the nested up-sampling layers are transmitted across scans for increased attention to smaller regions of interest (such as opacity in Lung-CT images). This layer propagation across scans enables multi-class semantic segmentation with only 10% of annotated images per 3D volume stack.

Another major family of Unet models that have been applied to volumetric image segmentation tasks in the medical imaging domain is the 3D Unet model variants, as shown in [16]. These models have significantly higher computational complexity when compared to the 2D Unet model and its variants due to the 3D convolutions in each layer, but they achieve superior segmentation performance for pathological sites in 3D image stacks. Another work in [28] combined the Resnet backbone with the 3D Unet model to improve the resolution of segmentation for small ROIs in Lung-CT images. As additional variants of the 3D Unet model, the encoder architecture can be modified with the VGG19, 3D ResNet152 or DenseNet201 backbone to achieve 80–98% *Dice* scores for multi-class semantic segmentation tasks [16]. However, these 3D Unet models are difficult to train and may need around 1700 epochs and 1.8 h to train on single-GPU systems. Besides 3D Unets, another recent work that implemented a 3D fully convolutional neural network model for volumetric segmentation is shown in [29], where MRI stacks are segmented with about an 86% *Dice* score with over 48 h of training time. It is noteworthy that 3D Unet models have been preferred for cardiac CT segmentation so far, with the work in [15] applying a two-stage 3D Unet model for voxel-level segmentation of the heart. Another work in [30] implemented a deeply supervised 3D Unet model with a multi-branch residual network and deep feature fusion along with focal loss to achieve 86–96% *Dice* scores for the semantic segmentation of small and large ROIs. Our work aimed to perform 2D semantic segmentation and achieve a comparable segmentation performance to 3D model variants with under 10 min of training time on a single GPU system.

3. Materials and Methods
3.1. Data: Lung-CT and Heart-CT Stacks

In this work, we analyze two kinds of single-plane volumetric CT image stacks. In the first category, Lung-CT image stacks were collected from the Italian Society of Medical and Interventional Radiology. The first Lung-CT (Lung-med) volumetric stack [31] contains 829 images from a single 3D image stack with [512 × 512]-dimension images. Out of these 829 scans, 373 are annotated. The second dataset (Lung-rad) contains 9 axial volume chest CT scans with 39–418 images per stack. All Lung-CT images are annotated for 3 ROIs, namely, ground-glass opacity (GGO), consolidations and the lung region as the foreground and can be downloaded from [32].

In the second category, the Heart-CT image dataset is from the MICCAI 2017 Multi-Modality Whole Heart Segmentation (MM-WHS) challenge [15,30], from which we selected the first 10 training CT image stacks of the heart region for analysis. This dataset contains coronal volumetric stacks with 116–358 images per volume and multi-class semantic segmentation annotations for up to 7 heart-specific ROIs represented by label-pixel values of [205, 420, 500, 550, 600, 820, 850], respectively. These pixel regions represent the left ventricle blood cavity (LV), myocardium of the left ventricle (Myo), right ventricle blood cavity (RV), left atrium blood cavity (LA), right atrium blood cavity (RA), ascending aorta (AA) and pulmonary artery (PA), respectively. It is noteworthy that for the Heart-CT dataset, only 10–15% of the images per stack contain annotated ROIs. Thus, when selecting the ordered training dataset, it was ensured that at least 50% of the training samples contained annotations. Some examples of the Lung-CT and Heart-CT images and their respective annotations are shown in Figure 2.

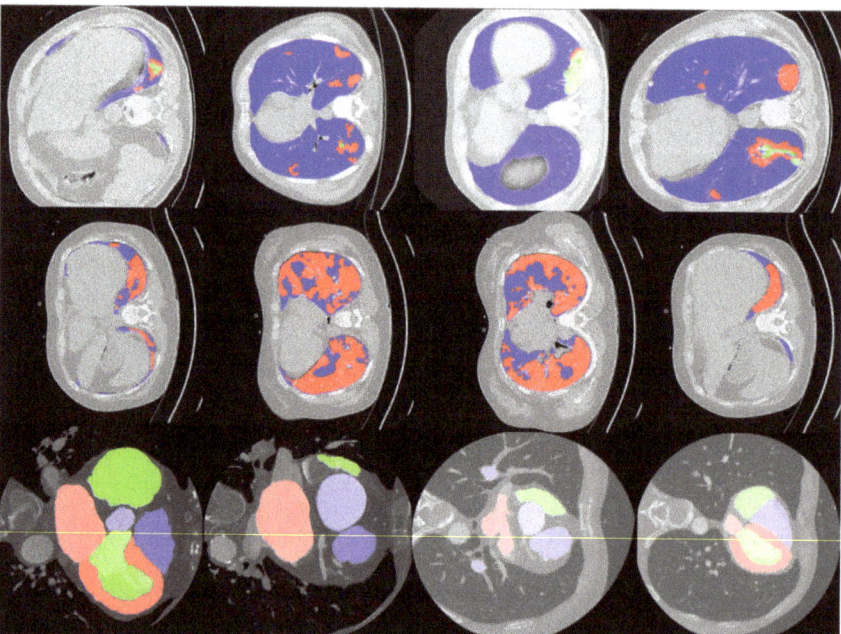

Figure 2. Examples of multi-class segmentation datasets used in this work. **Row 1**: Lung-med dataset. **Row 2**: Lung-rad dataset. For **Row 1** and **Row 2** the regional color coding is as follows. Blue: lung region; Red: GGO; Green: consolidation regions. **Row 3**: Heart-CT dataset. The ROIs are color-coded as follows. Red plane: label pixels 205 and 420. Blue plane: label pixels 500 and 550. Green plane: label pixels 600, 820 and 850.

3.2. Image Data Pre-Processing

Each image from the data stacks under analysis here was pre-processed for the Unet and variant models. First, each input image was resized to [256 × 256 × 1] for ease of processing. Next, the resized image I was re-scaled to the range [0,1], thereby resulting in image I', using min–max normalization, as shown in (1), where min_I and max_I refer to the minimum and maximum pixel values in I. This is followed by the generation of multi-dimensional label vectors [256 × 256 × d] per image, where d represents the number of classes that each pixel can be classified into. These label vectors are generated as binary images for each class. For example, the Heart-CT stack images contain up to 7 different annotated regions depicted by a certain pixel value pix_i, $\forall i$ = [1:7]. Thus, the ground-truth label vector (G') generated per image contains 7 planes, where each plane G'_i is generated as a binary mask from the label masks (G), as shown in (2). This process defines the ground-truth G' such that the Unet decision-making function (f_i) proceeds to analyze whether each pixel belongs to a particular class i or not. Finally, the output is a d-dimensional binary image (P), where each image plane (P_i) is thresholded at a pixel value $\tau = 0.5$, as shown in (3).

$$I' = \frac{I - min_I}{max_I - min_I}. \tag{1}$$

$$\forall i \in [1:d], G'_i = [G == pix_i], \tag{2}$$

$$and, P_i = [f_i(I') > \tau]. \tag{3}$$

Once the datasets are pre-processed, the next step is to separate the data stacks into training, validation and test sets. There are two ways in which the training/validation/test datasets are sampled for each volume stack. The first is the random sampling method, where 10% of the scans per volume are randomly selected in ascending order for training, 1% of the remaining images are randomly selected for validation, and all remaining images are used for testing. The second is the sequential sampling method, which starts from a reference scan in the volumetric stack. This reference scan can either be the first or middle scan in the stack. We sample 10% of the total number of images in the stack starting from the reference scan in sequence, and these become the training set of images. From the remaining images, 1% can be randomly selected for validation, while all remaining scans are test set images in sequence. Using these methods, we generated training sets with the sizes [82 × 256 × 256 × 1], [84 × 256 × 256 × 1] and [363 × 256 × 256 × 1] for the Lung-med, Lung-rad and Heart-CT stacks, respectively.

3.3. Unet Model Variant Model Implementation

To date, Unet and its variants, such as wUnet and Unet++ models, have been applied to improve foreground segmentation precision for small ROIs, as shown in [14,30]. One major difference between the Unet++ and Unet models [3] is the presence of nested layers that combine the convolved and pooled layers with the up-sampling (transposed convolutional) layers at the same level. Thus, for a Unet with a depth of 4, a Unet++ model results in 6 additional nested layers, shown as [X(1,2), X(1,3) X(1,4), X(2,2), X(2,3), X(3,2)] in Figure 3. These additional layers increase the signal strength at each depth level and amplify the segmentation decisions around boundary regions of ROIs [14]. We selected an optimal depth of 4 for our analysis of Unet and variant models based on the prior work in [33], which showed superior semantic segmentation at a depth of 4 when compared to shallower Unet models. Additionally, depth-4 Unet and variant models are preferred for an appropriate comparative analysis with previous works.

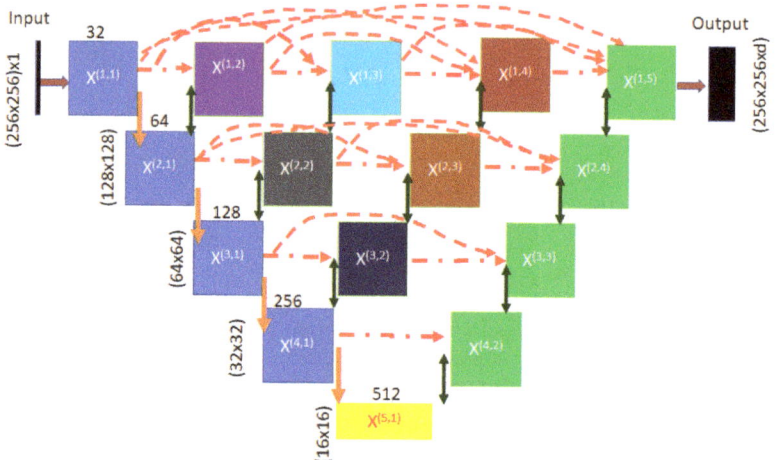

Figure 3. Example of a Unet++ model with a depth of 4. The global feature layer is X(5,1), and the depth is associated with the distance of each layer from the global feature layer. The blue layers correspond to convolved and pooled layers. The green layers correspond to merged transposed convolutions, followed by convolution outcomes from the same depth layers. The 6 additional nested color-coded layers (purple, cyan, red, gray, orange, dark and blue, corresponding to [X(1,2), X(1,3), X(1,4), X(2,2), X(2,3), X(3,2)], respectively) contain spatial pixel neighborhood information, that can be transmitted temporally across images/scans for an increased accuracy of semantic segmentation.

A Unet model comprises encoder and decoder layers, where the encoder layers perform convolution followed by a max-pooling operation, while the decoder layers perform concatenation followed by up-sampling and convolution operations. Starting with the input image I', the encoder layers are [X(1,1), X(2,1), X(3,1), X(4,1)], respectively. The output of each encoder layer results in an image with half the input dimensions but with additional feature planes. For example, the input to layer X(1,1) is an image with the size [256 × 256 × 1], while the output has dimensions of [128 × 128 × 32] due to convolution with a [3 × 3] kernel with a width of 32 and max-pooling with a [2 × 2] kernel. Thus, at the final level (X(5,1)), a global feature vector with the size [16 × 16 × 512] is generated. At this point, the decoder layers [X(4,2), X(3,3), X(2,4), X(1,5)] convert the dense features back to the segmented image planes. The decoder layers concatenate the up-sampled features with the encoder layer outputs from the same level to promote a better distinction between foreground pixels (scaled value of 1) versus background pixels (scaled value of 0). For example, at depth level 1 from the global feature layer, the output from layer X(4,1) is concatenated with the up-sampled image from layer (5,1), resulting in image features with dimensions of [32 × 32 × 512] that are then subjected to convolutions in layer (4,2), thereby resulting in image features with dimensions of [32 × 32 × 256].

The Unet++ model, on the other hand, was developed to enhance the boundary regions for relatively small ROIs by introducing nested decoder layers at each depth level, as shown in Figure 3. The 6 additional nested/hidden decoder layers that are introduced in the skip connection pathway are [X(1,2), X(1,3), X(1,4), X(2,2), X(2,3), X(3,2)] in Figure 3. The 2D weights for each decoder layer X in image n with encoder layer index i' and decoder layer index j' (i.e., $x^n(i', j')$) are generated using Equation (4), as shown in [14]. Here, $\zeta(.)$ refers to the convolution operation, $v(.)$ refers to the up-sampling operation and $[.]$ refers to concatenation.

$$x^n(i', j') = \begin{cases} \zeta(x^n(i'-1, j')) & j' = 1 \\ \zeta([[x^n(i', k')]_{k'=1}^{j'-1}, v(x^n(i'+1, j'-1))]) & j' > 1. \end{cases} \quad (4)$$

For example, the decoder layer outcome $x^n(4,2) = \zeta[[x^n(4,1), v(5,1)]]$ using Equation (4). This ensures additional skip connections that lead to improved region boundary detection.

The primary parameters that need to be tuned to ensure the optimal training of the Unet or variant model are the following: data augmentation methods, batch size, loss function, learning rate and reported metric per epoch. In this work, we applied image data augmentation using the tensorflow keras library by augmenting images randomly to ensure a rotation range, width shift range, height shift range and shear range of 0.2 and a zoom range of [0.8, 1] per image. Since the training dataset has few samples, we implemented a training batch size of 5 for the Lung-CT images and a batch size of 10 for Heart-CT images. It is noteworthy that the batch size should scale with the number of detection classes; thus, we used additional images per batch for the Heart-CT stack. For all Unet and variant models, we used the Adam optimizer with a learning rate of 10^{-4}. Finally, the metrics under analysis are shown in (5)–(8) based on the work in [34]. For each image with l pixels and d image planes for the ground-truth (G'_i), the intersection over union (IoU) or Jaccard metric in (5) represents the average fraction of correctly identified ROI pixels. Precision (Pr) in (6) and recall (Re) in (7) denote the average fraction of correctly detected ROI pixels per predicted image and per ground-truth image plane, respectively. The $Dice$ coefficient in (8) further amplifies the fraction of correctly classified foreground pixels. The $Dice$ coefficient can also be derived from the precision (Pr_i) and recall (Re_i) metrics per image plane, as shown in (8).

$$IoU = \sum_{i=1}^{d}\sum_{j=1}^{l} \frac{|P_i(j) \cap G'_i(j)|}{P_i \cup G'_i}, \tag{5}$$

$$Pr = \sum_{i=1}^{d}\sum_{j=1}^{l} \frac{P_i(j) \cap G'_i(j)}{P_i(j)}, \tag{6}$$

$$Re = \sum_{i=1}^{d}\sum_{j=1}^{l} \frac{P_i(j) \cap G'_i(j)}{G'_i(j)}, \tag{7}$$

$$Dice = \sum_{i=1}^{d}\sum_{j=1}^{l} \frac{2*|P_i(j) \cap G'_i(j)| + 1}{P_i(j) + G'_i(j) + 1} = \sum_{i=1}^{d} \frac{2*Pr_i*Re_i}{Pr_i + Re_i}. \tag{8}$$

The loss functions under analysis are shown in (9)–(11). The $Dice$ coefficient loss (DL) in (9) is the inverse of the $Dice$ coefficient, so it ensures that the average fraction of correctly detected foreground regions increases for each epoch. The binary cross-entropy loss (BCL) in (10) is a standard entropy-based measure that decreases as the predictions and ground-truth become more alike. Finally, the binary cross-entropy-Dice loss (BDL) in (11) is a combination of BCL and DL based on the work in [14].

$$DL = -D, \tag{9}$$

$$BCL = -\sum_{i=1}^{d}\sum_{j=1}^{l}[P_i(j)log(G'_i(j))], \tag{10}$$

$$BDL = \frac{BCL}{2} + DL. \tag{11}$$

Finally, we analyze the loss function curves per epoch using the deep-supervision feature from the Unet++ model [14] in Figure 4. Here, we assessed convergence rates for outputs at each depth level. In Figure 4, we observe that the curves for the convergence of outputs from depths 4 and 3 (i.e., layers X(1,5) and the resized output of X(2,4)) are relatively similar and better than the loss curves at depth 1 (resized output of layer X(4,2)). This implies that as the transposed convolutions move farther away from the global feature layer X(5,1), additional local feature-level information gets added to the semantic segmentation output. Thus, for a *well-trained* Unet++ model, the initial transposed convolution layers closer to the global feature layer X(5,1) add less value to the semantic segmentation task when compared to the layers farther away from it. This variation in loss curves at the different depth levels, based on the work in [35], demonstrates the importance of the additional nested up-sampling layers to the final multi-class segmented image.

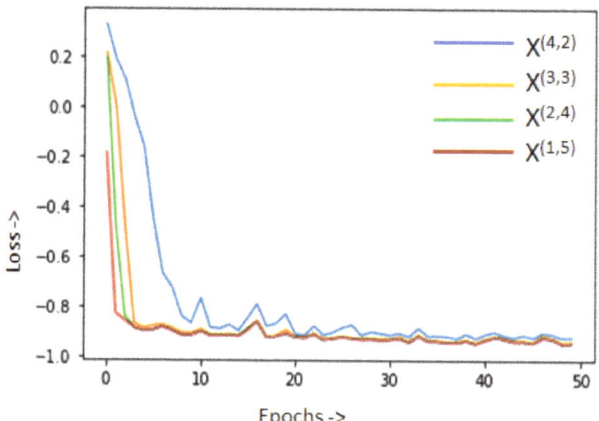

Figure 4. Example of loss functions per depth layer in Unet++ model using the deep-supervision feature on the Lung-med training dataset. The resized image outcome from X(4,2) achieves lower segmentation resolution when compared to the outcome from X(1,5). Thus, nested layers enhance local boundary-region-specific features for segmentation.

3.4. The NUMSnet Model

While the Unet and variant models are efficient in the 2D segmentation of each scan, segmenting volume stacks requires further intervention wherein pixel neighborhood information can be transmitted to the next ordered scan, thereby allowing better resolution of semantic segmentation while training on few images. The NUMSnet model is a 3D extension of the Unet++ model, wherein the outcomes of the nested Unet++ layers are transmitted to subsequent scans. As a first step for an image n, the 2D weights for the decoder layers are computed using Equation (4). Next, the 2D weights of the nested layers are transmitted using Equation (12), where the final 3D weight for each hidden layer ($X^n(i', j')$) is computed by concatenating the weights of the same layer (i', j') from the previous scan, followed by the convolution operation. For the first image in each stack, the hidden layers are concatenated with themselves, followed by convolution, as shown in Equation (12).

$$X^n(i', j') = \begin{cases} \zeta([x^n(i', j'), x^n(i', j')]) & n = 1 \\ \zeta([x^{n-1}(i', j'), x^n(i', j')]) & n > 1, \forall i <= j. \end{cases} \quad (12)$$

From the implementation perspective, for the NUMSnet model, we applied batch normalization to encoder layers only and dropout at layers X(4,1) and X(5,1) only (GitHub code available at https://github.com/sohiniroych/NUMSnet, accessed on 12 June 2023). In addition, the widths of kernels per depth layer for the NUMSnet model are [5, 70, 140, 280, 560], similar to those of the wUnet model. This process of transmitting and concatenating layer-specific features with those of the subsequent ordered images generates finer boundaries for ROIs. This variation in the Unet++ model to generate the NUMSnet model is shown in Figure 5. The additional layers generated in this process are shown in the model diagrams in Appendix A Figure A1.

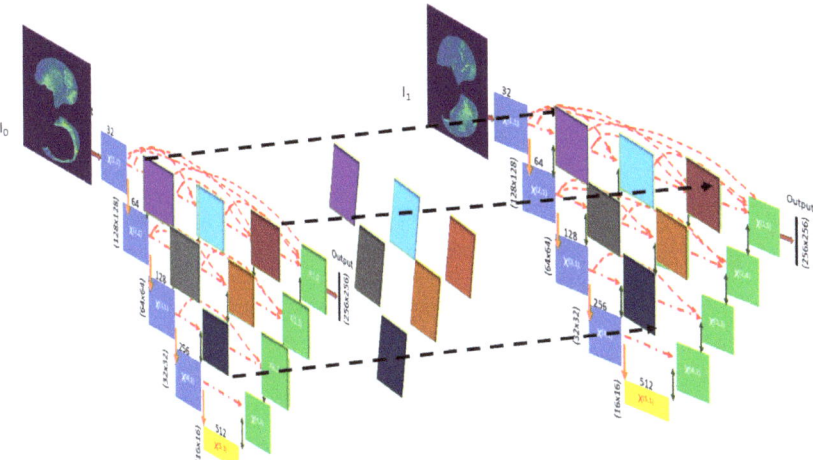

Figure 5. The proposed NUMSnet, which propagates the image features from the 6 nested layers across scans. The outcome of each nested layer is concatenated and convolved with the equivalent layer of the subsequent ordered image in the 3D stack.

The NUMSnet model has two key hyper-parameters. First, the relative location of the training scans in the 3D volume stack impacts the training phase. Since layer information is transmitted to the subsequent ordered scans, selecting training scans that contain ROIs in several subsequent scans is important. We analyze this sensitivity to the training data location in a 3D stack by varying the location of the reference training frame from the beginning to the middle of the stack, followed by selecting the subsequent or randomly selected frames in order. For example, this ensures that in the Heart-CT stacks, if an aortic region is detected for the first time in a scan, the ROI first increases and then decreases in size as training progresses. The second hyper-parameter for the NUMSnet model is the number of decoder layers that can be transmitted across scans. If all 10 decoder layers [X(1,2), X(1,3), X(1,4), X(1,5), X(2,2), X(2,3), X(2,4), X(3,2), X(3,3), X(4,2)] in Figure 3 are transmitted to the subsequent scans, this would incur high computational complexity (14.5 million trainable parameters). Thus, we analyze the segmentation performance using this NUMSnet variant (called NUMS-all), where features from all 10 up-sampling layers are transmitted. The primary reason for transmitting only up-sampling layers is that up-sampling generates image feature expansion based on pixel neighborhood estimates. Thus, information added during the up-sampling process further aids in the foreground versus background decision-making process per image plane.

4. Experiments and Results

In this work, we analyze the performance of the Unet model and its variants for the multi-class semantic segmentation of volumetric scans using only 10% of the annotated data for training. To analyze the importance of nested layer propagation across subsequent images, we performed five sets of experiments. First, we comparatively analyze the segmentation performance per ROI for the NUMSnet when compared to the Unet [3] model and its variants [14] for the Lung-CT image stacks. Second, we analyze the sensitivity of the NUMSnet model to the relative position and selection of training data for randomly ordered sampling versus sequential sampling from the beginning or middle of the volumetric stack. Third, we analyze the semantic segmentation performance of the NUMSnet model when only nested layer features are transmitted versus when all up-sampling layer features are transmitted (NUMS-all). Fourth, we assessed the semantic segmentation capability of the

NUMSnet in comparison with Unet variants for the transfer learning of weights and biases from segmenting three ROIs (in Lung-CT stacks) to segmenting seven ROIs (in Heart-CT stacks). Finally, we performed an ablation study, in which we assessed the importance of each hidden layer to the superior semantic segmentation performance of the NUMSnet model. We compared the segmentation performance when the selected hidden layers per level are propagated. We also comparatively analyze the performance of the NUMSnet with respect to state-of-the-art models that were trained on higher volumes of data.

It is noteworthy that while the training samples are ordered, the test samples may be out of order, starting at the other end of the stack or starting at a new volumetric stack. In the testing phase, the nested layer outputs and model layer weights and biases are collected per test image and passed to the next image. Once the NUMSnet model is optimally trained, the out-of-order scans in the test stacks do not significantly impact the segmentation outcomes. All other parameters, including data augmentation, loss functions, batch size, compiler, learning rate and reported metrics, are kept similar to those of the Unet model and variants to realize the segmentation enhancements per epoch.

An additional consideration for segmenting medical images is that relative variations in pixel neighborhoods are significantly less than those in regular camera-acquired images, such as those used for autonomous driving or satellite imagery [4]. Thus, feature-level propagation across scans through the NUMSnet model enhances the decision making around boundary regions, especially for smaller ROIs. However, the additional nested layer transmission introduces a higher number of parameters in the Unet variant models, which leads to a slower training time and higher GPU memory requirements for model training. In this work, we used Nvidia RTX 3070 with 8GB of GPU RAM on an Ubuntu Laptop and tensorflow/keras libraries to train and test the volume segmentation performance. In instances where models have a high number of parameters, keeping a small batch size of 5–10 ensures optimal model training. We collectively analyzed the segmentation performance along with the computational complexities incurred by each model to demonstrate the ease of use and generalization to new datasets and use cases.

4.1. Multi-Class Segmentation Performance of Unet Variants

For any multi-class semantic segmentation model, it is important to assess the computational complexity introduced by additional layers in terms of the number of trainable parameters jointly with the semantic segmentation performance. Table 1 shows the variations in the number of trainable and non-trainable parameters for all 2D Unet variants analyzed in this work. Here, we found that Unet is the fastest model, while NUMS-all has almost twice the number of trainable parameters when compared to Unet. In addition, the NUMSnet model is preferable to NUMS-all with regard to computational complexity, as it has less of a chance of overfitting [36]. Since the NUMSnet model performs 2D operations in encoder and decoder layers, we comparatively analyzed its performance with the 2D model variants only.

Table 1. Variations in the number of parameters in Unet model variants.

Model	Total Params	Trainable Params	Non-Trainable Params
Unet	7,767,523	7,763,555	3968
wUnet	9,290,998	9,286,658	4340
Unet++	9,045,507	9,043,587	1920
NUMSnet	11,713,943	11,711,843	2100
NUMS-all	14,526,368	14,524,268	2100

It is noteworthy that the base 3D Unet model, as shown in [16,28], has 19,069,955 total parameters, which increases rapidly with modifications to the encoder–decoder block backbones. Next, we analyze the multi-class semantic segmentation performance of the NUMSnet and Unet model variants. In Table 2, the average semantic segmentation across five randomly ordered training dataset selections of the three ROIs in the Lung-med dataset is presented. Here, we observe that the performance of lung segmentation is the best and similar across all Unet variants, with a *Dice* score ranging between 92 and 96%. This is intuitive since the lung is the largest region that is annotated in most images. The Unet and variant models preferentially extract this ROI with minimal training data. We also observe that for the segmentation of opacity (GGO) and consolidation (Con) regions, the NUMSnet model has the best combination of Pr and Re, thereby resulting in 2–8% higher *Dice* scores than all Unet variants. The Unet++ model, on the other hand, achieves superior overall Pr metrics but low Re metrics, which leads to lower *Dice* and *IoU* scores. Some examples of Unet and variant model segmentation are shown in Figure 6. Here, we observe that for small as well as large ROIs, the NUMSnet has better segmentation resolution when compared to all other Unet variants.

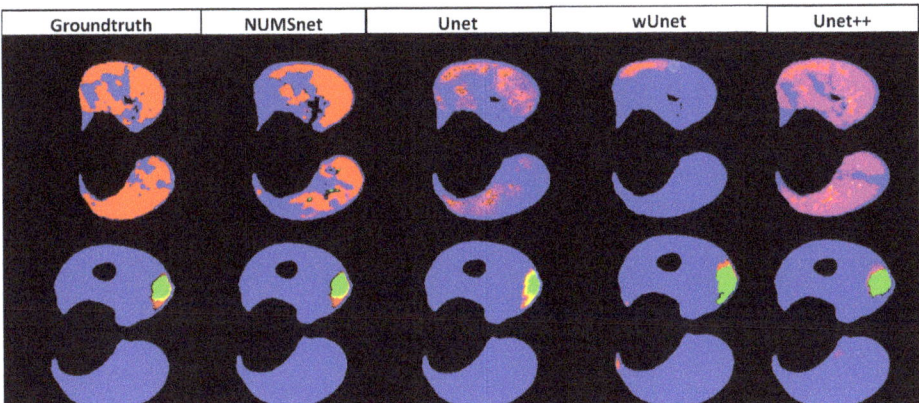

Figure 6. Example of Lung-CT segmentation by the Unet variant models. **Row 1** represents poor segmentation results. **Row 2** represent good segmentation results since the major ROI is the lung. The color coding is as follows. Blue: lung regions; Red: GGO regions; Green: consolidation regions; Magenta: over-detection of consolidation regions.

For all Unet variants under analysis, the number of epochs is 60, and the optimal loss function is the BDL with the *Dice* coefficient as the reported metric. We observe poor convergence with the DL loss function since the large lung regions are weighted more by the DL, thereby resulting in the high accuracy of lung segmentation but poor performance for GGO and consolidation segmentation.

Next, we analyze the segmentation performance on smaller Lung-CT stacks from radiopedia (Lung-rad), and the results are shown in Table 3. For the lung region segmentation, we have similar observations on this dataset to those on the Lung-med dataset. All Unet variants models achieve 95–96% *Dice* scores for the segmentation of the large lung region. However, for segmenting GGO and Con regions, the NUMSnet model achieves higher Re and up to 10% improvement in *Dice* coefficients over the other Unet variant models. Examples of good and bad selected segmentation on this dataset are shown in Figure 7. Here, we observe that the lung region is well detected by all Unet model variants, but Unet misclassifies the GGO as consol (in row 2, red regions are predicted as green), while the NUMSnet under-predicts the GGO regions. The reason for the lower performance for the Lung-rad stacks when compared to the Lung-med stack is that the number of frames in the sequence for training per stack is lower when compared to the Lung-med stack. Thus, for denser volumetric stacks, the NUMSnet has better multi-class segmentation performance when compared to shorter stacks with few images.

Table 2. Comparative performance of Unet and variant models on the Lung-med stack averaged over 5 runs. The best values for each metric are highlighted.

Task	Pr	Re	IoU	Dice
NUMSnet, Con	82.06	65.86	**57.43**	**61.25**
NUMSnet, GGO	89.86	85.87	**78.76**	**81.29**
NUMSnet, Lung	97.35	**94.96**	**92.94**	**95.9**
Unet, Con	**91.91**	32.48	30.43	33.84
Unet, GGO	90.56	73.69	68.26	70.92
Unet, Lung	91.66	94.31	86.59	92.2
wUnet, Con	64.02	**77.85**	53.42	53.66
wUnet, GGO	81.92	**95.29**	78.33	80.43
wUnet, Lung	99.27	91.47	90.94	94.35
Unet++, Con	71.67	57.14	42.21	45.36
Unet++, GGO	**92.87**	71.54	68.06	71.18
Unet++, Lung	**99.61**	90.41	90.17	93.89

Table 3. Averaged performance of Unet and variant models on 10 Lung-rad CT stacks across 5 runs. The best values for each metric are highlighted.

Task	Pr	Re	IoU	Dice
NUMSnet, Con	68.22	**79.1**	**57.08**	**59.42**
NUMSnet, GGO	85.1	**91.86**	**80.31**	**83.0**
NUMSnet, Lung	**99.36**	93.29	92.76	95.22
Unet, Con	64.2	49.93	31.2	31.28
Unet, GGO	92.33	79.11	75.06	77.99
Unet, Lung	98.52	93.75	92.41	95.11
wUnet, Con	**83.31**	47.68	42.18	46.26
wUnet, GGO	89.41	86.61	79.4	81.99
wUnet, Lung	97.15	**95.71**	**93.22**	**95.8**
Unet++, Con	71.51	62.08	47.27	50.48
Unet++, GGO	**94.14**	71.92	69.83	73.03
Unet++, Lung	98.36	94.3	92.84	95.4

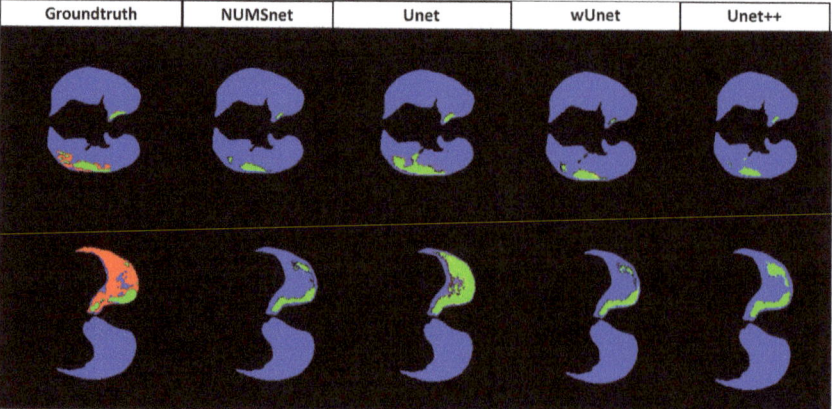

Figure 7. Example of Lung-CT segmentation by Unet variant models. **Row 1**: Best-case detection. **Row 2**: Worst-case detection. The color coding is as follows. Blue: lung regions; Red: GGO regions; Green: consolidation regions.

4.2. Sensitivity to Training Data

In this experiment, we modified the training dataset sequence and observed the segmentation performance variations. We comparatively analyze the performance for three sets of variations in training and test sequences. The first set comprised a training dataset that started with the first scan in the image stack as the reference image, followed by 10% of sequential images extracted per stack for training. All remaining images in the sequence were considered test samples, while 1% of the images from the test samples were withheld for hyper-parameterization as a validation dataset. This is called the [$Initial, Seq$] set. The second set comprised training images that started with the middle scan per 3D stack. Then, 10% of the subsequent scans were randomly selected while maintaining the order of images to generate the training sequence. All remaining images were used as test data, with 1% of the images randomly removed as the validation dataset. This is called the [$Mid, Rand$] set. The third set started with training images from the middle scan per stack, and 10% of the frames in a sequence were selected as training data. All remaining images were test data, with 1% of the images separated for validation tasks. This is called the [Mid, Seq] set. The variations in the multi-class semantic segmentation of the Lung-med and Lung-rad scans for all three training/test stacks are shown in Table 4.

Table 4. Comparative performance of NUMSnet on Lung-CT stacks when varying the training dataset, averaged over 5 runs. The best values for each metric are highlighted.

Task	Pr	Re	IoU	$Dice$
Data:	Lung-med			
Initial, Seq, Con	**82.5**	35.05	26.1	29.34
Initial, Seq, GGO	**85.78**	69.13	59.30	62.21
Initial, Seq, Lung	88.85	**93.45**	82.98	89.90
Mid, Rand, Con	60.38	96.52	**57.97**	**57.97**
Mid, Rand, GGO	70.15	**99.46**	**69.75**	**69.75**
Mid Rand, Lung	**99.27**	89.19	**88.62**	**92.94**
Mid, Seq, Con	60.37	**97.32**	58.91	58.91
Mid, Seq, GGO	70.15	93.17	68.01	68.01
Mid, Seq, Lung	98.73	89.28	88.27	92.59
Data:	10 Lung-rad	Stacks		
Initial, Seq, Con	**87.74**	44.24	38.94	43.13
Initial, Seq, GGO	**92.23**	75.69	72.46	75.19
Initial, Seq, Lung	95.44	**96.74**	**92.87**	**95.79**
Mid, Rand, Con	62.05	**99.1**	60.91	60.91
Mid, Rand, GGO	72.22	**99.0**	70.22	70.22
Mid Rand, Lung	**99.79**	91.74	91.6	94.57
Mid, Seq, Con	59.15	98.51	59.49	59.76
Mid, Seq, GGO	82.22	**99.0**	**80.22**	**80.22**
Mid, Seq, Lung	99.0	90.74	90.6	93.8

Here, we observe that the IoU and $Dice$ scores for segmentation using the [$Initial, Seq$] training/test stack are consistently worse than those obtained using training sets that begin in the middle of each volume stack. This is intuitive since the initial layers often contain no annotations or minimal ROIs, being a precursor to the intended ROIs. Thus, using the [$Initial, Seq$] training dataset, the NUMSnet model does not learn enough to discern the small ROIs in this stack. We also observe that the performance of the [$Mid, Rand$] and [Mid, Seq] training stacks are similar to that of the Lung-med stack. In addition, we observe a 10% improvement in Pr and D for [Mid, Seq] over [$Mid, Rand$] for GGO segmentation only. Thus, selecting training images in the middle of 3D stacks with randomly ordered selection is important for training the multi-class NUMSnet model.

4.3. Performance Analysis for NUMSnet Variants

In the third experiment, we analyze the number of up-sampling layers that should be propagated to subsequent training scans for optimal multi-class segmentation tasks per volume. In Table 5, we report the segmentation performance of NUMS-all for Lung-CT stacks, where all 10 up-sampling layers are transmitted. Comparing the *Dice* scores for the Lung-med stack for NUMS-all with those of NUMSnet in Table 2, we observe that NUMS-all improves segmentation *Re* for the smaller ROIs of GGO and Con, but the overall segmentation performance across all ROIs remains comparable. We make similar observations for the 10 Lung-rad stacks when comparing Table 5 and Table 3. Thus, given that NUMS-all has higher computational complexity without a significant improvement in the overall segmentation performance, the NUMSnet model can be considered superior to NUMS-all while training with limited images.

Table 5. Performance of Lung-CT segmentation with NUMS-all model averaged across 5 runs.

Data	Lung-Med			
Task	*Pr*	*Re*	*IoU*	*Dice*
NUMS-all, Con	66.81	72.63	53.08	54.86
NUMS-all, GGO	83.11	91.06	78.09	81.02
NUMS-all, Lung	99.67	90.93	90.74	94.64
Data	10 Lung-rad	Stacks		
NUMS-all, Con	64.14	96.04	63.05	63.06
NUMS-all, GGO	86.97	92.34	81.82	84.34
NUMS-all, Lung	99.63	92.89	92.56	95.1

4.4. Transfer Learning for Heart-CT Images

In this experiment, we analyze the transfer learning capabilities of pre-trained Unet and variant models from the Lung-CT stack to the Heart-CT stack. The trained models from the Lung-med image stack were saved, all layers before the final layer were unfrozen, and the final layer dimensions were altered to be retrained on the Heart-CT dataset. The only difference in the Unet and variant models between the Lung-CT and the Heart-CT image sets is the final number of classes in the last layer X(1,5). Re-using the weights and biases of all other layers provides a warm start to the model and aids in faster convergence while training with randomly selected ordered images. For this experiment, the performance of each Unet variant in segmenting regions with the label pixel values [205, 420, 500, 550, 600, 820, 850] are represented by the model name and [pix_{205}, pix_{420}, pix_{500}, pix_{550}, pix_{600}, pix_{820}, pix_{850}], respectively, in Table 6. Here, we observe that the NUMSnet has superior segmentation performance for the smaller ROIs with the pixel values [500, 550, 600, 820, 850], respectively, with 2–16% improvements in *Dice* scores for these regions over the Unet++ model. Thus, the NUMSnet model aids in transfer learning across anatomical image stacks and across label types and yields higher precision when segmenting smaller ROIs.

Table 6. Averaged performance of the Unet and variant models on 10 Heart-CT stacks across 5 runs. The best values for each metric are highlighted.

Task	*Pr*	*Re*	*IoU*	*Dice*
NUMSnet, pix_{205}	**96.2**	78.83	75.53	78.01
NUMSnet, pix_{420}	**96.89**	86.2	83.42	85.04
NUMSnet, pix_{500}	94.84	**98.16**	**93.29**	**95**
NUMSnet, pix_{550}	**96.61**	86.23	83.4	85.8
NUMSnet, pix_{600}	94.95	80.26	76.03	79.28
NUMSnet, pix_{820}	**98.42**	**96.84**	**95.55**	**96.88**
NUMSnet, pix_{850}	90.41	81.55	73.03	75.05

Table 6. Cont.

Task	Pr	Re	IoU	Dice
Unet, pix_{205}	95.01	**79.17**	75.48	**79.3**
Unet, pix_{420}	95.54	88.39	85.31	**87.78**
Unet, pix_{500}	94.8	95.08	91.06	93.34
Unet, pix_{550}	92.27	82.5	76.44	80.49
Unet, pix_{600}	90.09	**83.1**	74.84	79.23
Unet, pix_{820}	97.53	80.95	79.43	81.93
Unet, pix_{850}	88.1	46.81	44.01	46.81
wUnet, pix_{205}	95.93	75.18	72.37	76.02
wUnet, pix_{420}	94.64	**91.75**	87.37	89.96
wUnet, pix_{500}	94.42	95.05	90.73	93.11
wUnet, pix_{550}	89.27	64.52	57.46	61.54
wUnet, pix_{600}	90.93	80.84	72.93	77.22
wUnet, pix_{820}	95.3	88.77	84.91	87.99
wUnet, pix_{850}	84.37	69.65	60.09	62.74
Unet++, pix_{205}	96.11	67.93	65.01	68.82
Unet++, pix_{420}	94.69	88.92	84.59	86.91
Unet++, pix_{500}	**97.06**	92.21	89.93	92.46
Unet++, pix_{550}	88.46	73.42	63.44	67.36
Unet++, pix_{600}	94.21	73.17	69.7	73.09
Unet++, pix_{820}	96.07	88.15	85.06	86.96
Unet++, pix_{850}	65.06	**99.95**	65.07	65.07

Some examples of good and average segmentation using the Unet model variants on the Heart-CT stack are shown in Figure 8. Here, we observe significant variations for smaller ROIs across the Unet model variants.

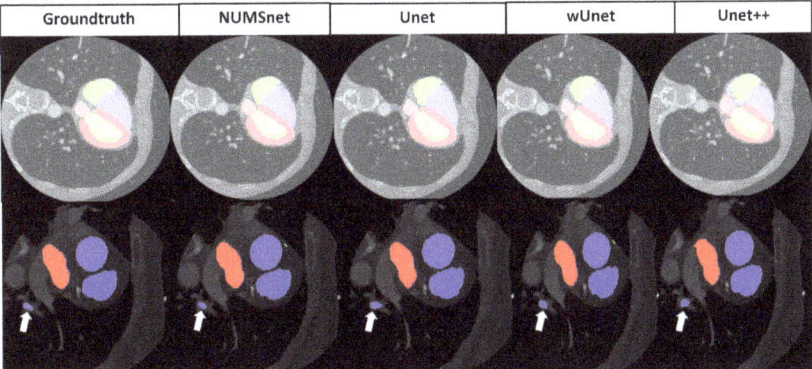

Figure 8. Examples of Heart-CT segmentation by the Unet variant models. **Row 1**: Good segmentation. **Row 2**: Average segmentation. In Row 2, we observe variations in the small ROI across Unet variants shown by the white arrow.

4.5. Ablation Study and Comparative Assessment

Finally, we analyze the importance of each hidden layer to the superior performance of the NUMSnet model when compared to the other Unet variant models. In this ablation study, we compared the performance of NUMSnet, with 11,713,943 total parameters, with its versions when only one hidden layer from the first level from the global feature layer (i.e., layer X(3,2) in Figure 3) is transmitted. This NUMSnet version is called $NUMSnet_{l1}$, and it has 11,349,628 parameters, of which 11,347,528 are trainable. Next, we generated a NUMSnet version in which the first two levels from the global feature level, i.e., layers (X(2,2), X(2,3) and X(3,2) from Figure 3), are transmitted. This is called $NUMSnet_{l12}$, and it has 11,614,508 parameters, of which 11,612,408 are trainable. The comparative performance of NUMSnet$_{l1}$ and NUMSnet$_{l12}$ on the Lung-CT and Heart-CT datasets is shown in Table 7. Here, we observe that for the Lung-med stack, Re improves as more hidden layers are transmitted. However, for the shorter Lung-rad stacks, there is a small significant improvement in segmentation performance when increasing the number of transmitted layers from NUMSnet$_{l1}$ to NUMSnet$_{l12}$. We also observe that for the Heart-CT stacks, transmitting more hidden layers significantly enhances Re and the overall segmentation performance. Thus, by comparing NUMSnet$_{l1}$ and NUMSnet$_{l12}$ in Table 7 with the NUMSnet performance in Table 2, Table 3 and Table 6 for the Lung-CT and Heart-CT stacks, respectively, we conclude that the transmission of all six hidden layers in the NUMSnet model ensures superior segmentation performance across datasets.

Table 7. Comparative multi-class segmentation performance of the NUMSnet model variants.

Data	Lung-Med			
Task	Pr	Re	IoU	Dice
NUMSnet$_{l1}$, Con	70.48	71.34	51.14	53.1
NUMSnet$_{l1}$, GGO	91.11	80.6	75.62	78.48
NUMSnet$_{l1}$, Lung	99.61	90.55	90.24	93.99
NUMSnet$_{l12}$, Con	66.82	86.12	58.86	60.3
NUMSnet$_{l12}$, GGO	78.56	97.75	77.56	79.8
NUMSnet$_{l12}$, Lung	98.5	92.61	91.38	94.61
Data	10 Lung-rad	Stacks		
NUMSnet$_{l1}$, Con	67.66	75.28	51.86	53.67
NUMSnet$_{l1}$, GGO	89.67	88.22	80.63	83.38
NUMSnet$_{l1}$, Lung	99.51	93.16	92.72	95.2
NUMSnet$_{l12}$, Con	68.42	75.53	53.51	55.35
NUMSnet$_{l12}$, GGO	88.76	88.95	80.14	82.88
NUMSnet$_{l12}$, Lung	99.52	93.42	93.0	95.36
Data	Heart-CT			
NUMSnet$_{l1}$, pix$_{205}$	97.38	67.21	65.51	68.85
NUMSnet$_{l1}$, pix$_{420}$	94.92	88.71	84.42	86.03
NUMSnet$_{l1}$, pix$_{500}$	97.29	94.56	92.34	94.31
NUMSnet$_{l1}$, pix$_{550}$	90.03	87.87	78.95	82.43
NUMSnet$_{l1}$, pix$_{600}$	90.9	75.95	68.3	71.9
NUMSnet$_{l1}$, pix$_{820}$	97.91	87.58	85.82	87.43
NUMSnet$_{l1}$, pix$_{850}$	89.96	75.67	68.12	70.17
NUMSnet$_{l12}$, pix$_{205}$	96.63	78.18	75.65	78.36
NUMSnet$_{l12}$, pix$_{420}$	95.9	83.1	80.24	81.93
NUMSnet$_{l12}$, pix$_{500}$	97.44	90.48	88.44	90.33
NUMSnet$_{l12}$, pix$_{550}$	94.49	78.9	74.98	77.97
NUMSnet$_{l12}$, pix$_{600}$	93.76	76.93	71.15	74.16
NUMSnet$_{l12}$, pix$_{820}$	98.52	90.13	88.84	90.19
NUMSnet$_{l12}$, pix$_{850}$	89.07	86.02	76.42	78.34

Finally, the comparative performance of the NUMSnet model and previous works that trained deep learning models on larger training datasets is shown in Table 8. Here, we assessed the number of training images and training time on standalone GPU machines as an indicator of computational complexity, along with the segmentation performance or $Dice$ scores for each output class category i. In addition, the previous works are identified as 2D vs. 3D based on the nature of convolutions in the implementations.

We observe that the proposed NUMSnet model achieves comparable or improved semantic segmentation performance across a variety of anatomical CT image stacks with only a fraction of the training images. This demonstrates the importance of nested layer transmission for enhanced boundary segmentation, especially for relatively small ROIs. For the Lung-CT stacks, the work by Voulodimos et al. [21] introduced a few-shot method using a Unet backbone for GGO segmentation only, and while this method achieved high precision and accuracy, it had low recall and *Dice* scores. In addition, for the same dataset, the work by Saood et al. [13] used a small fraction of the images for training and achieved better binary segmentation performance than multi-class segmentation performance. It is noteworthy that no prior works have bench-marked the segmentation performance for the Lung-rad image stacks. For the Heart-CT stacks, most works have trained 3D Unet or 3D-segmentation models for voxel-level convolutions and trained on 20 CT stacks while testing on another 20 stacks for the high precision of segmentation per ROI. Our work is one of the few implementations of 2D convolutions on dense Heart-CT scans and the only work that evaluates the Heart-CT stacks in [30].

Table 8. Comparative performance of NUMSnet with respect to previous works.

Method	Data	#Training Images	Metrics	Epochs/Training Time
Saood et al. (2D) [13]	Lung-med	72	$D_i = [22.5–60]\%$	160/25 min
Voulodimos (2D) [21]	Lung-med	418	$D_i = [65–85]\%$ (GGO)	$\sim$210 s
Roychowdhury (2D) [35]	Lung-med	40	$D_i = 64\%$ (GGO)	40/$\sim$70 s
NUMSnet (2D)	Lung-med	82	$D_i = [61–96\%]$	40/224 s
Payer et al. (3D) [22]	Heart-CT	7831	$D_i = [84–93\%]$	30,000/3–4 h
Wang et al. (3D) [15]	Heart-CT	7831	$D_i = [64.82–90.44\%]$	12,800/(Azure cloud)
Ye et al. (3D) [30]	Heart-CT	7831	$D_i = [86–96\%]$	60,000/$\sim$2–4 h
NUMSnet (Ours) (2D)	Heart-CT	363	$D_i = [75–97\%]$	60/362 s

In Table 8, it is noteworthy that for Heart-CT segmentation, we applied a pre-trained model on Lung-CT and fine-tuned it on 4.6% of all hHeart-CT images to obtain similar segmentation performance. Additionally, we observe that the 3D-segmentation models yield stable *Dice* scores in a narrower range of 84–96% for Heart-CT data while taking several thousand epochs and several hours to train when compared to our work, which has a wider range of *Dice* scores but comparable performance for smaller ROIs to that in [15,22] and a training time of seconds. In addition, the work in [15] implemented 3D convolutions in a virtual machine in Azure cloud, so the training time is not comparable to those of standalone systems.

5. Discussion

The proposed NUMSnet model aims to reproduce the segmentation performance of 3D encoder–decoder models with 2D encoder–decoder equivalents, with the intention to scale the method across medical imaging modalities and scan densities. The current implementation is a NUMSnet model with a depth of 4, based on all the previous comparative works in Table 8, but the depth can be increased in future works based on the growing complexity, overlap and number of ROIs in medical image use cases. Additionally, the NUMSnet only uses 2D concatenations and convolution operations to ensure low additional computational complexity. However, for future works and specific complex use cases where the training time and computational complexity are not bottlenecks, some of the following three enhancements can be made. First, additional skip connections between scans can be added to combine up-sampled outcomes from previous scans to the current scans based on the underlying complexities of segmentation. Such skip connections will still have less training time and complexity when compared to 3D operations. Second, the encoder and decoder layers can be further enhanced with Resnet, Densenet and Retinanet backbones for segmentation enhancements in future works. Third, a combination of loss functions can be used at the block and scan levels for optimal parameterization.

Most existing deep learning models for multi-class semantic segmentation tasks have been developed at the image level to scale across imaging modalities [37]. However, for 3D medical image stacks, segmentation at a stack level minimizes irregularities related to varying imaging conditions, thereby resulting in superior region boundaries for small and large ROIs. It is noteworthy that one key limiting condition for all semantic segmentation models is when the medical scans include written text on them. These irregularities can interfere with the segmentation of the outermost ROIs. In such situations, an overall mask can be generated and centered around all ROI regions and superimposed on the original image before passing it to the Unet and variant models, thus eliminating the written text region. Another alternative for reliable end-to-end segmentation in these cases, if enough annotated images are available, is to train two Unet or variant models to first detect the foreground region in the first Unet variant model, followed by segmenting the ROIs in the second Unet model, as shown in [15].

It is noteworthy that the single-stage Unet model and its variants are easily trainable with few annotated images, and they typically do not overfit. However, for high-resolution images, such as whole-slide images (WSI), where the dimensions of the medical images are a few thousand pixels per side, resizing such images to smaller dimensions to fit a Unet model or its variants may result in poor segmentation results [38]. In such scenarios, splitting the images into smaller patches, followed by training the Unet model and its variants, can improve the segmentation performance, as shown in [21].

A key consideration for multi-class segmentation using Unet variant models is the disparity between the ROI sizes, which can significantly impact the training stages when only a few annotated training images are available. For example, in the Lung-CT image stacks, the lung regions are larger than the GGO and consolidation areas, and because of this, using few training images and *Dice* coefficient loss over hundreds of epochs can bias the model to segment the lung region only. This occurs because the relative variation in pixel neighborhoods for larger ROIs is smaller than in pixel neighborhoods for smaller ROIs. In such situations, it is crucial to ensure that more training images are selected that have the smaller ROIs annotated and that the Unet variant models are run for about 40–60 epochs with region-sensitive loss functions.

Finally, for transfer learning applications, full image network weights transfer better when compared to Unet model variants trained on image patches, such as in [21]. This aligns with the works in [39,40], which demonstrate the ability of pre-trained models from one medical image modality to scale to other medical image stacks. Future efforts can be directed toward the transfer learning capabilities of the proposed NUMSnet model on WSI and patch image sets.

6. Conclusions

In this work, we present a novel NUMSnet model, which is a variation of the Unet++ model specifically for the multi-class semantic segmentation of 3D medical image stacks using only 10% of the images per stack, selected randomly in an ordered manner around the central scan of the 3D stacks. The novelty of this model lies in the temporal transmission of spatial pixel and neighborhood feature information across scans through nested layers. The proposed model enhances *Dice* scores over Unet++ and other Unet model variants by 2–9% in Lung-CT stacks and 2–16% in Heart-CT stacks. In addition, the NUMSnet is the only model that applies 2D convolutions for Heart-CT stack segmentation for the [30] dataset.

Additionally, in this work, we analyzed a variety of sampling methods to optimally select the minimal 10% training set. We conclude that the random selection of ordered scans is the optimal mechanism to select a minimal training set. Further, we analyzed the optimal number of up-sampling layers that should be transmitted for the best semantic segmentation performance. Here, we conclude that all six nested layers of a Unet++ model are significant for transmission, while adding additional up-sampling layers for transmission increases the overall computational complexity of the NUMSnet model while not significantly contributing to the segmentation performance for sparse training image sets.

Finally, we assessed the transfer learning capabilities of the NUMSnet model after it was pre-trained on Lung-CT stacks and fine-tuned on only 5% of available annotated Heart-CT images. We conclude that the NUMSnet model aids in transfer learning for similar medical image modalities, even if the number of classes and ROIs change significantly. Future work can be directed toward extending the NUMSnet model to additional medical image modalities, such as X-rays, OCT, MRI stacks and RGB videos from dental to colonoscopy use cases.

Funding: This research received no external funding.

Data Availability Statement: Not applicable.

Conflicts of Interest: The authors declare no conflict of interest.

Appendix A. Model Graphs

The proposed NUMSnet model layers and interconnections are shown in Figure A1. The layer interconnections from the NUMS-all model are shown in Figure A2.

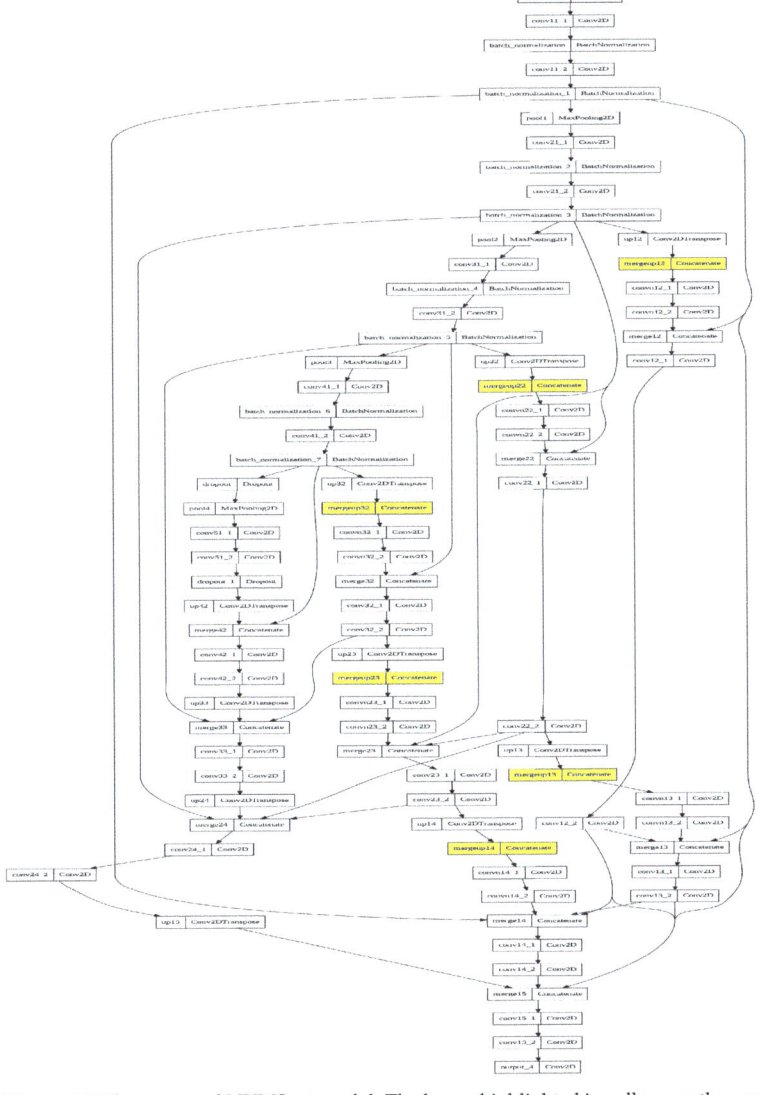

Figure A1. The proposed NUMSnet model. The layers highlighted in yellow are the new concatenation layers introduced by NUMSnet. All other layers are from the Unet++ model.

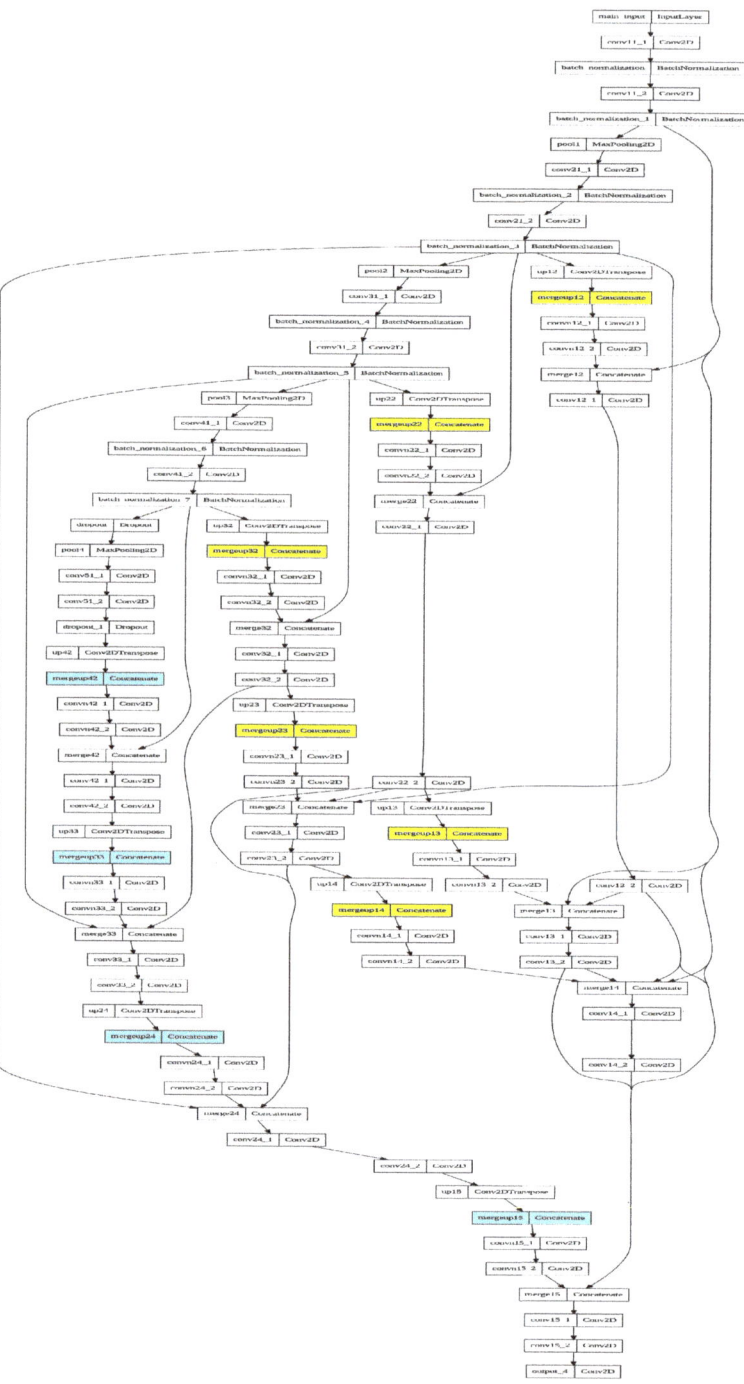

Figure A2. The NUMS-all model with all up-sampled layer features transmitted. The layers highlighted in yellow are the new NUMSnet concatenation layers. The layers highlighted in blue are the additional up-sampling layers in the NUMS-all model. All remaining layers are from the Unet++ model.

References

1. Zhao, Z.Q.; Zheng, P.; Xu, S.T.; Wu, X. Object detection with deep learning: A review. *IEEE Trans. Neural Netw. Learn. Syst.* **2019**, *30*, 3212–3232. [CrossRef]
2. Chai, J.; Zeng, H.; Li, A.; Ngai, E.W. Deep learning in computer vision: A critical review of emerging techniques and application scenarios. *Mach. Learn. Appl.* **2021**, *6*, 100134. [CrossRef]
3. Ronneberger, O.; Fischer, P.; Brox, T. U-net: Convolutional networks for biomedical image segmentation. In *Medical Image Computing and Computer-Assisted Intervention*; Springer: Berlin/Heidelberg, Germany, 2015; pp. 234–241.
4. Nezla, N.; Haridas, T.M.; Supriya, M. Semantic segmentation of underwater images using unet architecture based deep convolutional encoder decoder model. In Proceedings of the 2021 7th International Conference on Advanced Computing and Communication Systems (ICACCS), Coimbatore, India, 19–20 March 2021; Volume 1, pp. 28–33.
5. Darapaneni, N.; Raj, P.; Paduri, A.R.; Anand, E.; Rajarathinam, K.; Eapen, P.T.; Krishnamurthy, S. Autonomous car driving using deep learning. In Proceedings of the 2021 2nd International Conference on Secure Cyber Computing and Communications (ICSCCC), Jalandhar, India, 21–23 May 2021; pp. 29–33.
6. Sampathila, N.; Chadaga, K.; Goswami, N.; Chadaga, R.P.; Pandya, M.; Prabhu, S.; Bairy, M.G.; Katta, S.S.; Bhat, D.; Upadya, S.P. Customized Deep Learning Classifier for Detection of Acute Lymphoblastic Leukemia Using Blood Smear Images. *Healthcare* **2022**, *10*, 1812. [CrossRef]
7. Chadaga, K.; Prabhu, S.; Sampathila, N.; Nireshwalya, S.; Katta, S.S.; Tan, R.S.; Acharya, U.R. Application of Artificial Intelligence Techniques for Monkeypox: A Systematic Review. *Diagnostics* **2023**, *13*, 824. [CrossRef] [PubMed]
8. Ait Nasser, A.; Akhloufi, M.A. A Review of Recent Advances in Deep Learning Models for Chest Disease Detection Using Radiography. *Diagnostics* **2023**, *13*, 159. [CrossRef] [PubMed]
9. Sivagami, S.; Chitra, P.; Kailash, G.S.R.; Muralidharan, S. Unet architecture based dental panoramic image segmentation. In Proceedings of the 2020 International Conference on Wireless Communications Signal Processing and Networking (WiSPNET), Chennai, India, 4–6 August 2020; pp. 187–191.
10. Nguyen, H.T.; Luong, H.H.; Phan, P.T.; Nguyen, H.H.D.; Ly, D.; Phan, D.M.; Do, T.T. HS-UNET-ID: An approach for human skin classification integrating between UNET and improved dense convolutional network. *Int. J. Imaging Syst. Technol.* **2022**, *32*, 1832–1845. [CrossRef]
11. Safarov, S.; Whangbo, T.K. A-DenseUNet: Adaptive densely connected UNet for polyp segmentation in colonoscopy images with atrous convolution. *Sensors* **2021**, *21*, 1441. [CrossRef]
12. Renard, F.; Guedria, S.; Palma, N.D.; Vuillerme, N. Variability and reproducibility in deep learning for medical image segmentation. *Sci. Rep.* **2020**, *10*, 1–16. [CrossRef]
13. Saood, A.; Hatem, I. COVID-19 lung CT image segmentation using deep learning methods: U-Net versus SegNet. *BMC Med. Imaging* **2021**, *21*, 1–10. [CrossRef]
14. Zhou, Z.; Rahman Siddiquee, M.M.; Tajbakhsh, N.; Liang, J. Unet++: A nested u-net architecture for medical image segmentation. In *Deep Learning in Medical Image Analysis and Multimodal Learning for Clinical Decision Support*; Springer: Berlin/Heidelberg, Germany, 2018; pp. 3–11.
15. Wang, C.; MacGillivray, T.; Macnaught, G.; Yang, G.; Newby, D. A two-stage 3D Unet framework for multi-class segmentation on full resolution image. *arXiv* **2018**, arXiv:1804.04341.
16. Asnawi, M.H.; Pravitasari, A.A.; Darmawan, G.; Hendrawati, T.; Yulita, I.N.; Suprijadi, J.; Nugraha, F.A.L. Lung and Infection CT-Scan-Based Segmentation with 3D UNet Architecture and Its Modification. *Healthcare* **2023**, *11*, 213. [CrossRef]
17. Hashemi, A.; Pilevar, A.H.; Rafeh, R. Mass detection in lung CT images using region growing segmentation and decision making based on fuzzy inference system and artificial neural network. *Int. J. Image Graph. Signal Process.* **2013**, *5*, 16.
18. Liu, C.; Pang, M. Automatic lung segmentation based on image decomposition and wavelet transform. *Biomed. Signal Process. Control.* **2020**, *61*, 102032. [CrossRef]
19. Ranjbarzadeh, R.; Jafarzadeh Ghoushchi, S.; Bendechache, M.; Amirabadi, A.; Ab Rahman, M.N.; Baseri Saadi, S.; Aghamohammadi, A.; Kooshki Forooshani, M. Lung infection segmentation for COVID-19 pneumonia based on a cascade convolutional network from CT images. *Biomed Res. Int.* **2021**, *2021*, 1–16. [CrossRef] [PubMed]
20. He, K.; Gkioxari, G.; Dollár, P.; Girshick, R. Mask r-cnn. In Proceedings of the IEEE international Conference on Computer Vision, Venice, Italy, 22–29 October 2017; pp. 2961–2969.
21. Voulodimos, A.; Protopapadakis, E.; Katsamenis, I.; Doulamis, A.; Doulamis, N. Deep learning models for COVID-19 infected area segmentation in CT images. In Proceedings of the 14th PErvasive Technologies Related to Assistive Environments Conference, Corfu, Greece, 29 June–2 July 2021; pp. 404–411.
22. Payer, C.; Štern, D.; Bischof, H.; Urschler, M. Multi-label whole heart segmentation using CNNs and anatomical label configurations. In Proceedings of the Statistical Atlases and Computational Models of the Heart, ACDC and MMWHS Challenges: 8th International Workshop, STACOM 2017, Held in Conjunction with MICCAI 2017, Quebec City, QC, Canada, 10–14 September 2017; Revised Selected Papers; Springer: Berlin/Heidelberg, Germany, 2018; pp. 190–198.
23. Amyar, A.; Modzelewski, R.; Li, H.; Ruan, S. Multi-task deep learning based CT imaging analysis for COVID-19 pneumonia: Classification and segmentation. *Comput. Biol. Med.* **2020**, *126*, 104037. [CrossRef]
24. Gunraj, H.; Wang, L.; Wong, A. Covidnet-ct: A tailored deep convolutional neural network design for detection of COVID-19 cases from chest ct images. *Front. Med.* **2020**, *7*, 608525. [CrossRef]

25. Fan, D.P.; Zhou, T.; Ji, G.P.; Zhou, Y.; Chen, G.; Fu, H.; Shen, J.; Shao, L. Inf-net: Automatic COVID-19 lung infection segmentation from ct images. *IEEE Trans. Med. Imaging* **2020**, *39*, 2626–2637.
26. Liu, K.; Xie, J.; Chen, M.; Chen, H.; Liu, W. MA-UNet++: A multi-attention guided U-Net++ for COVID-19 CT segmentation. In Proceedings of the 2022 13th Asian Control Conference (ASCC), Jeju, Republic of Korea, 4–7 May 2022; pp. 682–687.
27. Huang, C. CT image segmentation of COVID-19 based on UNet++ and ResNeXt. In Proceedings of the 2021 11th International Conference on Information Technology in Medicine and Education (ITME), Vancouver, BC, Canada, 27–28 May 2023; pp. 420–424.
28. Xiao, Z.; Liu, B.; Geng, L.; Zhang, F.; Liu, Y. Segmentation of lung nodules using improved 3D-UNet neural network. *Symmetry* **2020**, *12*, 1787. [CrossRef]
29. Milletari, F.; Navab, N.; Ahmadi, S.A. V-net: Fully convolutional neural networks for volumetric medical image segmentation. In Proceedings of the 2016 Fourth International Conference on 3D Vision (3DV), Stanford, CA, USA, 25–28 October 2016; pp. 565–571.
30. Ye, C.; Wang, W.; Zhang, S.; Wang, K. Multi-depth fusion network for whole-heart CT image segmentation. *IEEE Access* **2019**, *7*, 23421–23429. [CrossRef]
31. Yang, X.; He, X.; Zhao, J.; Zhang, Y.; Zhang, S.; Xie, P. COVID-CT-dataset: A CT scan dataset about COVID-19. *arXiv* **2020**, arXiv:2003.13865.
32. Ministry for Primary Industries. COVID-19 CT Segmentation Dataset. 2020. Available online: http://medicalsegmentation.com/covid19/ (accessed on 9 January 2022).
33. Girish, G.; Thakur, B.; Chowdhury, S.R.; Kothari, A.R.; Rajan, J. Segmentation of intra-retinal cysts from optical coherence tomography images using a fully convolutional neural network model. *IEEE J. Biomed. Health Inform.* **2018**, *23*, 296–304. [CrossRef]
34. Jadon, S. A survey of loss functions for semantic segmentation. In Proceedings of the 2020 IEEE Conference on Computational Intelligence in Bioinformatics and Computational Biology (CIBCB), Viña del Mar, Chile, 27–29 October 2020; pp. 1–7. [CrossRef]
35. Roychowdhury, S. QU-net++: Image Quality Detection Framework for Segmentation of Medical 3D Image Stacks. *arXiv* **2022**, arXiv:2110.14181.
36. Zhang, Q.; Ren, X.; Wei, B. Segmentation of infected region in CT images of COVID-19 patients based on QC-HC U-net. *Sci. Rep.* **2021**, *11*, 22854. [CrossRef] [PubMed]
37. Asgari Taghanaki, S.; Abhishek, K.; Cohen, J.P.; Cohen-Adad, J.; Hamarneh, G. Deep semantic segmentation of natural and medical images: A review. *Artif. Intell. Rev.* **2021**, *54*, 137–178. [CrossRef]
38. Yu, H.; Sharifai, N.; Jiang, K.; Wang, F.; Teodoro, G.; Farris, A.B.; Kong, J. Artificial intelligence based liver portal tract region identification and quantification with transplant biopsy whole-slide images. *Comput. Biol. Med.* **2022**, *150*, 106089. [CrossRef] [PubMed]
39. Yu, X.; Wang, J.; Hong, Q.Q.; Teku, R.; Wang, S.H.; Zhang, Y.D. Transfer learning for medical images analyses: A survey. *Neurocomputing* **2022**, *489*, 230–254. [CrossRef]
40. Alzubaidi, L.; Fadhel, M.A.; Al-Shamma, O.; Zhang, J.; Santamaría, J.; Duan, Y.; R. Oleiwi, S. Towards a better understanding of transfer learning for medical imaging: A case study. *Appl. Sci.* **2020**, *10*, 4523. [CrossRef]

Disclaimer/Publisher's Note: The statements, opinions and data contained in all publications are solely those of the individual author(s) and contributor(s) and not of MDPI and/or the editor(s). MDPI and/or the editor(s) disclaim responsibility for any injury to people or property resulting from any ideas, methods, instructions or products referred to in the content.

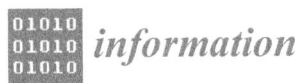

Article

A Comparison of Machine Learning Techniques for the Detection of Type-2 Diabetes Mellitus: Experiences from Bangladesh

Md. Jamal Uddin [1], Md. Martuza Ahamad [1], Md. Nesarul Hoque [1], Md. Abul Ala Walid [2], Sakifa Aktar [1], Naif Alotaibi [3], Salem A. Alyami [3], Muhammad Ashad Kabir [4] and Mohammad Ali Moni [5,*]

1. Department of Computer Science and Engineering, Bangabandhu Sheikh Mujibur Rahman Science and Technology University, Gopalganj 8100, Bangladesh; jamal.bsmrstu@gmail.com (M.J.U.); martuza.cse@bsmrstu.edu.bd (M.M.A.); mnhshisir@gmail.com (M.N.H.); sakifa.cse@bsmrstu.edu.bd (S.A.)
2. Department of Computer Science and Engineering, Bangladesh Army University of Engineering & Technology (BAUET), Natore 6431, Bangladesh; abulalawalid@gmail.com
3. Department of Mathematics and Statistics, Faculty of Science, Imam Mohammad Ibn Saud Islamic University (IMSIU), Riyadh 13318, Saudi Arabia; nmaalotaibi@imamu.edu.sa (N.A.); saalyami@imamu.edu.sa (S.A.A.)
4. School of Computing, Mathematics, and Engineering, Charles Sturt University, Bathurst, NSW 2795, Australia; akabir@csu.edu.au
5. Artificial Intelligence & Data Science, School of Health and Rehabilitation Sciences, Faculty of Health and Behavioural Sciences, The University of Queensland, St Lucia, QLD 4072, Australia
* Correspondence: m.moni@uq.edu.au; Tel.: +61-414-701-759

Citation: Uddin, M.J.; Ahamad, M.M.; Hoque, M.N.; Walid, M.A.A.; Aktar, S.; Alotaibi, N.; Alyami, S.A.; Kabir, M.A.; Moni, M.A. A Comparison of Machine Learning Techniques for the Detection of Type-2 Diabetes Mellitus: Experiences from Bangladesh. *Information* 2023, *14*, 376. https://doi.org/10.3390/info14070376

Academic Editors: Sidong Liu, Cristián Castillo Olea and Shlomo Berkovsky

Received: 13 May 2023
Revised: 25 June 2023
Accepted: 26 June 2023
Published: 2 July 2023

Copyright: © 2023 by the authors. Licensee MDPI, Basel, Switzerland. This article is an open access article distributed under the terms and conditions of the Creative Commons Attribution (CC BY) license (https://creativecommons.org/licenses/by/4.0/).

Abstract: Diabetes is a chronic disease caused by a persistently high blood sugar level, causing other chronic diseases, including cardiovascular, kidney, eye, and nerve damage. Prompt detection plays a vital role in reducing the risk and severity associated with diabetes, and identifying key risk factors can help individuals become more mindful of their lifestyles. In this study, we conducted a questionnaire-based survey utilizing standard diabetes risk variables to examine the prevalence of diabetes in Bangladesh. To enable prompt detection of diabetes, we compared different machine learning techniques and proposed an ensemble-based machine learning framework that incorporated algorithms such as decision tree, random forest, and extreme gradient boost algorithms. In order to address class imbalance within the dataset, we initially applied the synthetic minority oversampling technique (SMOTE) and random oversampling (ROS) techniques. We evaluated the performance of various classifiers, including decision tree (DT), logistic regression (LR), support vector machine (SVM), gradient boost (GB), extreme gradient boost (XGBoost), random forest (RF), and ensemble technique (ET), on our diabetes datasets. Our experimental results showed that the ET outperformed other classifiers; to further enhance its effectiveness, we fine-tuned and evaluated the hyperparameters of the ET. Using statistical and machine learning techniques, we also ranked features and identified that age, extreme thirst, and diabetes in the family are significant features that prove instrumental in the detection of diabetes patients. This method has great potential for clinicians to effectively identify individuals at risk of diabetes, facilitating timely intervention and care.

Keywords: diabetes mellitus; machine learning; survey; feature selection; feature importance

1. Introduction

Diabetes is a lifelong disease that prevents the body from obtaining energy from food sources due to a deficiency insulin, an influential factor in enhancing the cells' ability to absorb glucose and produce energy [1]. There are three primary types of diabetes: type 1 diabetes mellitus (T1DM), type 2 diabetes mellitus (T2DM), and gestational diabetes mellitus (GDM). In this study, we focused on T2DM, as it accounts for approximately 90% of all occurrences of diabetes [2]: insulin resistance, in which the body does not respond adequately to insulin, is a defining characteristic. T2DM is diagnosed most frequently in elderly adults; however, it is becoming increasingly prevalent in children, teenagers, and young people due to rising rates of poor diet, physical inactivity, and obesity. Several risk factors, including diabetes in the family, excess weight, an unhealthy diet, a lack of exercise, increasing age, and higher blood pressure, are associated with T2DM.

Diabetes is the underlying cause of several associated diseases, including kidney disease, tuberculosis, cardiovascular disease, and eye management [3]. Patients with diabetes are susceptible to amputation, blindness, stroke, heart disease, kidney failure, and premature death [4]. According to the International Diabetes Federation (IDF), there were approximately 537 million diabetic patients worldwide—1 in 10 people—of whom 81% resided in low- and middle-income nations in 2021 [5]. In 2021, the IDF counted 6.7 million diabetes-related fatalities worldwide. In addition, the global cost of diabetes-related medical expenses in 2019 was USD 760 billion; this amount is set to grow to USD 825 billion by 2030 and to USD 845 billion by 2045 [6]. Chronic diseases induced by diabetes have imposed a financial burden on every nation [7].

The IDF estimates that in Bangladesh there are 7.1 million diabetics and approximately the same number of undiagnosed cases; this number is anticipated to double by 2025. In addition, the cost of diabetes imposes a significant burden on natural expenditures in low- and middle-income countries [8].

Our research focused on T2DM-type diabetes. Although this type of diabetes cannot be cured, most people can still avoid developing it. Early identification and lifestyle changes can minimize the chance of developing diabetes. T2DM risk can be accurately identified by doctors when treating an individual patient; however, clinicians encounter significant obstacles when screening thousands of patients with high-risk illnesses. In this situation, analytical methods are required for T2DM screening in the population.

Machine learning (ML) methods have been used to solve several problems recently, such as diagnosing cancer [9], COVID-19 [10], autism [11,12], meningitis, diabetes, and heart disease. Recent research suggests that ML can summarize patient characteristics and predict T2DM risk [13–17]. The authors of Haque and Alharbi [18] investigated 18 features of T2DM in Bangladesh. The principal contribution of this study was that the authors considered demographic and clinical data together and achieved the best output of 83.8% accuracy and 70% F1-score, using the LR model; however, the performance could be enhanced by including more features related to people's eating habits, lifestyle, and clinical diagnosis. In another work, Tasin et al. [19] specifically investigated females in Bangladesh. They developed a diabetes detection system with 81% accuracy using the XGBoost model with the ADASYN oversampling technique. They used an explainable AI approach with the LIME and Shapley additive explanations (SHAP) frameworks to provide feature weights relating to diabetes. They also deployed a website and an Android mobile application to detect diabetes in females. The authors only considered eight features in their detection system; therefore, the question of reliability arose. Nipa et al. [8] examined three datasets: the Sylhet Diabetes Hospital dataset (SDHD) of 520 samples; the pre-diagnosis diabetes dataset (PDD) of 558 samples; and the combined SDHD and PDD dataset (MDD). They tested 32 classifiers, where extra tree (ET), light gradient boosting machine (LGBM), stacking, multi-layer perceptron (MLP), histogram gradient boosting classifier (HGBC), RF, bagging, and gradient boosting classifier (GBC) presented more stable outputs. ET provided the best result of 97.11% accuracy for the SDHD dataset; MLP yielded the highest accuracy of 96.42%; and LGBM and HGBC showed the maximum output of 94.9% accuracy, separately. They applied the SHAP framework to find the features more responsible for diabetes. The authors of Kaur and Kumari [20] employed five ML models to identify a patient as diabetic or non-diabetic: linear SVM, radial bias SVM, k-NN, artificial neural network (ANN), and multi-factor dimensionality reduction (MDR). They obtained superior results with linear SVM and k-NN, where linear SVM displayed an accuracy of 89% and an F1-score of 87%, and k-NN exhibited an accuracy of 88% and an F1-score of 88%. Before applying the ML models, they filtered significant features using the Boruta wrapper feature selection method. In this research, the authors investigated the error analysis of the detection system. Zheng et al. [21] analysed the T2DM-related features and experimented with various ML models to identify diabetic patients. The authors observed that SVM, J48, and RF presented a more stable output than the other ML models such as LR, NB, and k-NN.

We found many research works on the Pima Indians Diabetes Database (PIDD) dataset [22–31]. The dataset comprises 768 female patients, of whom 268 have diabetes, and 500 do not. The dataset has eight input features and one target variable. Here, Yahyaoui et al. [27], Abdulhadi and Al-Mousa [28], Tigga and Garg [30], Pranto et al. [31], and Ali et al. [23] proposed RF classifiers, while Saha et al. [22] and Wei et al. [25] preferred neural network-based models to obtain the best performance. On the other hand, Birjais et al. [26], Battineni et al. [29], and Howlader et al. [24] achieved the maximum output by utilizing gradient boosting (GB), LR, and the generalized additive model using LOESS (GAMLOESS) models, respectively.

The authors of Sneha and Gangil [32] attempted to employ a predictive analysis in the early detection of diabetes mellitus, ensuring that all significant features were utilized. With an accuracy of 82.03%, naive Bayes (NB) was the most accurate of the five ML algorithms utilized in the study. The highest specificities of RF and DT were 98% and 98.2%, respectively. The authors of [33] utilized LR, classification [34], and regression trees (CART), ANN, SVM, RF, and gradient boosting machine (GBM) classifiers to determine the likelihood an individual would develop T2DM. The GBM model achieved the best among those considered. In addition, they identified the significance of factors based on each classifier and the Shapley additive explanations approach and demonstrated the relevant features such as sweet affinity, urine glucose, age, heart rate, creatinine, waist circumference, uric acid, pulse pressure, insulin, and hypertension.

Le et al. [35] presented a ML model to predict early onset diabetes in patients and employed grey wolf optimization (GWO) and adaptive particle swam optimization (APSO) to optimize the number of significant input attributes. Using their proposed strategy, their computational results indicated a higher degree of accuracy (96% for GWO-MLP and 97% for APGWO-MLP). Next, Islam et al. [36] utilized two statistical analyses to determine the diabetes risk factors. They used diabetes information from the 2011 Bangladesh Demographic and Health Survey. Six ML-based classifiers were used to predict and categorize diabetes. Eleven of the fifteen examined factors were found to be associated with diabetes, and the bagged CART model had the highest accuracy and area under the curve at 94.3% and 0.6, respectively. Using ML techniques, Haq et al. [37] developed a diagnostic system for diabetes. Furthermore, a filtering approach based on the DT algorithm was used to select the most critical features. Experiments showed that the proposed method for choosing features improved the accuracy of the classifying predictive models.

Shuja et al. [38] created a model for diabetes prognosis based on data mining categorization approaches using a dataset from the Kashmir Valley Clinical Institute. After performing SMOTE for data oversampling, the balanced dataset was fed to five ML algorithms: bagging, SVM, MLP, simple logistic, and DT. DT had the best accuracy of 94.7%, precision of 0.947, and sensitivity of 0.947. Then, Chatrati et al. [39] suggested developing a smart domestic system using five different supervised ML approaches to monitor a patient's glucose and blood pressure. The accuracy of all algorithms from SVM was 75%, from k-NN was 74%, from DT was 66.1%, LR was 74.5%, and DA was 74.7%. In another work, Islam et al. [40] identified risk variables for T2DM and offered an ML method to predict it. Next, five ML methods predicted T2DM. For 2009–2010, these researchers indicated six potential risks: age, learning, marital status, SBP, smoking, and BMI. For 2011–2012, they identified nine threat issues: age, race, martial status, SBP, DBP, direct cholesterol, bodily activity, smoking, and BMI. The RF-based classifier achieved a correctness of 95.9%, a sensitivity of 95.7%, an F-score of 95.3%, and an AUC of 0.946.

A significant number of diabetic patients in Bangladesh have gone undetected. Furthermore, inadequate healthcare equipment is incapable of accommodating for or treating an extensive number of diabetic patients, and the expense of diabetes carries an immense strain on the citizens of the country. Unfortunately, we have discovered very little research on the inhabitants of Bangladesh. Therefore, we must establish an automated system for the early diagnosis of T2DM. We have made the following contributions in this regard:

- We created a dataset of 508 study populations for diabetes.
- We applied and compared state-of-the-art clinically applicable ML models to conduct a benchmark analysis, aiming to contribute to further research in the field.
- We proposed a framework that utilizes ML techniques to detect diabetic patients.
- We ranked and identified significant features associated with diabetes mellitus.

2. Materials and Methods

The workflow of this study is depicted in Figure 1.

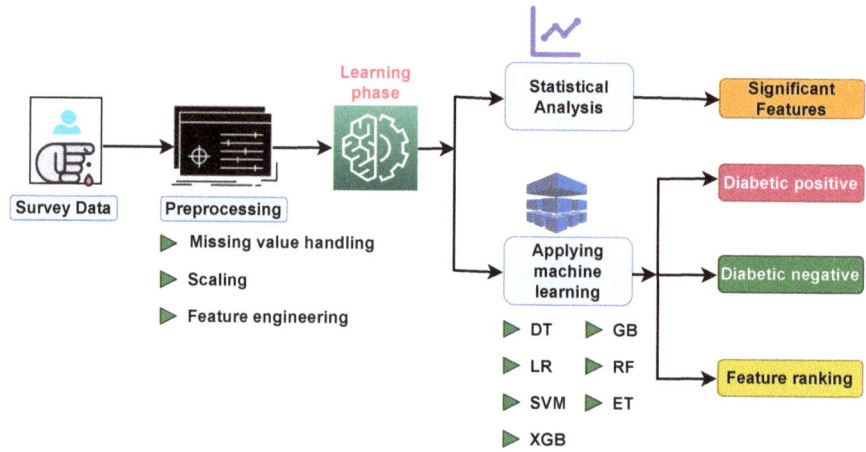

Figure 1. Workflow of this study.

The main dataset was gathered through surveys with closed-ended questions and direct interviews, also called in-person interviews. All respondents were from Bangladesh. In our study, we used the most commonly used variables (for preparing questionnaires) from recent articles on diabetes prediction models [33,35,41]. The primary dataset was converted into a secondary dataset in order to perform several mathematical operations. We performed an exploratory data analysis on our proposed Bangladeshi T2DM dataset to find out previously unknown information. Moreover, the dataset was processed through various stages, including missing value handling, data encoding, feature scaling, feature engineering, etc. Symmetrical analysis checked the amount of skewness in the target class. Next, the dataset was segmented into training and testing sets based on the target class ratio, and the training set exhibited the same level of skewness as before. Initially, seven ML models were trained and evaluated with this preliminary training set. SMOTE and ROS were applied to the training set to resolve the skewness property in the target class and improve the results of the ML model. Furthermore, seven ML models were applied to the datasets, balanced using SMOTE and ROS techniques. A statistical method known as the chi-squared test was also applied in order to identify any associative features, and several ML models were employed to detect any significant feature sets.

2.1. Data Collection and Description

In order to perform this research, we constructed a dataset from the perspective of the Bangladeshi population. Based on an analysis of the relevant studies, 33 questionnaires were made to obtain first-hand information. There were 508 respondents. The primary dataset was acquired by means of both online surveys and in-person interviews. Furthermore, we also collected the respective information about the participants' locations. Therefore, it is seen that the study covered all 64 districts of Bangladesh with no selection bias. This dataset was turned into secondary data so that it could be used to build a model for ML. Each property is organized and briefly explained in Table 1, displaying the possible values for each attribute.

Table 1. Dataset description.

ID	Attribute Name	Feature Description	Count (N = 508), n (%) or Avg., Min, Max, Median
1	Age	Identifying age groups	1–18: 244 (48.03%) 19–40: 95 (18.7%) 40–65: 99 (19.49%) 65 or more: 70 (13.78%)
2	Gender	Gender of the respondent	Male: 249 (49.01%) Female: 259 (50.99%)
3	Education Level	Level of education can be no education, primary, secondary or higher	Primary: 52 (10.36%) Secondary: 95 (18.7%) Higher: 305 (60.03%) No education: 51 (10.03%)
4	Diabetes in the family	Respondent's ancestors or parents suffered from the disease or not	Yes: 298 (58.66%) No: 210 (41.34%)
5	Occupation	Respondent can be unemployed, employed or find job	Looking work: 56 (11.02%) Not working: 189 (37.20%) Working: 260 (51.18%)
6	Household monthly income	Household monthly income of the respondent	Avg.: 30,477 Max: 300,000 Min: 1000 Median: 30,000
7	Wealth index	Wealth index can be low, middle or upper class	Poor: 46 (0.09%) Middle: 406 (79.91%) Rich: 58 (11%)
8	Place of residence	Place of residence indicates in which area the respondent usually lives	Urban: 233 (45.86%) Rural: 276 (54.14%)
9	Walk/ Run/ Physical exercise	How much jogging or walking the respondent did	None: 43 (8.46%) Less half: 90 (17.71%) More half: 151 (29.72%) One hour or More: 224 (44.09%)
10	BMI	Calculated from Height and Weight	Avg.: 23.2 Max: 58.44 Min: 12 Median: 23.12
11	Smoking	Whether the respondent smokes or not	Yes: 53 (10.44%) No: 455 (89.56%)
12	Alcohol consumption	Whether or not the respondent drinks alcohol	Yes: 22 (4.33%) No: 486 (95.67%)
13	Hours of sleep	Total hour of sleep each day	Avg.: 7.77 Max: 12 Min: 1 Median: 8
14	Regular intake of medicine (Except insulin)	Regular medication use, excluding insulin	Yes: 233 (45.86%) No: 275 (54.14%)
15	Junk food consumption	Prevalence of junk food consumption	Yes: 194 (38.18%) No: 314 (61.82%)

Table 1. Cont.

ID	Attribute Name	Feature Description	Count (N = 508), n (%) or Avg., Min, Max, Median
16	Stress	Stress level of respondent	Not at all: 66 (13%) Sometimes: 329 (64.76%) Often: 60 (11.8%) Always: 55 (10.82%)
17	Blood pressure level	Average level of blood pressure	High: 83 (16.33%) Normal: 383 (75.4%) Low: 43 (8.26%)
18	Hypertension	Whether or not the respondent has hypertension	Yes: 269 (52.95%) No: 239 (47.05%)
19	Frequency of urination	Frequency of urination each day	Not much: 360 (70.86%) Quite much: 148 (29.14%)
20	Extreme thirst	Whether or not the respondent is extremely thirsty	Yes: 253 (49.8%) No: 255 (50.2%)
21	Sudden weight loss	Whether the respondent ever noticed sudden weight loss	Yes: 110 (21.65%) No: 334 (65.74%) May be: 64 (12.6%)
22	Weakness	Whether the respondent feels more vulnerable	Yes: 225 (44.29%) No: 187 (36.81%) May be: 96 (18.9%)
23	More appetite	Whether the respondent feels more hungry	Yes: 151 (29.72%) No: 250 (49.21%) May be: 106 (20.86%)
24	Irritability	Whether the respondent feels irritability	Yes: 250 (49.2%) No: 258 (50.8%)
25	Delayed healing	Whether the respondent notices delayed healing of the wound	Yes: 213 (41.92%) No: 295 (58.08%)
26	Muscle stiffness	Whether the respondent notices muscle stiffness of their body	Yes: 234 (46.06%) No: 274 (53.94%)
27	Partial paralysis.	Partial paralysis of any part of the body is noticed or not	Yes: 69 (13.58%) No: 396 (77.95%) May be: 33 (8.46%)
28	Hair loss	Whether the respondent notices gradually losing hair or not	Yes: 231 (45.47%) No: 203 (39.76%) May be: 70 (14.76%)
29	Other diseases	Whether the respondent has other serious diseases	Yes: 260 (51.18%) No: 248 (48.82%)
30	Number of dependent family members	Total number of dependent family members	Avg.: 3.43 Max: 15 Min: 0 Median: 3
31	Living house type	Respondent home can be rental or owned	Owned: 409 (80.51%) Rented: 99 (19.49%)
32	Anxiety	Whether the respondent has extreme anxiety or not	Yes: 293 (57.67%) No: 215 (42.33%)
33	Diabetes (output factor)	Diabetes, non-diabetes	Yes: 275 (54.14%) No: 233 (45.86%)

2.2. Explanatory Data Analysis

Exploratory data analysis was conducted on our dataset in an attempt to reveal buried information. This dataset comprised 508 samples, and the output variable contained two distinct categories: Diabetes (affected with diabetes) and non-diabetes (not affected with diabetes). A property of imbalance was observed by analysing the distribution of output classes. There were 275 (54.14%) observations belonging to the majority class named diabetes, and the rest belonged to the minority class, non-diabetes. The maximum age of the individuals was 78 years, with a minimum of 18 years, and a median of 41 years. A total of 49.01% were men and 50.99% were women in our dataset. Two hundred and fifty-three individuals suffered from extreme thirst, while 148 had a high frequency of urination. A total of 576.7% of the population suffered from anxiety, whereas 51.8% suffered from other diseases.

The number of people with diabetes who had a family history of the disease was significantly higher than the number of those without a family history of diabetes. Diabetes affected 223 individuals whose ancestors or parents had the condition, but only 52 individuals whose ancestors or parents did not have the disease. Figure 2 represents the correlation between the features. We found no significant correlation between the features. Therefore, we did not remove any characteristics from the dataset. Figure 3 depicts the association between the category of the output variable non-diabetes and the walk/run/physical exercise variable, indicating that a person has a higher likelihood of falling into the category of non-diabetes if they are physically active for at least one hour. We also saw that most diabetic observations involved higher blood pressure levels compared to non-diabetic observations.

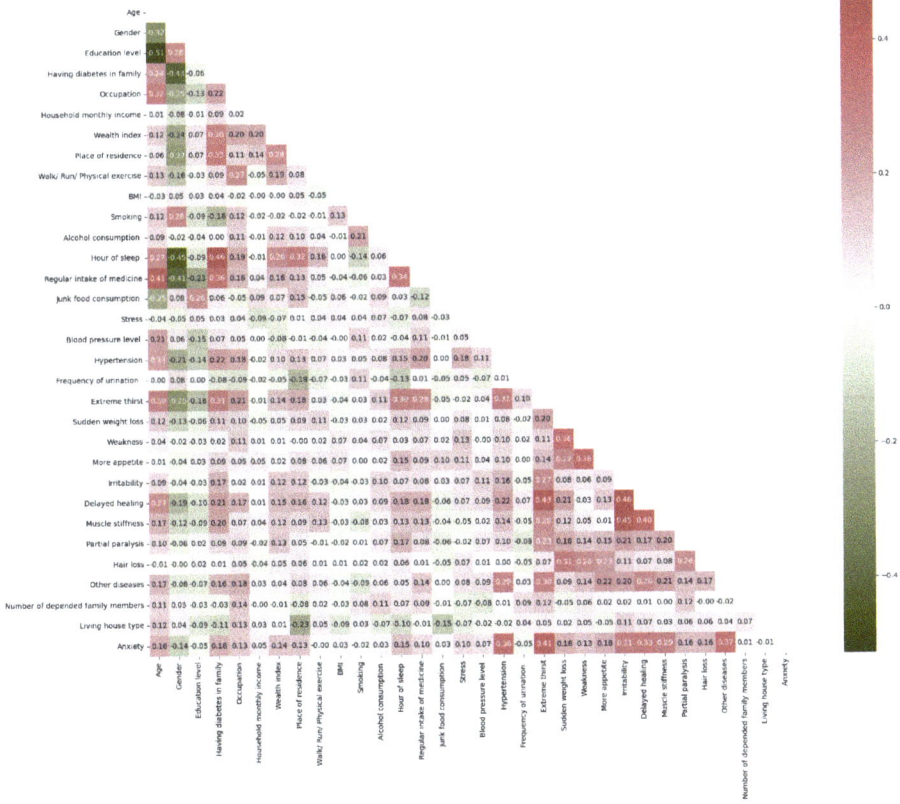

Figure 2. Heatmap between each of the features, representing the correlations between them.

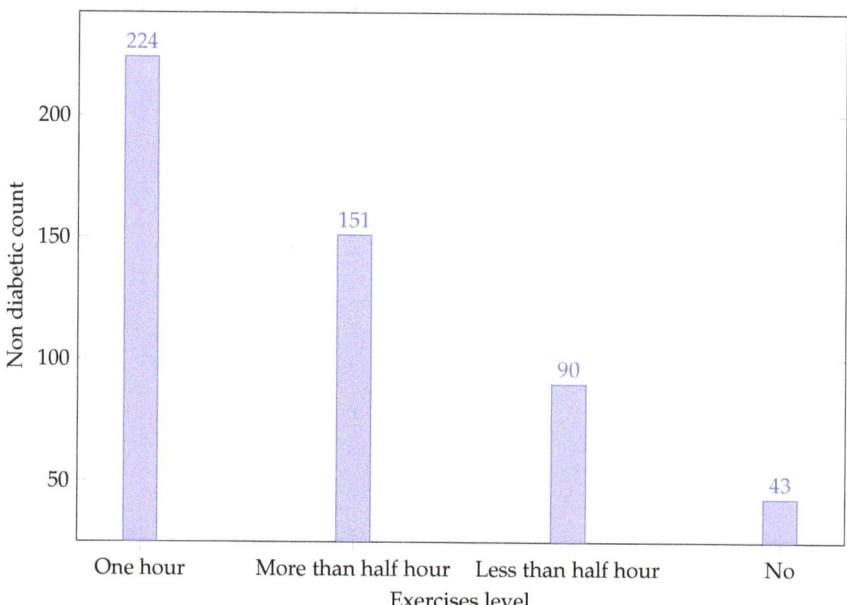

Figure 3. Relation between the output variable (non-diabetes) and the walk/run/physically active variable.

2.3. Data Preprocessing

We used the mean instead of the missing values for age and monthly household income found in our dataset. The BMI attribute was derived from the height and weight attributes. To scale the dataset, we also employed the standard scalar technique. The most important characteristic was determined using the recursive feature elimination technique. We rectified the class disparity using the SMOTE and ROS techniques.

2.4. Data Balancing Technique

In particular, when working with medical datasets, class imbalance is a prominent issue. This issue arises when instances are not distributed uniformly throughout the classes. As a result, the classifications of the classifiers become skewed, and the minority class is ignored. This problem can be resolved through either oversampling or undersampling. We utilized two oversampling techniques: the SMOTE and the ROS technique.

SMOTE is a method of oversampling in which the data points of minority classes are oversampled in order to balance the dataset [42]. It generates synthetic samples from minority classes and prevents duplication of samples, unlike standard oversampling algorithms. It randomly selects examples of the minority class, identifies their k nearest minority class neighbours, and then selects one of the neighbours [43].

On the other hand, ROS is a technique for balancing an unbalanced dataset prior to feeding it to ML classifiers in order to improve the performance and eliminate bias towards the majority class of the classifiers. Typically, it substantially increases the size of the dataset. It is a non-heuristic strategy that achieves data balancing by duplicating or replicating minority class samples at random [44].

2.5. Feature Transformation

The standard scalar is a process for scaling characteristics that removes the mean of every feature and normalizes its variance to one. It offers many benefits, including being smooth, bidirectional, swift, and highly scalable. The standard scalar's equation is presented below:

$$\hat{X}_i = \frac{X_i - \bar{X}}{\sigma} \quad (1)$$

where the standard scalar is represented as $\hat{X}_i$, each observation as X_i, the mean as $\bar{X}$, and the standard deviation as σ [45].

2.6. Feature Selection

Feature selection is the primary data dimension reduction procedure. It increases the accuracy of the classifier's predictions by identifying a collection of attributes that strongly contribute to the target class. It shortens the procedure and reduces the cost of computation. We used the recursive feature elimination (RFE) technique in our work. It is an iterative method for selecting features based on the model's accuracy. In each iteration, it calculates the ranking score metric and eliminates low-ranking characteristics. Until the required number of attributes has been reached, the recursive operation continues [46].

2.7. Statistical Methods Identifying the Most Significant and Associative Diabetes Features

The chi-square test employs the p value to determine the significance of a dependent variable-related characteristic. H_0 is a "null hypothesis", denoting that the target variable and categorical feature have nothing in common. H_1 is an alternative hypothesis that says there is a strong link between the categorical feature and target variable. If the p value is greater than 0.05, the null hypothesis cannot be rejected because there is no connection between the target variable and categorical features. If the p value is less than 0.05, the null hypothesis is rejected as there is evidence of a connection between the categorical characteristics and the target variable. All of these features are then used in the next step of the ML pipeline [47]. The equation for $\tilde{\chi}^2$ is given below:

$$\chi^2 = \sum_{k=1}^{n} \frac{(O_k - E_k)^2}{E_k} \quad (2)$$

where the observed frequencies is denoted as O_k, the expected frequencies as E_k, and the number of samples as n [46].

2.8. Machine Learning Model

In our work, we applied multiple ML algorithms to predict diabetes, including DT, LR, SVM, GBs, XGBs, RF, and our custom ETs.

- DT is a white box concept that has an effective learning component. Numerous leaf nodes, multiple internal nodes, and a central root node constitute DT. Each leaf node is labelled according to its class and linked to the root of the tree via internal nodes. A DT's root node serves as its beginning point, and the route from this node to its leaf nodes produces the classification rules [48].
- LR is an excellent method for predicting the probability of a result in a variety of classification situations. Commonly, the LR model is used when people can make predictions about health or illness. The LR algorithm predicts the probability of the target category dependent variable by applying the training examples to a logistic sigmoid activation function. In LR, the target attribute's calculated probability ranges from 0 to 1. Additionally, a threshold is established to classify an event into a certain target class. The predicted probability is input into a certain target category based on the threshold value [49,50].
- The SVM [51,52] is a type of linear generalized classifier that sorts binary data using supervised learning. It is appropriate for small data collections with minimal outliers. The goal is to identify a hyperplane that can be used to connect data points. This hyperplane divides the space into separate domains, each of which holding different kinds of data. There are numerous hyperplanes from which to choose to split the two groups of data. Our objective was to find the plane with the largest margin. The

margin is the distance between the hyperplane and two data points that are closest to it that represent two subclasses. The SVM attempts to optimize the algorithm by increasing this margin value, thereby determining the optimal superplane to divide the dataset into two layers. The nearest data points to the hyperplane are referred to as support vectors.

- GB is a prominent supervised ML method for disease forecasting since it creates an ensemble forecasting model using weak classifiers based on a DT. It constructs DTs using a gradient decent iterative optimization technique to discover the best parameter values, unlike RF. Then, we use the weighted majority votes from each DT to forecast the predicted value [53,54].
- XGBoost [55,56] constructs multiple new algorithms and merges them into a single ensemble model. First, the inaccuracy the of residuals for every observation is determined based on an established model. Based on previous errors, a revised model is developed to predict the residuals. The predictions of this model are then incorporated into the ensemble models. XGBoost is superior to GB algorithms because it finds a balance between bias and variation.
- RF is an ML algorithm that uses a random subspace approach and bagging ensemble learning. In the training stage, RF builds several DTs for arbitrarily partitioning data. For each node in the root DT, a subset of K attributes is chosen at random from the node's attribute set. From this subset, an effective attribute is then chosen for partitioning. Each tree submits a classification as a vote for the other trees, and the RF selects the classification with the most votes [29,57].
- ET is a procedure for data mining that combines multiple methods into a single optimal predictive model to improve predictions. This technique provides superior predictive performance when compared to a single model. We combined DT, XGB, and RF to benefits from all the algorithms to improve the overall predictive performance. By uniting the strengths of multiple models, ETs can provide enhanced generalization, increased robustness, and enhanced precision. It can help reduce individual model biases and improve model performance overall [58].

2.9. Model Evaluation

Employing accuracy, precision, recall, ROC-AUC, F1-score, geometric mean (GM), and log-loss, we assessed the ML classifiers. The entire dataset was divided into 10 parts using a 10-fold cross-validation technique. One part was utilized for model testing, while the other parts were employed for training the model in each fold. The evaluation procedure was performed 10 times [59]. Accuracy provides an accurate rating of the categorization. It is calculated as the ratio of the summation of the true positive (TPS) and true negative (TNG) in the whole population [60]. Precision is the percentage of predicted positives that are real [61]. Recall measures the models ability to categorize samples inside a class [62]. The F1-score maintains a balance between the classifier's precision and recall [63]. The log-loss computes the ambiguity of the method's probability by evaluating its exact labels [64]. A lower log-loss number suggests a more accurate forecast. ROC-AUC demonstrates the link between sensitivity and specificity as well as reflecting the model's capacity for discrimination. TPSs are those in which the model correctly recognizes the positive class. A TNG is a result which the model forecasts the negative class properly. When the model wrongly predicts the positive class, a false positive (FPS) is generated. False negatives (FNG) occur when models incorrectly predict the negative class.

$$Accuracy = \frac{TPS + TNG}{TPS + TNG + FPS + FNG} \quad (3)$$

$$Precision = \frac{TPS}{TPS + FPS} \quad (4)$$

$$Recall = \frac{TPS}{FNG + TPS} \tag{5}$$

$$FS = 2 * \frac{Precision * Recall}{Precision + Recall} \tag{6}$$

$$Log - loss = -\frac{1}{N}\sum_{i=1}^{N}(y_i, \log(p(y_i)) + (1 - y_i)\log(1 - \log(p(y_i)))) \tag{7}$$

$$GM = \sqrt{\frac{TPS}{TPS + FNG} * \frac{TNG}{TNG + FPS}} \tag{8}$$

3. Results and Discussion

We implemented seven ML models: DT, LR, SVM, GB, XGBoost, RF, and custom-built ET on the diabetes dataset. First, we discuss the experimental setup and hardware configuration. After this, we present the implementation output of each model with a comparative analysis. Finally, we provide a detailed discussion of our detection system.

3.1. Experimental Setup

We used the Google Co-laboratory platform, which provides the Jupyter Notebook Python language editor (version 3.7.13) and offers many built-in Python modules and packages through which we applied every ML model. In addition, we generated every plot and figure using 'matplotlib' in Python and 'ggplot2' within the R language. To determine the significance of a variable for the DT, GB, XGB, RF, and ET methods, we used the 'feature_importance_' approach; for SVM and LR, we used the 'coef_' technique. Various evaluation indicators were employed to assess their performance. We used a 10-fold cross-validation method on the dataset to produce a more reliable detection system.

3.2. Result Analysis

The experiment outcome for the primary dataset is displayed in Table 2. All classifiers had an accuracy between 80 and 90%. However, ET provided the best results with an accuracy of 87.60%. Then, GB, XGB, SVM, LR, and DT successively delivered the best results.

Table 2. Performance analysis of the various classifiers using the main diabetes dataset.

Classifier	DT	LR	SVM	XGB	GB	RF	ET
Accuracy	0.813	0.8386	0.8602	0.8661	0.8681	0.874	0.876
Precision	0.8409	0.8459	0.8864	0.8791	0.8741	0.8809	0.8926
Recall	0.8073	0.8582	0.8509	0.8727	0.8836	0.8873	0.8764
ROC-AUC	0.8135	0.8368	0.8611	0.8655	0.8667	0.8728	0.8760
F1-Score	0.8237	0.852	0.8683	0.8759	0.8788	0.8841	0.8844
Geometric Mean	0.8135	0.8365	0.861	0.8655	0.8665	0.8727	0.8759
Log-Loss	6.7404	5.8181	5.0376	4.8247	4.7538	4.5409	4.47

The classification results for the balanced dataset using SMOTE are subsequently displayed in Table 3. ET had the highest accuracy of 87.45%, precision of 87.05%, recall of 88%, ROC-AUC of 0.8745, F1-score of 87.52%, GM of 87.45%, and the lowest log-loss of 4.5218 in this scenario. DT, on the other hand, yielded the lowest results across all evaluation metrics. Therefore, the results demonstrate that GB, XGB, and SVM produce are clearly better than DT and LR.

Table 3. Performance analysis of the different classifiers using SMOTE.

Classifier	DT	LR	SVM	XGB	GB	RF	ET
Accuracy	0.8018	0.8509	0.8655	0.8691	0.8673	0.8636	0.8745
Precision	0.8029	0.8561	0.8708	0.8664	0.8686	0.8676	0.8705
Recall	0.8	0.8436	0.8582	0.8727	0.8655	0.8582	0.88
ROC-AUC	0.8018	0.8509	0.8655	0.8691	0.8673	0.8636	0.8745
F1-Score	0.8015	0.8498	0.8645	0.8696	0.867	0.8629	0.8752
Geometric Mean	0.8018	0.8509	0.8654	0.8691	0.8673	0.8636	0.8745
Log-Loss	7.1432	5.3738	4.8495	4.7184	4.784	4.915	4.5218

Table 4 shows the results of different classifiers in the balanced dataset using the ROS technique. In this scenario, ET had the best accuracy of 89.27%, precision of 89.71%, recall of 88.73%, ROC-AUC of 0.8927, F1-score of 89.21%, GM of 89.27%, and the lowest log-loss of 3.8665. DT, on the other hand, produced the worst results across all the evaluation metrics. XGB and RF all produced results that were very close for all evaluation metrics.

Table 4. Performance analysis of the different classifiers using the ROS technique.

Classifier	DT	LR	SVM	XGB	GB	RF	ET
Accuracy	0.8473	0.8527	0.8691	0.8873	0.8764	0.8891	0.8927
Precision	0.8577	0.8514	0.883	0.8959	0.8906	0.8934	0.8971
Recall	0.8327	0.8545	0.8509	0.8764	0.8582	0.8836	0.8873
ROC-AUC	0.8473	0.8527	0.8691	0.8873	0.8764	0.8891	0.8927
F1-Score	0.845	0.853	0.8667	0.886	0.8741	0.8885	0.8921
Geometric Mean	0.8471	0.8527	0.8689	0.8872	0.8762	0.8891	0.8927
Log Loss	5.5048	5.3082	4.7184	4.0631	4.4563	3.9976	3.8665

Table 5 depicts the outcomes of several classifiers using 20 significant features. All of them had an accuracy greater than 80%. ET displayed a maximum accuracy of 88.18%, precision of 89.77%, ROC-AUC of 0.8818, F1-score of 87.94%, GM of 88.16%, and a minimum log-loss of 3.8665. On the other hand, SVM generated the highest recall of 87.27% in comparison with other classifiers. However, XGB produced the second-best outcome. Furthermore, the other classifiers, such as SVM, GB, and RF, also produced excellent outcomes.

Table 5. Classification results (evaluation metrics) with 20 important features.

Classifier	DT	LR	SVM	XGB	GB	RF	ET	ET (Tuning)
Accuracy	0.8364	0.8545	0.8673	0.8782	0.8655	0.8764	0.8818	0.9927
Precision	0.8627	0.847	0.8633	0.891	0.8764	0.8848	0.8977	1
Recall	0.8	0.8655	0.8727	0.8618	0.8509	0.8655	0.8618	0.9855
ROC-AUC	0.8364	0.8545	0.8673	0.8782	0.8655	0.8764	0.8818	0.9927
F1-Score	0.8302	0.8561	0.868	0.8762	0.8635	0.875	0.8794	0.9927
Geometric Mean	0.8356	0.8545	0.8673	0.878	0.8653	0.8763	0.8816	0.9927
Log-Loss	5.8981	5.2427	4.784	4.3908	4.8495	4.4563	4.2597	0.2621

In addition, we optimized the hypeparameters of the ET algorithm for the highest performance. ET exhibited 99.27% accuracy, 100% precision, 98.55% recall, 0.9927 ROC-AUC, 99.27% F1-score, 99.27% GM, and 0.2621 log-loss.

Figure 4 illustrates the associative features with T2DM using $-log_{10}(P)$. The $-log_{10}(P)$ function changes the p value into a range of positive numbers that can be used to make good decisions for each feature. If the value of $-log_{10}(P)$ is greater than 1.301, then the feature is considered significant. Furthermore, a high $-log_{10}(P)$ value indicates a highly significant feature. The results show that age is the most significant element, whereas smoking is the least significant component. Other significant factors include extreme thirst, gender, regular intake of medicine, and having diabetes in the family; while stress and living house type are less significant.

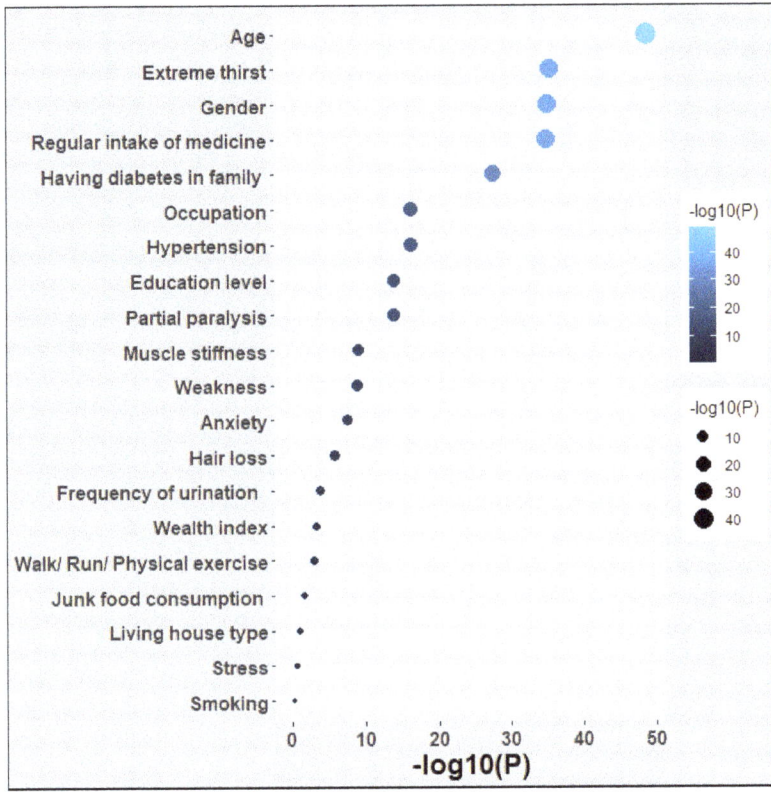

Figure 4. Significance of the features, *p* values with negative 10 base logarithm. The lighter and larger bubbles represent more significance.

Our research also revealed the significance of features, estimated based on the mean coefficient value of every classifier employed. We calculated feature significance values for every method and then normalized them by applying the min–max technique to ensure that they ranged between 0 and 1. Next, we determined the mean scores for every characteristic. In Table 6, we examined the significance of the diabetic features and found that age was the most significant attribute (average coefficient value 0.99). Other crucial elements included having diabetes in the family, regular intake of medicine, extreme thirst, etc. The least important characteristics included muscle stiffness, living house type, stress, wealth index, etc. The ROC curves [65] for each classification method are shown in Figure 5. We observed that the ET classifier performed better than the rest of the classifiers in the ROC curves.

Table 6. Feature ranking using ML techniques based on coefficient values.

Feature Name	DT	SVM	LR	RF	XGB	GB	ET	Avg.	Rank
Age	1	0.95	1	1	1	1	1	0.99	1
Having diabetes in family	0.26	1	0.94	0.45	0.34	0.23	0.23	0.49	2
Regular intake of medicine	0.08	0.89	0.79	0.48	0.13	0.2	0.19	0.39	3
Extreme thirst	0.08	0.82	0.75	0.39	0.15	0.13	0.19	0.36	4
Occupation	0.06	0.77	0.67	0.17	0.03	0.04	0.06	0.26	5
Frequency of urination	0.04	0.66	0.57	0.06	0.05	0.04	0.04	0.21	6
Walk/ Run/ Physically exercise	0.06	0.62	0.56	0.13	0.01	0.02	0.03	0.21	6

Table 6. Cont.

Feature Name	DT	SVM	LR	RF	XGB	GB	ET	Avg.	Rank
Weakness	0.06	0.57	0.58	0.11	0.01	0.02	0.05	0.2	7
Smoking	0.05	0.67	0.66	0	0.01	0	0.01	0.2	7
Junk food consumption	0.05	0.64	0.6	0.02	0.03	0	0.01	0.19	8
Partial paralysis	0	0.6	0.58	0.06	0.05	0.02	0.03	0.19	8
Education level	0.08	0.36	0.37	0.22	0.02	0.04	0.09	0.17	9
Hypertension	0.01	0.51	0.53	0.09	0	0.01	0.02	0.17	9
Gender	0.18	0	0	0.48	0.21	0.14	0.21	0.17	9
Hair loss	0.05	0.43	0.38	0.12	0.01	0.01	0.04	0.15	10
Anxiety	0.02	0.43	0.37	0.05	0.01	0	0.02	0.13	11
Wealth index	0.01	0.34	0.33	0.04	0.02	0	0.02	0.11	12
Stress	0.04	0.25	0.25	0.1	0.03	0.02	0.04	0.11	12
Living house type	0.02	0.38	0.34	0	0	0	0	0.11	12
Muscle stiffness	0.04	0.26	0.27	0.06	0.01	0.01	0.05	0.1	13

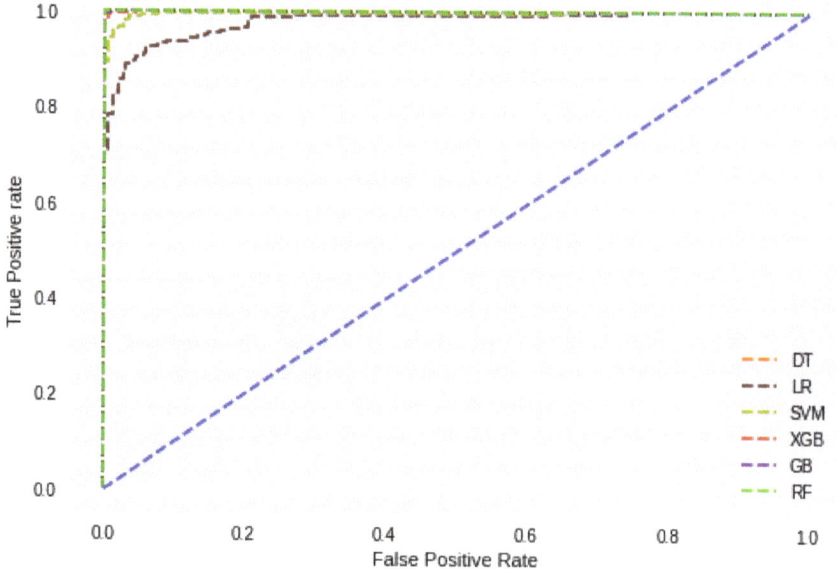

Figure 5. Comparison of the ROC curves obtained by using the seven ML classifiers.

3.3. Discussion

The detection of diabetes may play a crucial role in the management of this disease. Initially, we preprocessed the dataset and then normalized the entire dataset using scaling techniques. We independently applied statistical and ML algorithms to the dataset. In the statistical study, the most relevant characteristics were found, but in the ML classification approaches, the patients were divided into diabetic and non-diabetic. We ordered the characteristics of diabetes according to their significance.

ML techniques are widely accepted as a way to display disease-related characteristics as distinguishing indicators in predicting disease diagnoses such as diabetes [66–68]. The potential of ML methods to uncover hidden trends in data by analysing a set of attributes might result in a deeper comprehension. The classification results with a high degree of precision imply a reliable prognosis and ensure practical applicability. The majority of models studied here are capable of making correct predictions since their accuracy, precision, recall, ROC-AUC, F1-score, and GM were all greater than 80%. Excellent model performance was shown by a small log-loss value in binary classification. In comparison to other models, the ET model reached the highest degree of accuracy.

Our findings imply a number of crucial and relevant characteristics. Depending on the log-based association, the most significant characteristics include age, extreme thirst, and gender. In the ML models, the most essential features are age, having diabetes in the family, regular intake of medicine, and extreme thirst. Our analysis reveals that significant features are adequate for detecting diabetes, and this will aid in the implementation of diagnosing diabetes.

We also compared our findings to prior research based on ML techniques, represented in Table 7. Pranto et al. [31] utilized female diabetic patients from Bangladesh to predict an accuracy of 81.2%, precision of 80%, and an F1-score of 88%. In another study, Syed and Khan [69] developed a data-driven predictive model to screen for T2DM in the western region of Saudi Arabia, achieving 82.1% accuracy, 77.6% precision, 89% recall, 0.867 ROC-AUC, and 82.9% F1-score. Next, Chou et al. [70] predicted the onset of diabetes using ML methods, achieving 95.3% accuracy, 92.7% precision, 93.1% recall, 0.991 ROC-AUC, and 92.9% F1-score. Then, Laila et al. [71] used an ensemble-based ML model to predict diabetes with an accuracy of 97.11%, precision of 97.1%, recall of 97.1%, and an F1-score of 97.1%. In contrast, our proposed framework outperformed the previous studies, achieving an accuracy of 99.27%, precision of 100%, ROC-AUC of 0.9927, and an F1-score of 99.27%. Additionally, we computed a GM of 99.27% and a log-loss of 0.2621. We also determined the most significant characteristic using both log-based correlations and ML models. It is important to note that this study was conducted with a limited sample size, restricting the generalizability of the findings. Nevertheless, this approach shows promise as a predictive method for real-world applications and could greatly assist practitioners in prompt diabetes diagnosis.

Table 7. Comparing the performance of the proposed model with existing studies.

Reference	Dataset	Accuracy	Precision	Recall	ROC-AUC	F1-Score	Geometric Mean	Log-Loss
Pranto et al. [31]	PIMA, Kurmitola Hospital, Dhaka	0.8120	0.8	1	0.84	0.88	–	–
Syed and Khan [69]	Western Region of Saudi Arabia	0.821	0.776	0.89	0.867	0.829	–	–
Chou et al. [70]	Taipei Municipal Medical Center	0.953	0.927	0.931	0.991	0.929	–	–
Laila et al. [71]	UCI Repository	0.9711	0.971	0.971	–	0.971	–	–
This study	Bangladesh, 2022	0.9927	1	0.9855	0.9927	0.9927	0.9927	0.2621

The proposed framework for diabetes detection, utilizing an ensemble-based ML approach, offers several advantages compared to the existing gold standard methods. This is particularly crucial in Bangladesh, where there is a shortage of diabetologists relative to the country's population. While the gold standard relies on costly and time-consuming lab-based diagnostics and manual interpretation of clinical data by diabetologists, our automated approach can help alleviate the burden on healthcare providers, allowing them to efficiently screen a larger number of individuals for diabetes risk. Through the application of statistical and ML techniques, this study identified age, extreme thirst, and family history of diabetes as key features that play instrumental roles in diabetes detection. By implementing the proposed framework in clinical settings, healthcare providers can proactively identify individuals at risk of diabetes based on their risk factors. This prompt identification enables timely intervention and personalized care, helping to mitigate the risks and severity associated with diabetes.

4. Conclusions

Our proposed ET with hyperparameter tuning outperformed the other ML models to identify T2DM patients in this region. We obtained an outstanding accuracy of 99.27% and an F1-score of 99.27%. In addition, using various statistical and ML models we determined four key factors: age, having diabetes in the family, regular intake of medicine, and extreme thirst, highly associated with diabetes. Since our proposed diabetes detection system has a high degree of precision, physicians and clinicians may use our proposed framework to assess diabetes risk. In Bangladesh, the ratio of diabetic patients to physicians is insufficient, and there are less detection instruments available across the country. Therefore, a fast diagnosis system based on ML is effective for patients and diabetologists. In this study, we found that a number of lifestyle factors are associated with the development of diabetes; therefore, sustaining a lifestyle that includes the observance of these factors could reduce the rate of diabetes progression. The quantity of data was a primary limitation in our study. In the future, we will use additional data to investigate diabetes as well as other medical conditions such as kidney disease, heart disease, and breast cancer. We will also incorporate our proposed system into intuitive web and mobile application platforms. Finally, we will concentrate on diabetes mellitus disease prevention and recovery strategies.

Author Contributions: Conceptualization, M.J.U. and M.M.A.; methodology, M.J.U.; software, M.J.U. and M.M.A.; validation, M.J.U., M.A.K. and M.M.A.; formal analysis, M.J.U., S.A. and M.M.A.; investigation, M.J.U., N.A, S.A.A. and M.M.A.; resources, M.J.U., N.A, and S.A.A.; data curation, M.J.U.; writing—original draft preparation, M.J.U., S.A, M.N.H., M.A.A.W., N.A. and M.M.A.; writing—review and editing, S.A.A., N.A, M.A.K. and M.A.M.; visualization, M.J.U., M.A.A.W., M.A.K. and M.M.A.; supervision, M.A.M.; project administration, S.A.A., N.A and M.A.M.; funding acquisition, S.A.A. All authors have read and agreed to the published version of the manuscript.

Funding: The authors extend their appreciation to the Deanship of Scientific Research at Imam Mohammad Ibn Saud Islamic University (IMSIU) for funding and supporting this work through Research Partnership Program no RP-21-09-09.

Informed Consent Statement: Written informed consent has been obtained from the patient(s) to publish this paper.

Data Availability Statement: Data will be available only for research purposes. Please email to the corresponding author for further information.

Acknowledgments: The authors would like to thank all the participants who participated in this survey. Furthermore, we also give thanks to Bangabandhu Sheikh Mujibur Rahman Science and Technology University Research Cell for supporting the data collection.

Conflicts of Interest: The authors declare no conflict of interest.

Abbreviations

The following abbreviations are used in this manuscript:

ML	Machine learning
DT	Decision tree
RF	Random forest
LR	Logistic regression
SVM	Support vector machine
GB	Gradient boosting

References

1. Association, A.D. Diagnosis and classification of diabetes mellitus. *Diabetes Care* **2014**, *37*, S81–S90. [CrossRef] [PubMed]
2. IDF. Type 2 Diabetes. Available online: https://www.idf.org/aboutdiabetes/type-2-diabetes.html (accessed on 7 May 2023).
3. John, J.E.; John, N.A. Imminent risk of COVID-19 in diabetes mellitus and undiagnosed diabetes mellitus patients. *Pan Afr. Med. J.* **2020**, *32874422*. [CrossRef] [PubMed]
4. Gahlan, D.; Rajput, R.; Singh, V. Metabolic syndrome in north indian type 2 diabetes mellitus patients: A comparison of four different diagnostic criteria of metabolic syndrome. *Diabetes Metab. Syndr.* **2019**, *13*, 356–362. [CrossRef] [PubMed]

5. Atlas, I.D. Diabetes around the World in 2021. Available online: https://diabetesatlas.org/ (accessed on 7 May 2023).
6. Williams, R.; Karuranga, S.; Malanda, B.; Saeedi, P.; Basit, A.; Besançon, S.; Bommer, C.; Esteghamati, A.; Ogurtsova, K.; Zhang, P.; et al. Global and regional estimates and projections of diabetes-related health expenditure: Results from the International Diabetes Federation Diabetes Atlas. *Diabetes Res. Clin. Pract.* **2020**, *162*, 108072. [CrossRef] [PubMed]
7. Htay, T.; Soe, K.; Lopez-Perez, A.; Doan, A.H.; Romagosa, M.A.; Aung, K. Mortality and cardiovascular disease in type 1 and type 2 diabetes. *Curr. Cardiol. Rep.* **2019**, *21*, 45. [CrossRef]
8. Nipa, N.; Riyad, M.M.H.; Satu, M.S.; Walliullah, M.; Howlader, K.C.; Moni, M.A. Clinically Adaptable Machine Learning Model To Identify Early Appreciable Features of Diabetes In Bangladesh. *Intell. Med.* **2023**. [CrossRef]
9. Huang, Y.; Roy, N.; Dhar, E.; Upadhyay, U.; Kabir, M.A.; Uddin, M.; Tseng, C.L.; Syed-Abdul, S. Deep Learning Prediction Model for Patient Survival Outcomes in Palliative Care Using Actigraphy Data and Clinical Information. *Cancers* **2023**, *15*, 2232. [CrossRef]
10. Panday, A.; Kabir, M.A.; Chowdhury, N.K. A survey of machine learning techniques for detecting and diagnosing COVID-19 from imaging. *Quant. Biol.* **2022**, *10*. [CrossRef]
11. Uddin, M.J.; Ahamad, M.M.; Sarker, P.K.; Aktar, S.; Alotaibi, N.; Alyami, S.A.; Kabir, M.A.; Moni, M.A. An Integrated Statistical and Clinically Applicable Machine Learning Framework for the Detection of Autism Spectrum Disorder. *Computers* **2023**, *12*, 92. [CrossRef]
12. Hossain, M.D.; Kabir, M.A.; Anwar, A.; Islam, M.Z. Detecting autism spectrum disorder using machine learning techniques: An experimental analysis on toddler, child, adolescent and adult datasets. *Health Inf. Sci. Syst.* **2021**, *9*, 17. [CrossRef]
13. Aguilera-Venegas, G.; López-Molina, A.; Rojo-Martínez, G.; Galán-García, J.L. Comparing and tuning machine learning algorithms to predict type 2 diabetes mellitus. *J. Comput. Appl. Math.* **2023**, *427*, 115115. [CrossRef]
14. Zhao, M.; Wan, J.; Qin, W.; Huang, X.; Chen, G.; Zhao, X. A machine learning-based diagnosis modelling of type 2 diabetes mellitus with environmental metal exposure. *Comput. Methods Programs Biomed.* **2023**, *235*, 107537. [CrossRef] [PubMed]
15. Xia, S.; Zhang, Y.; Peng, B.; Hu, X.; Zhou, L.; Chen, C.; Lu, C.; Chen, M.; Pang, C.; Dai, Y.; et al. Detection of mild cognitive impairment in type 2 diabetes mellitus based on machine learning using privileged information. *Neurosci. Lett.* **2022**, *791*, 136908. [CrossRef] [PubMed]
16. Ejiyi, C.J.; Qin, Z.; Amos, J.; Ejiyi, M.B.; Nnani, A.; Ejiyi, T.U.; Agbesi, V.K.; Diokpo, C.; Okpara, C. A robust predictive diagnosis model for diabetes mellitus using Shapley-incorporated machine learning algorithms. *Healthc. Anal.* **2023**, *3*, 100166. [CrossRef]
17. Hennebelle, A.; Materwala, H.; Ismail, L. HealthEdge: A Machine Learning-Based Smart Healthcare Framework for Prediction of Type 2 Diabetes in an Integrated IoT, Edge, and Cloud Computing System. *Procedia Comput. Sci.* **2023**, *220*, 331–338. [CrossRef]
18. Haque, M.; Alharbi, I. A Dataset-Specific Machine Learning Study for Predicting Diabetes (Type-2) in a Developing Country Context. *Indian J. Sci. Technol.* **2022**, *15*, 1932–1940. [CrossRef]
19. Tasin, I.; Nabil, T.U.; Islam, S.; Khan, R. Diabetes prediction using machine learning and explainable AI techniques. *Healthc. Technol. Lett.* **2022**, 1684017. [CrossRef]
20. Kaur, H.; Kumari, V. Predictive modelling and analytics for diabetes using a machine learning approach. *Appl. Comput. Inform.* **2022**, *18*, 90–100. [CrossRef]
21. Zheng, T.; Xie, W.; Xu, L.; He, X.; Zhang, Y.; You, M.; Yang, G.; Chen, Y. A machine learning-based framework to identify type 2 diabetes through electronic health records. *Int. J. Med. Inform.* **2017**, *97*, 120–127. [CrossRef]
22. Saha, P.K.; Patwary, N.S.; Ahmed, I. A widespread study of diabetes prediction using several machine learning techniques. In Proceedings of the 2019 22nd International Conference on Computer and Information Technology (ICCIT), Dhaka, Bangladesh, 18–20 December 2019; IEEE: Piscataway NJ, USA, 2019; pp. 1–5.
23. Ali, M.S.; Islam, M.K.; Das, A.A.; Duranta, D.; Haque, M.; Rahman, M.H. A novel approach for best parameters selection and feature engineering to analyze and detect diabetes: Machine learning insights. *Biomed Res. Int.* **2023**, 8583210. [CrossRef]
24. Howlader, K.C.; Satu, M.S.; Awal, M.A.; Islam, M.R.; Islam, S.M.S.; Quinn, J.M.; Moni, M.A. Machine learning models for classification and identification of significant attributes to detect type 2 diabetes. *Health Inf. Sci. Syst.* **2022**, *10*, 2. [CrossRef] [PubMed]
25. Wei, S.; Zhao, X.; Miao, C. A comprehensive exploration to the machine learning techniques for diabetes identification. In Proceedings of the 2018 IEEE 4th World Forum on Internet of Things (WF-IoT), Singapore, 5–8 February 2018; IEEE: Piscataway NJ, USA, 2018; pp. 291–295.
26. Birjais, R.; Mourya, A.K.; Chauhan, R.; Kaur, H. Prediction and diagnosis of future diabetes risk: A machine learning approach. *SN Appl. Sci.* **2019**, *1*, 1112. [CrossRef]
27. Yahyaoui, A.; Jamil, A.; Rasheed, J.; Yesiltepe, M. A decision support system for diabetes prediction using machine learning and deep learning techniques. In Proceedings of the 2019 1st International Informatics and Software Engineering Conference (UBMYK), Ankara, Turkey, 6–7 November 2019; IEEE: Piscataway NJ, USA, 2019; pp. 1–4.
28. Abdulhadi, N.; Al-Mousa, A. Diabetes detection using machine learning classification methods. In Proceedings of the 2021 International Conference on Information Technology (ICIT), Amman, Jordan, 14–15 July 2021; IEEE: Piscataway NJ, USA, 2021; pp. 350–354.
29. Battineni, G.; Sagaro, G.G.; Nalini, C.; Amenta, F.; Tayebati, S.K. Comparative machine-learning approach: A follow-up study on type 2 diabetes predictions by cross-validation methods. *Machines* **2019**, *7*, 74. [CrossRef]

30. Tigga, N.P.; Garg, S. Prediction of Type 2 Diabetes using Machine Learning Classification Methods. *Procedia Comput. Sci.* **2020**, *167*, 706–716. [CrossRef]
31. Pranto, B.; Mehnaz, S.M.; Mahid, E.B.; Sadman, I.M.; Rahman, A.; Momen, S. Evaluating machine learning methods for predicting diabetes among female patients in Bangladesh. *Information* **2020**, *11*, 374. [CrossRef]
32. Sneha, N.; Gangil, T. Analysis of diabetes mellitus for early prediction using optimal features selection. *J. Big Data* **2019**, *121*, 54–64. [CrossRef]
33. Zhang, L.; Wang, Y.; Niu, M.; Wang, C.; Wang, Z. Machine learning for characterizing risk of type 2 diabetes mellitus in a rural Chinese population: The Henan Rural Cohort Study. *Sci. Rep.* **2020**, *10*, 4406. [CrossRef]
34. Bonifazi, G.; Enrico Corradini, D.U.; Virgili, L. Defining user spectra to classify Ethereum users based on their behavior. *J. Big Data* **2022**, *9*, 37. [CrossRef]
35. Le, T.M.; Vo, T.M.; Pham, T.N.; Dao, S.V.T. A novel wrapper–based feature selection for early diabetes prediction enhanced with a metaheuristic. *IEEE Access* **2020**, *9*, 7869–7884. [CrossRef]
36. Islam, M.M.; Rahman, M.J.; Roy, D.C.; Maniruzzaman, M. Automated detection and classification of diabetes disease based on Bangladesh demographic and health survey data, 2011 using machine learning approach. *Diabetes Metab. Syndr. Clin. Res. Rev.* **2020**, *14*, 217–219. [CrossRef]
37. Haq, A.U.; Li, J.P.; Khan, J.; Memon, M.H.; Nazir, S.; Ahmad, S.; Khan, G.A.; Ali, A. Intelligent machine learning approach for effective recognition of diabetes in E-healthcare using clinical data. *Sensors* **2020**, *20*, 2649. [CrossRef] [PubMed]
38. Shuja, M.; Mittal, S.; Zaman, M. Effective Prediction of Type II Diabetes Mellitus Using Data Mining Classifiers and SMOTE. In *Proceedings of the Advances in Computing and Intelligent Systems*; Sharma, H., Govindan, K., Poonia, R.C., Kumar, S., El-Medany, W.M., Eds.; Springer: Singapore, 2020; pp. 195–211.
39. Chatrati, S.P.; Hossain, G.; Goyal, A.; Bhan, A.; Bhattacharya, S.; Gaurav, D.; Tiwari, S.M. Smart home health monitoring system for predicting type 2 diabetes and hypertension. *J. King Saud Univ. Comput. Inf. Sci.* **2022**, *34*, 862–870. [CrossRef]
40. Islam, M.M.; Rahman, M.J.; Menhazul Abedin, M.; Ahammed, B.; Ali, M.; Ahmed, N.F.; Maniruzzaman, M. Identification of the risk factors of type 2 diabetes and its prediction using machine learning techniques. *Health Syst.* **2022**, *12*, 243–254. [CrossRef] [PubMed]
41. Islam, S.M.S.; Islam, M.T.; Uddin, R.; Tansi, T.; Talukder, S.; Sarker, F.; Mamun, K.A.A.; Adibi, S.; Rawal, L.B. Factors associated with low medication adherence in patients with Type 2 diabetes mellitus attending a tertiary hospital in Bangladesh. *Lifestyle Med.* **2021**, *2*, e47. [CrossRef]
42. Nnamoko, N.; Korkontzelos, I. Efficient treatment of outliers and class imbalance for diabetes prediction. *Artif. Intell. Med.* **2020**, *104*, 101815. [CrossRef] [PubMed]
43. Ganie, S.M.; Malik, M.B. An ensemble Machine Learning approach for predicting Type-II diabetes mellitus based on lifestyle indicators. *Healthc. Anal.* **2022**, *2*, 100092. [CrossRef]
44. Petmezas, G.; Haris, K.; Stefanopoulos, L.; Kilintzis, V.; Tzavelis, A.; Rogers, J.A.; Katsaggelos, A.K.; Maglaveras, N. Automated atrial fibrillation detection using a hybrid CNN-LSTM network on imbalanced ECG datasets. *Biomed. Signal Process. Control* **2021**, *63*, 102194. [CrossRef]
45. Mehedi Hassan, M.; Mollick, S.; Yasmin, F. An unsupervised cluster-based feature grouping model for early diabetes detection. *Healthc. Anal.* **2022**, *2*, 100112. [CrossRef]
46. Deberneh, H.M.; Kim, I. Prediction of Type 2 Diabetes Based on Machine Learning Algorithm. *Int. J. Environ. Res. Public Health* **2021**, *18*, 3317. [CrossRef]
47. Aktar, S.; Ahamad, M.M.; Rashed-Al-Mahfuz, M.; Azad, A.; Uddin, S.; Kamal, A.; Alyami, S.A.; Lin, P.I.; Islam, S.M.S.; Quinn, J.M.; et al. Machine learning approach to predicting COVID-19 disease severity based on clinical blood test data: Statistical analysis and model development. *JMIR Med. Inform.* **2021**, *9*, e25884. [CrossRef]
48. Azad, C.; Bhushan, B.; Sharma, R.; Shankar, A.; Singh, K.K.; Khamparia, A. Prediction model using SMOTE, genetic algorithm and decision tree (PMSGD) for classification of diabetes mellitus. *Multimed. Syst.* **2022**, *28*, 1289–1307. [CrossRef]
49. Maniruzzaman, M.; Rahman, M.; Al-MehediHasan, M.; Suri, H.S.; Abedin, M.; El-Baz, A.; Suri, J.S. Accurate diabetes risk stratification using machine learning: Role of missing value and outliers. *J. Med. Syst.* **2018**, *42*, 92. [CrossRef]
50. Ahlqvist, E.; Storm, P.; Käräjämäki, A.; Martinell, M.; Dorkhan, M.; Carlsson, A.; Vikman, P.; Prasad, R.B.; Aly, D.M.; Almgren, P.; et al. Novel subgroups of adult-onset diabetes and their association with outcomes: A data-driven cluster analysis of six variables. *Lancet Diabetes Endocrinol.* **2018**, *6*, 361–369. [CrossRef]
51. Boubin, M.; Shrestha, S. Microcontroller implementation of support vector machine for detecting blood glucose levels using breath volatile organic compounds. *Sensors* **2019**, *19*, 2283. [CrossRef] [PubMed]
52. Muhammad, L.; Algehyne, E.A.; Usman, S.S. Predictive supervised machine learning models for diabetes mellitus. *SN Comput. Sci.* **2020**, *1*, 240. [CrossRef] [PubMed]
53. Islam, M.M.; Rahman, M.J.; Roy, D.C.; Tawabunnahar, M.; Jahan, R.; Ahmed, N.F.; Maniruzzaman, M. Machine learning algorithm for characterizing risks of hypertension, at an early stage in Bangladesh. *Diabetes Metab. Syndr. Clin. Res. Rev.* **2021**, *15*, 877–884. [CrossRef] [PubMed]
54. Ahamad, M.M.; Aktar, S.; Rashed-Al-Mahfuz, M.; Uddin, S.; Liò, P.; Xu, H.; Summers, M.A.; Quinn, J.M.; Moni, M.A. A machine learning model to identify early stage symptoms of SARS-Cov-2 infected patients. *Expert Syst. Appl.* **2020**, *160*, 113661. [CrossRef] [PubMed]

55. Dutta, A.; Hasan, M.K.; Ahmad, M.; Awal, M.A.; Islam, M.A.; Masud, M.; Meshref, H. Early prediction of diabetes using an ensemble of machine learning models. *Int. J. Environ. Res. Public Health* **2022**, *19*, 12378. [CrossRef]
56. Kibria, H.B.; Nahiduzzaman, M.; Goni, M.O.F.; Ahsan, M.; Haider, J. An ensemble approach for the prediction of diabetes mellitus using a soft voting classifier with an explainable AI. *Sensors* **2022**, *22*, 7268. [CrossRef] [PubMed]
57. Ijaz, M.F.; Alfian, G.; Syafrudin, M.; Rhee, J. Hybrid prediction model for type 2 diabetes and hypertension using DBSCAN-based outlier detection, synthetic minority over sampling technique (SMOTE), and random forest. *Appl. Sci.* **2018**, *8*, 1325. [CrossRef]
58. Amelio, A.; Bonifazi, G.; Corradini, E.; Di Saverio, S.; Marchetti, M.; Ursino, D.; Virgili, L. Defining a deep neural network ensemble for identifying fabric colors. *Appl. Soft Comput.* **2022**, *130*, 109687. [CrossRef]
59. Islam, S.M.S.; Talukder, A.; Awal, M.A.; Siddiqui, M.M.U.; Ahamad, M.M.; Ahammed, B.; Rawal, L.B.; Alizadehsani, R.; Abawajy, J.; Laranjo, L.; et al. Machine Learning Approaches for Predicting Hypertension and Its Associated Factors Using Population-Level Data From Three South Asian Countries. *Front. Cardiovasc. Med.* **2022**, *9*, 839379. [CrossRef] [PubMed]
60. Akter, T.; Ali, M.H.; Khan, M.I.; Satu, M.S.; Uddin, M.J.; Alyami, S.A.; Ali, S.; Azad, A.; Moni, M.A. Improved transfer-learning-based facial recognition framework to detect autistic children at an early stage. *Brain Sci.* **2021**, *11*, 734. [CrossRef] [PubMed]
61. Ahamad, M.M.; Aktar, S.; Uddin, M.J.; Rahman, T.; Alyami, S.A.; Al-Ashhab, S.; Akhdar, H.F.; Azad, A.; Moni, M.A. Early-Stage Detection of Ovarian Cancer Based on Clinical Data Using Machine Learning Approaches. *J. Pers. Med.* **2022**, *12*, 1211. [CrossRef]
62. Ahamad, M.M.; Aktar, S.; Uddin, M.J.; Rashed-Al-Mahfuz, M.; Azad, A.; Uddin, S.; Alyami, S.A.; Sarker, I.H.; Khan, A.; Liò, P.; et al. Adverse effects of COVID-19 vaccination: Machine learning and statistical approach to identify and classify incidences of morbidity and postvaccination reactogenicity. *Healthcare* **2022**, *11*, 31. [CrossRef]
63. Akter, T.; Khan, M.I.; Ali, M.H.; Satu, M.S.; Uddin, M.J.; Moni, M.A. Improved machine learning based classification model for early autism detection. In Proceedings of the 2021 2nd International Conference on Robotics, Electrical and Signal Processing Techniques (ICREST), Dhaka, Bangladesh, 5–7 January 2021; IEEE: Piscataway, NJ, USA, 2021; pp. 742–747.
64. Akter, T.; Satu, M.S.; Khan, M.I.; Ali, M.H.; Uddin, S.; Lio, P.; Quinn, J.M.; Moni, M.A. Machine learning-based models for early stage detection of autism spectrum disorders. *IEEE Access* **2019**, *7*, 166509–166527. [CrossRef]
65. Xiong, Y.; Lin, L.; Chen, Y.; Salerno, S.; Li, Y.; Zeng, X.; Li, H. Prediction of gestational diabetes mellitus in the first 19 weeks of pregnancy using machine learning techniques. *J. Matern. Fetal Neonatal Med.* **2022**, *35*, 2457–2463. [CrossRef]
66. Olisah, C.C.; Smith, L.; Smith, M. Diabetes mellitus prediction and diagnosis from a data preprocessing and machine learning perspective. *Comput. Methods Programs Biomed.* **2022**, *220*, 106773. [CrossRef]
67. Wei, H.; Sun, J.; Shan, W.; Xiao, W.; Wang, B.; Ma, X.; Hu, W.; Wang, X.; Xia, Y. Environmental chemical exposure dynamics and machine learning-based prediction of diabetes mellitus. *Sci. Total Environ.* **2022**, *806*, 150674. [CrossRef]
68. Rawat, V.; Joshi, S.; Gupta, S.; Singh, D.P.; Singh, N. Machine learning algorithms for early diagnosis of diabetes mellitus: A comparative study. *Mater. Today Proc.* **2022**, *56*, 502–506.
69. Syed, A.H.; Khan, T. Machine learning-based application for predicting risk of type 2 diabetes mellitus (T2DM) in Saudi Arabia: A retrospective cross-sectional study. *IEEE Access* **2020**, *8*, 199539–199561. [CrossRef]
70. Chou, C.Y.; Hsu, D.Y.; Chou, C.H. Predicting the Onset of Diabetes with Machine Learning Methods. *J. Pers. Med.* **2023**, *13*, 406. [CrossRef] [PubMed]
71. Laila, U.E.; Mahboob, K.; Khan, A.W.; Khan, F.; Taekeun, W. An ensemble approach to predict early-stage diabetes risk using machine learning: An empirical study. *Sensors* **2022**, *22*, 5247. [CrossRef] [PubMed]

Disclaimer/Publisher's Note: The statements, opinions and data contained in all publications are solely those of the individual author(s) and contributor(s) and not of MDPI and/or the editor(s). MDPI and/or the editor(s) disclaim responsibility for any injury to people or property resulting from any ideas, methods, instructions or products referred to in the content.

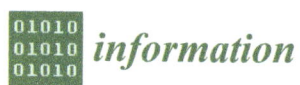 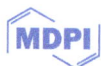

Article

Public Health Implications for Effective Community Interventions Based on Hospital Patient Data Analysis Using Deep Learning Technology in Indonesia

Lenni Dianna Putri [1], Ermi Girsang [1], I Nyoman Ehrich Lister [1], Hsiang Tsung Kung [2], Evizal Abdul Kadir [2,*] and Sri Listia Rosa [3]

1. Department of Public Health, Faculty of Health Science, Universitas Prima Indonesia, Medan 20118, Indonesia; lennidiannaputri@unprimdn.ac.id (L.D.P.); ermigirsang@unprimdn.ac.id (E.G.); nyoman@unprimdn.ac.id (I.N.E.L.)
2. Department of Computer Science, Harvard University, Cambridge, MA 02134, USA
3. Department of Informatics, Faculty of Engineering, Universitas Islam Riau, Pekanbaru 28284, Indonesia; srilistiarosa@eng.uir.ac.id
* Correspondence: evizal@eng.uir.ac.id

Citation: Putri, L.D.; Girsang, E.; Lister, I.N.E.; Kung, H.T.; Kadir, E.A.; Rosa, S.L. Public Health Implications for Effective Community Interventions Based on Hospital Patient Data Analysis Using Deep Learning Technology in Indonesia. *Information* **2024**, *15*, 41. https://doi.org/10.3390/info15010041

Academic Editors: Sidong Liu, Cristián Castillo Olea and Shlomo Berkovsky

Received: 7 December 2023
Revised: 8 January 2024
Accepted: 9 January 2024
Published: 11 January 2024

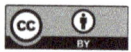

Copyright: © 2024 by the authors. Licensee MDPI, Basel, Switzerland. This article is an open access article distributed under the terms and conditions of the Creative Commons Attribution (CC BY) license (https://creativecommons.org/licenses/by/4.0/).

Abstract: Public health is an important aspect of community activities, making research on health necessary because it is a crucial field in maintaining and improving the quality of life in society as a whole. Research on public health allows for a deeper understanding of the health problems faced by a population, including disease prevalence, risk factors, and other determinants of health. This work aims to explore the potential of hospital patient data analysis as a valuable tool for understanding community implications and deriving insights for effective community health interventions. The study recognises the significance of harnessing the vast amount of data generated within hospital settings to inform population-level health strategies. The methodology employed in this study involves the collection and analysis of deidentified patient data from a representative sample of a hospital in Indonesia. Various data analysis techniques, such as statistical modelling, data mining, and machine learning algorithms, are utilised to identify patterns, trends, and associations within the data. A program written in Python is used to analyse patient data in a hospital for five years, from 2018 to 2022. These findings are then interpreted within the context of public health implications, considering factors such as disease prevalence, socioeconomic determinants, and healthcare utilisation patterns. The results of the data analysis provide valuable insights into the public health implications of hospital patient data. The research also covers predictions for the patient data to the hospital based on disease, age, and geographical residence. The research prediction shows that, in the year 2023, the number of patients will not be considerably affected by the infection, but in March to April 2024 the number will increase significantly up to 10,000 patients due to the trend in the previous year at the end of 2022. These recommendations encompass targeted prevention strategies, improved healthcare delivery models, and community engagement initiatives. The research emphasises the importance of collaboration between healthcare providers, policymakers, and community stakeholders in implementing and evaluating these interventions.

Keywords: public health; hospital; patient; community; artificial intelligence

1. Introduction

Public health is an important field in optimising the quality of life and overall well-being of a community. The approach is to prevent diseases, improve health, and reduce health disparities in society through various well-planned interventions, policies, and programmes. In the effort to achieve these goals, health data become a crucial element in identifying health challenges, measuring the impacts of interventions and informing policy decision making. One promising source of data is hospital patient data. These data include detailed information about patients, including medical diagnoses, treatments provided, length of hospital stay, and treatment outcomes. With a deep understanding of these data, we can analyse health trends, identify pressing health issues, evaluate treatment effectiveness, and identify high-risk population groups. During the 2018–2022 period, hospital patient data became more affordable and easily accessible due to the advances in information technology and health information systems [1]. These data are now documented electronically and available in large and heterogeneous amounts. The utilisation of hospital patient data to inform public health policies and interventions has great potential to enhance the effectiveness and efficiency of health efforts.

Several studies have explored the benefits of hospital patient data in the context of public health; however, challenges need to be overcome to maximise their potential. First, hospital patient data from 2018 to 2022 may encompass various medical record systems that are not always standardised, leading to complexity and difficulties in data integration and analysis due to the COVID-19 pandemic, which during the years 2020 to 2022 saw human movement control. Second, previous research has not fully optimised the utilisation of advanced data analysis techniques, such as cluster analysis and machine learning, to gain deeper insights from the available patient data in hospitals. Third, hospital patient data may only reflect populations seeking medical care, limiting information about populations not accessible to the formal healthcare system. Therefore, this research aims to address these challenges by conducting a comprehensive and in-depth analysis of hospital patient data from 2018 to 2022, with a focus on implications for public health and more effective interventions. The objective of the research analysing hospital patient data related to public health is to identify patterns, trends, and risk factors related to specific health issues within the patient population. In analysing patient data, this research aims to understand the geographic distribution of health problems, disease prevalence, and characteristics of populations more vulnerable to certain health conditions. The information generated from this research is expected to provide in-depth insights into existing public health challenges, thus aiding in formulating and designing more effective and targeted health interventions. The objectives of this research also include the use of data to support better clinical decision making and a more holistic understanding of public health in specific regions. By extracting information from hospital patient data, this research is expected to contribute positively to disease prevention efforts, improve the quality of healthcare, and develop more effective health policies for the overall community.

The overall aim of the research analysing hospital patient data related to public health is to gain in-depth insights into various aspects of public health based on existing data in electronic medical records. This work analyses patient data collected from different regions and populations to identify patterns, trends, and risk factors related to the health issues under investigation. Through data analysis, this research is expected to yield important information about the disease prevalence, geographic distribution of health problems, and characteristics of populations vulnerable to specific health conditions. The results of this research can contribute to a better understanding of public health challenges, aid in designing more effective health interventions, and support improved clinical decision making. The research analysing hospital patient data is also directed towards supporting disease prevention efforts, evidence-based health policy development, and the overall improvement of healthcare service quality, with the ultimate goal of enhancing the health and well-being of a community at large. The general objective of research analysing hospital patient data related to public health is to gain in-depth insights into various aspects of public health based on existing data in electronic medical records. This analyses patient data collected from different regions and populations to identify patterns, trends, and risk factors related to the health issues being investigated. In conducting data analysis, this research is expected to produce important information regarding the disease prevalence, geographic distribution of health problems, and characteristics of populations vulnerable to specific health conditions. The findings can contribute to an enhanced understanding of public health challenges, aid in designing more effective health interventions, and support improved clinical decision making. Additionally, the research analysing hospital patient data is also directed towards supporting disease prevention efforts, evidence-based health policy development, and overall improvement of healthcare service quality, with the ultimate goal of enhancing the health and well-being of a community at large. Figure 1 shows how the relationship of public health to several segments that have an impact on the community and individual or family support structures [1].

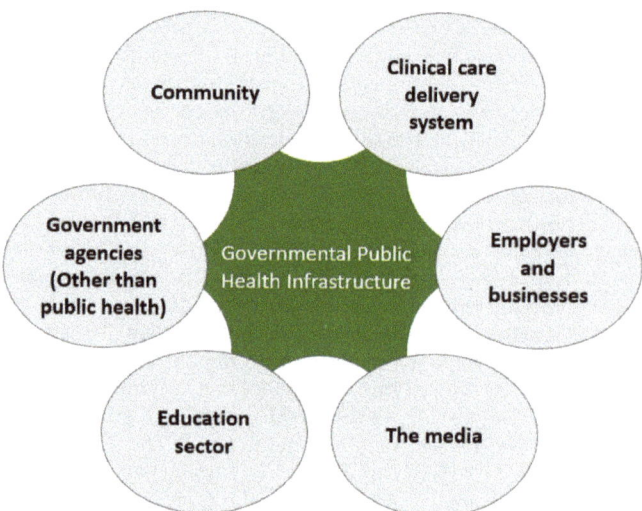

Figure 1. A sample model relationship of public health.

In achieving these objectives, this research is expected to provide valuable contributions to evidence-based health policy development and enhance the effectiveness of public health interventions. With a deeper understanding of public health and its implications for interventions, we hope that public health efforts can be more targeted and have a positive impact on improving the overall quality of life and well-being of a community.

2. Literature Review

The study of public health includes the analysis of factors influencing the health of populations, disease prevention efforts and health promotion, as well as the development and evaluation of evidence-based health interventions. The work is an essential aspect in achieving the goals of sustainable development, which are centred around improving global health and well-being [2]. The study of public health faces complex and varied challenges. Global health issues, such as infectious diseases, non-communicable diseases, reproductive health, and health inequalities, require holistic and evidence-based interventions. Efforts in public health research include improving the access to and quality of healthcare services, health promotion and prevention, research and development of innovations, community-based interventions, and global collaboration. To address these challenges, the study of public health plays a crucial role in improving the health and well-being of communities worldwide [3,4]. Public health in Indonesia is an essential aspect of national development and the well-being of society. The research and efforts of community health in Indonesia involve various aspects, including disease prevention efforts, health promotion, improving access to healthcare services, and the management of healthcare resources. As an archipelagic country with cultural and geographical diversity, Indonesia faces diverse and unique health challenges [5].

Mapping the patterns of the geographic distribution of diseases using hospital patient data, as discussed, can be performed through spatial approaches in public health [6]. This work highlights the importance of spatial analysis in mapping the patterns of the geographic distribution of diseases using hospital patient data. This study conducted research with a spatial analysis approach to identify specific disease hotspots within geographical areas. The study utilised hospital patient data from several hospitals in a metropolitan city to map the spatial distribution of infectious and noncommunicable diseases. The research findings indicate that spatial analysis approaches can help identify areas with high health risks and guide public health policies in effectively allocating resources. The contributing factors to health disparities among population groups have been analysed using data from hospitals [7,8]; in other words, an analysis using hospital patient data to identify socioeconomic factors contributing to variations in health outcomes among population groups was conducted. The study includes patient data from various demographic and economic groups. The research findings indicate that income level, educational attainment, and healthcare accessibility are some of the significant factors influencing public health outcomes. The work provides important insights into the socioeconomic aspects that need to be considered in designing public health interventions focusing on high-risk groups.

Evaluating the effectiveness of public health interventions based on patient data available in hospitals [9–11]: In this article, the effectiveness of several public health interventions conducted based on hospital patient data was evaluated. The study also compares treatment outcomes between the intervention group and the control group for some critical diseases. The research shows that some interventions have a significant impact on reducing readmission rates to the hospital and improving health outcomes. The results of this evaluation provide valuable guidance for healthcare decision makers in designing and implementing more effective interventions that have a positive impact on public health. Advanced data analysis techniques have been used in analysing data from available hospital patient records [12,13]. The utilisation of advanced analysis techniques, particularly machine learning, in analysing hospital patient data is explored. The team has reviewed various studies that apply machine learning methods to identify patterns and trends in hospital patient data. These studies include disease classification, health risk prediction, and the identification of high-risk population groups. This work guides the potential use of advanced analysis techniques in conducting more in-depth research on public health using hospital patient data. Hospital patient data have been used in public health research in developing countries [14–16]. The study conducted presents an overview of the utilisation of hospital patient data in public health in developing countries. The other articles present several studies conducted in developing countries, including the analysis of disease patterns, social and economic factors contributing to public health, and the effectiveness of public health interventions based on hospital patient data. The work provides a different perspective on understanding the potential of hospital patient data in developing countries and their relevance to health policies and interventions.

Spatial analysis has been used to enhance the quality of public health interventions [17–19]. This work discusses the role of spatial analysis in improving the quality of public health interventions. The article explores various studies that use spatial analysis to identify areas with high health risks, link disease patterns to environmental factors, and design more targeted interventions. The research provides insights into the benefits of spatial analysis in public health and its potential to enhance intervention effectiveness. Hospital patient data have been used to design disease prevention programmes [20,21]. The results also explore various hospital patient data to identify disease risk factors and develop more effective prevention strategies. This highlights the importance of involving hospital patient data in comprehensive and evidence-based disease prevention planning. Hospital patient data have been integrated with public health data to support integrated health policies [22–24]. They showed that hospital patient data should be integrated with public health data to provide a more comprehensive understanding of public health issues and aid in designing integrated, holistic, and effective health policies. The analysis of hospital patient data supports policy decision making [24,25]. Several discussions also present various examples of how hospital patient data can be utilised to identify pressing health issues, monitor the effectiveness of health policies, and inform health programme planning.

The literature provides valuable insights into how the use of hospital patient data can contribute to the development of effective and positively impactful health policies [26,27].

Machine learning has been used in analysing hospital patient data to enhance early disease detection and treatment [28], for which various examples of research are given that utilise machine learning algorithms to identify complex disease patterns, predict individual health risks, and assist in making more accurate clinical decisions. This work guides the potential of machine learning in enhancing healthcare diagnosis and treatment. Information technology has been applied in processing hospital patient data for public health [29–31]. This article highlights the application of information technology in the processing of hospital patient data for public health purposes. This study illustrates how integrated health information systems can be utilised to efficiently collect, store, and analyse hospital patient data. This work guides how the implementation of information technology can enhance the accessibility and quality of health data to support public health policies and interventions. The benefits of hospital patient data in supporting epidemiological research have been discussed in the literature [32,33]. The benefits of hospital patient data in supporting epidemiological research are discussed. The research team presents examples of studies that utilise hospital patient data to identify epidemiological trends, track the spread of infectious diseases, and inform public health interventions. The article provides insights into the potential of hospital patient data in supporting epidemiological research and overall public health.

Considering the diversity of the literature, the present study can strengthen the foundation of the knowledge and analysis methods used in understanding public health patterns, identifying factors contributing to health outcome variations and evaluating the effectiveness of public health interventions based on hospital patient data. This study can delve deeper into the use of hospital patient data, the role of information technology, and the application of machine learning techniques in supporting public health research. This research can provide a strong basis for optimising the utilisation of hospital patient data.

3. Methodology

The research methodology in public health serves as a strong foundation for data collection, information analysis, and decision making related to public health and wellbeing. One of the approaches used is a public health research plan (PHRP). This approach allows researchers to plan and conduct systematic, comprehensive research focused on relevant public health issues, especially during pandemics or major disease cases, after which preventive action has a guide for being enacted.

- Planning phase: In the planning phase of a PHRP, researchers will determine specific, relevant, and significant research topics in the context of public health. Here, research objectives must be clearly defined, and the research questions to be answered through the study must be formulated.
- Identifying scope and target population: Researchers must thoroughly understand the research scope and the population to be studied. In this regard, a PHRP requires identifying the health issues to be investigated and determining the relevant target population. Understanding the characteristics of this population is essential in designing data collection and analysis strategies.
- Data collection and measurement methods: After identifying the scope and target population, researchers need to plan appropriate data collection methods to gather the necessary information. Data collection methods may include surveys, interviews, observations, or the use of secondary data. Researchers also need to design valid and reliable measurement instruments with which to consistently collect data.
- Data analysis: Once data are collected, the data analysis phase becomes crucial in a PHRP. The collected data need to be analysed using appropriate statistical techniques to answer research questions. Data analysis helps identify patterns, relationships, and public health trends relevant to the research topic.

- Interpretation of results and implications for public health: After completing data analysis, researchers must interpret the research results carefully. Research findings should be connected back to the research objectives and research questions to draw valid and meaningful conclusions. Furthermore, the implications of research results for public health need to be clarified to make a real contribution to addressing existing health issues.
- Development of health interventions and policies: Based on research findings, a PHRP allows researchers to design evidence-based health interventions and policies. Consequently, research results can contribute to improving the quality and effectiveness of public health programmes.

The PHRP approach is a systematic research methodology for examining various relevant public health issues. Through this method, researchers can plan and conduct research with clear objectives, identify public health problems and formulate research questions that can be answered with appropriate methods. The research results can contribute to informing evidence-based public health policies and interventions, thereby enhancing overall public health and well-being.

3.1. Data Collection

The use of electronic systems or computers in patient data collection at hospitals, also known as electronic health records (EHRs), has become a common practice in healthcare. This system allows hospitals to store and access patient information digitally, improving data efficiency, accuracy, and interoperability. The process of patient data collection at hospitals using electronic systems or computers is as follows:

- Patient registration: The data collection process begins when patients come to the hospital for registration. Registration staff enter patient identification data, such as name, address, date of birth, and contact number, into the electronic system. This information serves as the starting point for creating a patient's electronic health record.
- Medical history: Next, doctors or nurses will conduct a medical history interview to gather a patient's health history. This includes complaints, past medical conditions, family history, allergies, and other relevant information. The collected data will be input into a patient's EHR.
- Test results: When patients undergo physical examinations or diagnostic tests, the results will be uploaded onto the electronic system; for example, laboratory test results, radiology results, and other diagnostic test results will be recorded in a patient's EHR digitally.
- Treatment notes: During a patient's hospitalisation, daily treatment notes will be input into the electronic system. These notes include information about a patient's condition, medical procedures performed, medications administered, and health progress during treatment.
- Specialist consultations: If necessary, patients may have consultations with specific specialists. The results of these consultations will also be uploaded onto a patient's EHR, allowing the attending doctor to access this information.
- Electronic health record: All collected data, including medical history, test results, treatment notes, and specialist consultations, will be stored in a patient's EHR. The EHR is integrated, enabling doctors and other medical staff to easily access and update the patient's medical information.
- Data security: EHR systems must be secured to protect patient medical information. Only authorised medical personnel have access to patient data, and the data must be encrypted to prevent unauthorised access.

Table 1 shows that using EHRs makes patient data collection at hospitals more efficient and accurate. Electronically collected data can be easily accessed by medical teams, facilitating precise clinical decision making and providing better as well as safer patient care. This system also allows hospitals to integrate data and track patients' complete health history, which are crucial for providing continuous and holistic care. The total number of patients was recorded within four years, resulting in more than 80,000 patients with complete data for analysis.

Table 1. Patient indicator data from hospital records (1).

Number	Patient Indicator in Hospital
1	Registration identity
2	Registration date
3	Patient name
4	Address
5	Identity card number
6	Date of birth
7	Gender
8	Clinic
9	Doctor
10	Ward room (if applicable)

In this patient data collection, the classified ranges of patient age, from infant to senior, were as follows:

- Toddlers → (0–4 years).
- Children → (5–10 years).
- Teenagers → (11–19 years).
- Adults → (20–39 years).
- Elderly → (40–65 years).
- Seniors → (66 years and above).

3.2. Data Analysis Technique

The method of analysing patient data at hospitals using electronic data involves the utilisation of information technology, particularly the EHR system. Electronic data allow hospitals to collect, store, and access patient information digitally, replacing manual processes that are time-consuming and prone to errors. With the EHR system, data analysis can be carried out efficiently and accurately. Patient data, such as medical history, test results, prescriptions, and treatment notes, can be easily analysed using various statistical techniques and data visualisation. The integration of data from various hospital systems also enables more accurate as well as holistic clinical decision making and facilitates more in-depth public health research; however, patient data security and privacy must be the top priority in the use of electronic data, and appropriate data security measures must always be followed to protect patients' personal information. The process of analysing patient data at hospitals using computer software applications involves several similar steps using the programming language Python. We will elaborate on the process of patient data analysis using computer programming, which is commonly used for data analysis and numerical processing. The steps in the process of analysing patient data at hospitals using Python programming are shown as follows (and in Figure 2):

- Data collection: Patient data are collected from an EHR system or other data sources and entered into a hospital information system. Data may include clinical data such as test results, diagnoses, treatment history, and other patient information.
- Data pre-processing: Data pre-processing involves data cleaning, handling missing or invalid data, and converting the data format into a suitable form for analysis.
- Statistical analysis: All datasets provide various built-in information functions that can be used for data analysis. These functions include average, median, standard deviation, and others.

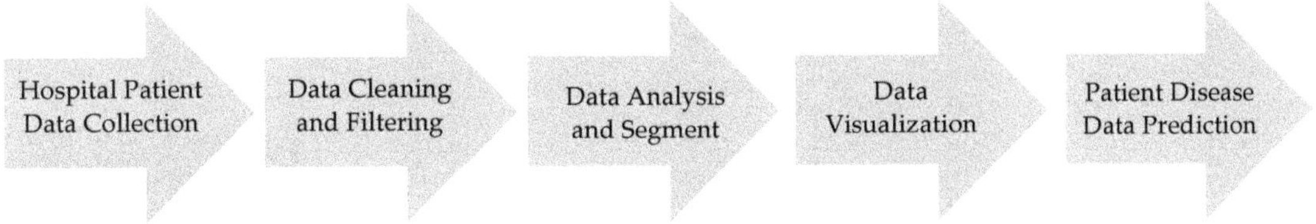

Hospital Patient Data Collection → Data Cleaning and Filtering → Data Analysis and Segment → Data Visualization → Patient Disease Data Prediction

Figure 2. The process of analysing patient data from a hospital.

The following functions facilitate the calculation of basic statistics from numerical data:

- Data visualisation: Python also offers various types of charts and graphs that can be used to create data visualisations. Bar charts, line graphs, pie charts, and others can be used to visualise data interactively.
- Pivot table and chart: Pivots are highly useful features in Python for analysing and summarising data quickly. A pivot table allows us to arrange data in a dynamic table, while a pivot chart enables us to create charts based on the pivot table.
- Data filtering and sorting: Python programming provides filtering and sorting features that allow us to easily filter and sort data. These features help us quickly identify patterns and trends in the data.
- Data validation: To ensure valid data, we can use data validation features in the computer program. This feature allows us to set validation rules for specific data columns, ensuring that the entered data comply with these rules.
- Interpretation of results: After conducting data analysis and obtaining findings, the results must be interpreted carefully. The results of data analysis should be used to provide useful insights for clinical decision making and hospital management.
- Data security: In the data analysis process, the security of patient data must be ensured. Patient data must be kept confidential and accessed only by authorised parties.

Computer software applications are versatile and capable of analysing data from various sources, including hospital data analysis. They are simple and user-friendly while still allowing for complex data analysis; however, in inpatient data analysis, we must adhere to ethical principles and comply with privacy as well as data security regulations. In this research, referring to a hospital with many sections according to patient disease, the data and information kept in the hospital management system are supported with digital data.

3.3. Python Programming and Deep Learning Algorithms

Python is one of the most popular programming languages and has a simple syntax, developed by Guido van Rossum in 1991 [34]. Python is also equipped with several powerful libraries and frameworks, such as NumPy, Pandas, Matplotlib, and TensorFlow, which make it convenient for developers to build complex solutions and applications quickly and efficiently. Extensive Python community support also makes it a valuable resource for developers, providing numerous tutorials, documentation, and discussion forums that can help them understand and solve various programming challenges. In the era of information technology and computers, many techniques and algorithms have been developed, with good results and faster processing times.

Deep learning algorithms are a method in artificial intelligence. One of the popular examples is long short-term memory (LSTM), which is an evolution of deep learning known as a recurrent neural network (RNN), first introduced by Sherstinsky [35]. The LSTM algorithm can analyse time series datasets to address problems. This algorithm is also capable of learning long-term dependencies in datasets and retaining information for extended periods by default. Figure 3 shows the basic architecture of a RNN–LSTM model, consisting of several main blocks called cells, such as the input gate, output gate, and forget gate. Figure 3 shows a sample of the RNN–LSTM algorithm structure in the Python programming application for this patient data in a hospital case.

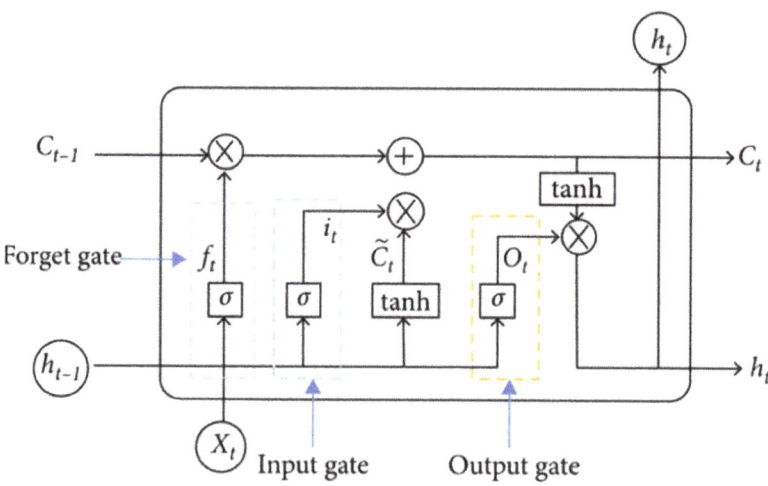

Figure 3. Sample of RNN–LSTM algorithm structure.

An LSTM model can be elaborate as short-term memory, which acts when the information is being acquired, retains that information for a few seconds, and then destines it to be kept for longer periods or discards it. Long-term memory, which permanently retains information, allows its recovery or recall. It contains all of our autobiographical data and all of our knowledge. Referring to the architecture of the LSTM model, which consists of three major cells, the calculation of each cell and the process can be written as Equations (1)–(6), as referred to in this research and publication [32]:

$$f_t = \sigma \left(W_f \cdot [h_{t-1}, x_t] + b_f \right) \tag{1}$$

$$i_t = \sigma \left(W_i \cdot [h_{t-1}, x_t] + b_i \right) \tag{2}$$

$$`C_t = \tanh \left(W_c \cdot [h_{t-1}, x_t] + b_c \right) \tag{3}$$

$$C_t = f_t * C_{t-1} + i_t * `C_t \tag{4}$$

$$o_t = \sigma \left(W_o [h_{t-1}, x_t] + b_o \right) \tag{5}$$

$$h_t = o_t * \tanh \left(C_t \right) \tag{6}$$

The deep learning LSTM algorithm model has the ability to handle problems with long-term RNN dependencies, while some other algorithms fail to achieve accurate results due to long histories and data variations. With a large amount of data and variations, conventional algorithms cannot accurately process information stored in long-term memory, but LSTM can provide more accurate predictions based on historical information. LSTM can be applied as a default to store data in the long term. It is commonly used for predicting, processing, and classifying time series data. A prediction model is used to calculate the number of future fire points using the LSTM algorithm, and the errors need to be justified. Several models can be used for forecasting, such as mean square error (MSE) to calculate the error squared and mean average error (MAE) to calculate the average error in a dataset. An additional method is R^2, which indicates the proportion of variance in a dataset. This method can be expressed as Equations (7)–(9) for *MSE*, *MAE*, and R^2, respectively [33]:

$$MSE = \frac{\sum_1^N (yi - y'_i)^2}{N} \tag{7}$$

$$MAE = \frac{\sum_1^N |yi - y'_i|}{N} \tag{8}$$

$$R^2 = 1 - \frac{\sum_1^N (yi - y'_i)^2}{\sum_1^N (yi - y_{avg})^2} \tag{9}$$

where y_i is the actual number of fire points at time i, y'_i is the predicted number of hotspots at time i^{th}, and y_{avg} is the total number of samples in the dataset as training data, while error figures are used as regression model metrics. All of the models used to calculate errors are used to check the forecasting performance of the dataset and can be utilised for future predictions, as well as calculating the average error in the simulation.

The LSTM algorithm model has a sigmoid function from W_f and b_f, presenting the weight matrix and bias, respectively, for the forget gate. This process is a step to determine and decide the input dataset, which is the new information, X_t, in the cell state, as well as to update the cell state. The next process of the sigmoid layer then determines whether the new dataset should be updated or ignored (0 or 1). The Tan_h function gives weight to the values that passed by deciding their level of importance (1 to 1). Figure 4 shows the neuron process of the LSTM model [34].

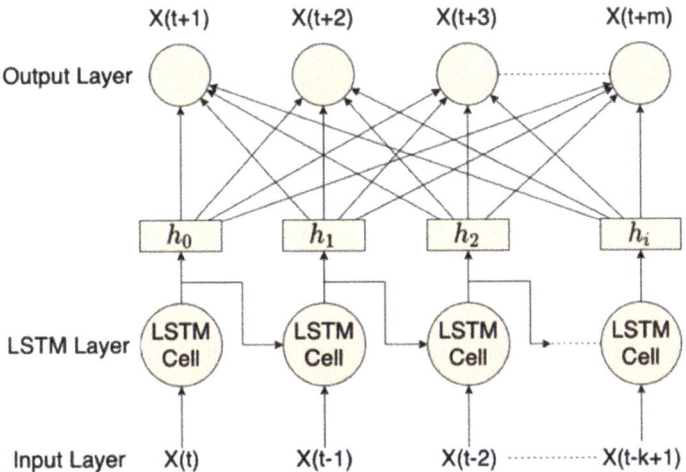

Figure 4. LSTM algorithm for internal cells in modern neurons.

The final step is to calculate the error from the available dataset for the forecasting results to examine the percentage of error. Many techniques can be used to calculate the error. For example, root mean square error (RMSE) is one statistical-based technique that is commonly used to compare forecasts with actual data values. RMSE is often used to evaluate how accurately forecasting results fit historical data values based on the relative range of a dataset. Equation (10) explains that X_i and X'_i present the actual hotspot dataset compared with the forecasted data at time t, X_i is the mean actual value of the hotspot dataset, and N is the total number of data points. When the RMSE value changes from a small number to zero, it implies that the LSTM algorithm produces reliable results:

$$RMSE = \sqrt{\frac{1}{N} \sum_{i=1}^{N} (X_i - X'_i)^2} \tag{10}$$

Among all of the methods for evaluating predictions or forecasting errors, RMSE and MAE evaluate based on short-term, hourly forecasts. The process of analysing patient data in a hospital using the Python computer program involves several important steps. The following are the steps in the process of patient data analysis in a hospital using Python.

3.4. Prediction Mathematical Modelling

The integration of LSTM with deep learning capability has the potential for the analysis of patient data by the permutation method, and the complex data on the hospital information system can be solved by numerical or approximate methods [36,37]. Once calculated, data simplification, calculation, and substitution can be obtained as in Equation (11):

$$\frac{L(t)}{\ln(\frac{L(t)}{A})} = C - e^{-Bt} \qquad (11)$$

where C and B are constants. In both sides of Equation (12), as an exponential function, L can be used to calculate the number of patient distribution data, as shown in Equation (6):

$$L(t) = A \cdot e^{e^{-Bt+C}} \qquad (12)$$

The differential equation refers to the Gompertz model of calculating human growth and development; it can be applied as a similar model to the growth of patient number visits and treatment in a hospital or medical centre, which describes the gradual contiguous rate of height with an increasing number of patients over time. Another model is the Bertalanffy model, which was proposed by the Austrian biologist and scientist Ludwig von Bertalanffy. It is a differential equation based on the growth model designed to describe the growth of a process in an institution that can comprise organisms or humans. This model assumes that the growth rate of patients with various backgrounds at different stages is influenced by several diseases during treatment. The specific differential equation of the Bertalanffy model is as follows:

$$\frac{dN}{dt} = r(N_\infty - N) \qquad (13)$$

where N denotes the number of patients registered in a medical centre or volumes of patients, t is the time, r is the growth rate constant, and N_∞ is the final number of patients in a medical centre or hospital. This model is commonly used to describe the growth process of the number of objects in calculating the growth that has been widely used in medical data analysis or medicine, environmental science, agriculture, and other fields.

The basic concept of artificial intelligence to calculate human or patients' data growth models takes into consideration many aspects, such as genetics, environments, clusters, and pandemics, of physical growth. These aspects can be modelled into sets to build differential equations with which to analyse and predict for the future indicators of mass pandemics and proportions of different kinds of disease. The models can also be applied to the studying of the changes in patient number development by the time points in medical centres and disease development, helping medical staff better analyse and diagnose diseases. The model has a significant impact on studying the development and prediction of disease infections in a community in an area. The mathematical models are very useful as a tool for predicting the growth and development of different types of environments and provide important reference information for medical scientists. Figure 5 shows a neural network model of artificial intelligence with a subset process to analyse patient data.

The k-th input sample, $x(k) = (x_1(k), \ldots, x_n(k))$, is randomly selected, and the corresponding expected outputs are $d_0(k) = (d_1(k), d_2(k), \ldots, d_q(k))$. The input and output of each neuron in the hidden layer are calculated, and the output is calculated as Equation (14):

$$\begin{aligned}
hi_h(k) &= \sum_{i=1}^{n} w_{ih} x_i(k) - b_h, h = 1, 2, \ldots, p \\
ho_h(k) &= f(hi_h(k)), h = 1, 2, \ldots, p \\
yi_o(k) &= \sum_{i=1}^{p} w_{ho} ho_h(k) - b_o, o = 1, 2, \ldots, q \\
yo_o(k) &= f(yi_o(k)), o = 1, 2, \ldots, p
\end{aligned} \qquad (14)$$

Then, the total error is computed as in Equation (9):

$$E = \frac{1}{2m}\sum_{k=1}^{m}\sum_{o=1}^{q}(d_o(k) - y_o(k))^2 \qquad (15)$$

The partial derivatives of the error function to each neuron in the output layer are calculated by using the expected output of the network, $\delta_o(k)$; then, the partial derivative of the error function to each neuron in the hidden layer is calculated by using the connection weights from the hidden layer to the output layer, $\delta_o(k)$, the output of the output layer, and $\delta_o(k)$, the output of the hidden layer [35]:

$$\begin{aligned}
\frac{\partial E}{\partial w_{ho}} &= \frac{\partial E}{\partial yi_o}\frac{\partial yi_o}{\partial w_{ho}} = -ho_h(k)(d_o(k) - yo_o(k))f'(yi_o(k)) = -ho_h\delta_o(k) \\
\Delta w_{ho}(k) &= -\mu\frac{\partial E}{\partial w_{ho}} = \mu\delta_o(k)ho_h(k) \\
w_{ho}^{N+1} &= w_{ho}^N + \eta\delta_o(k)ho_h(k) \\
\Delta w_{ih}(k) &= -\mu\frac{\partial E}{\partial hi_h(k)}\frac{\partial hi_h(k)}{\partial w_{ih}} = \delta_h(k)x_i(k) \\
w_{ih}^{N+1} &= w_{ih}^N + \eta\delta_h(k)x_i(k)
\end{aligned} \qquad (16)$$

The algorithm terminates when the error reaches the present accuracy or the number of learning is greater than the pre-specified set maximum number of times as set out in Equation (10). Otherwise, we select the next learning sample as well as the corresponding expected output and return to enter the next round of learning.

The process of retrieving electronic medical records (EMRs) from a hospital patient database involves a systematic flowchart that ensures efficient and secure access to patient information. The first step in this process is patient identification, where authorized personnel enter the system using secure login credentials. Once logged in, the system navigates to a central database where patient records are stored. The flowchart then branches into sections based on the type of information required, such as medical history, diagnostic reports, or treatment plans. Subsequently, the system validates the access rights of the user, ensuring that only authorized individuals can retrieve sensitive medical data. The flowchart includes encryption and security measures to safeguard patient confidentiality. Following this, the system retrieves the requested information and presents it to the authorized user in a comprehensible format. This comprehensive flowchart for EMR retrieval optimizes the efficiency of healthcare professionals while prioritizing the security and privacy of patient information. Figure 6 shows the flowchart of patient data retrieval, with the first step including the normalization that only valid and complete datasets transfer to the patient data analysis cloud system.

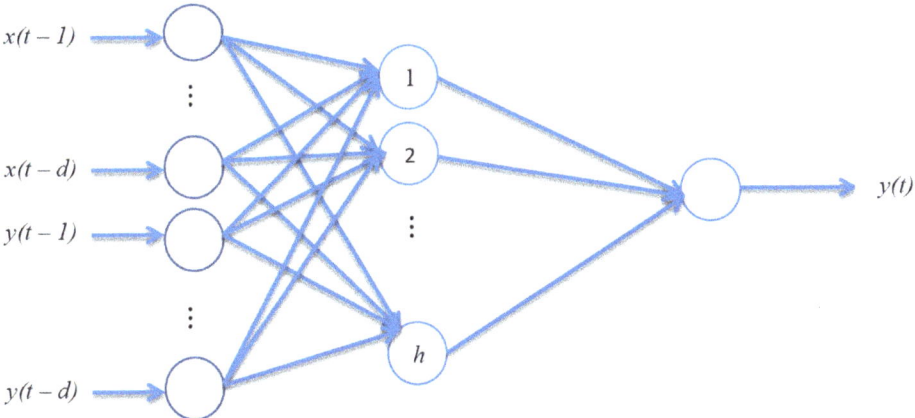

Figure 5. The architecture of the neural network for data analysis.

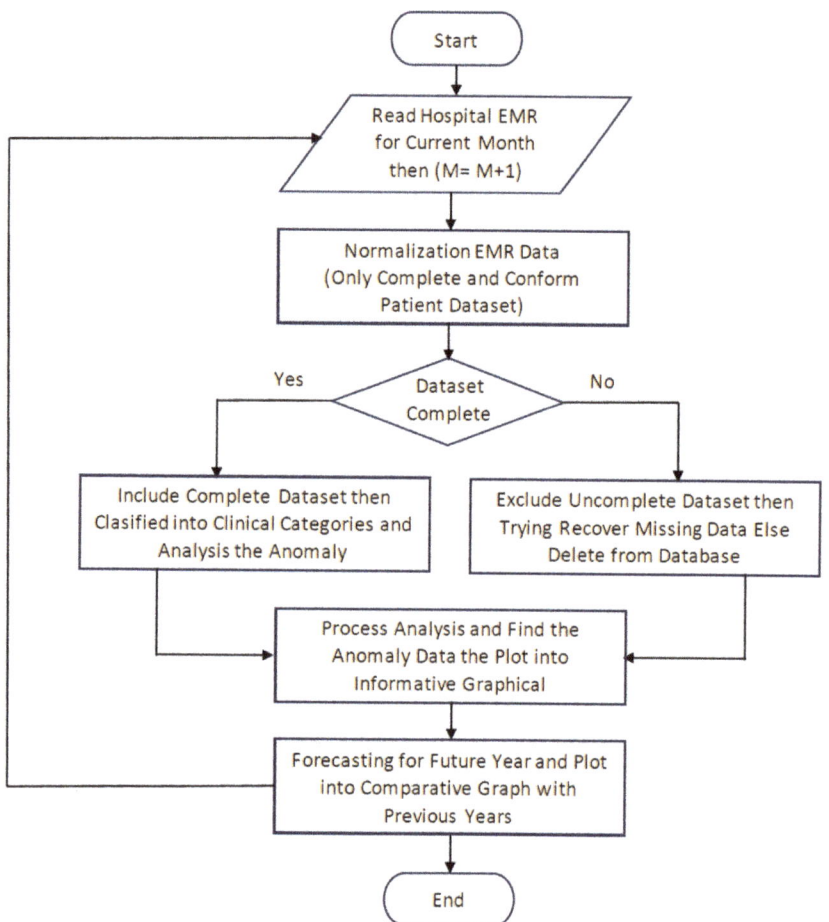

Figure 6. Process flow of patient data retrieval with a normalization dataset.

3.5. Ethics in Health Research

Ethical considerations play a central role in public health research. When conducting health research, researchers must always prioritise the rights and well-being of research participants. First and foremost, clear and voluntary informed consent from participants should be emphasised, ensuring that they have a full understanding of the risks and benefits involved in their participation. Additionally, the confidentiality and privacy of patient data must be strictly maintained to protect the identities and personal information of participants. Special protection is also necessary for vulnerable groups, such as children and pregnant women, to minimise potential risks and ensure that the benefits outweigh them. Ethical involvement in public health research also involves the obligation to report findings with integrity and transparency, ensuring clear social benefits for the community. Public health research that adheres to these ethical considerations can significantly contribute to improving the overall health and quality of life of society.

In public health research, several important ethical considerations should be observed and respected. Examples are as follows:

- Informed consent: Research participants should be provided with clear and comprehensive information about the research's purpose, procedures, potential benefits and risks, as well as their rights as participants. Participants should give voluntary consent after fully understanding the implications of their participation.

- Confidentiality and privacy: Participants' personal data and information must be kept confidential. Participant identities should be securely protected, and data should be processed in a way that prevents individual identification if possible.
- Protection of children and vulnerable groups: If research involves children, pregnant women or other vulnerable groups, special measures are needed to protect them. The potential risks should be minimised and the benefits should outweigh them.
- Non-maleficence: Public health research should prioritise the principle of non-maleficence, meaning not causing harm or endangering research participants. Risks should be carefully considered and efforts made to avoid them.
- Social benefits: Public health research should provide benefits to the community as a whole. Research findings should be used to improve public health and well-being.
- Transparency and integrity: Research should be conducted with transparency and integrity. All data and findings should be disclosed honestly, without manipulation or misrepresentation.
- Commitment to safety: The safety and health of research participants should be a top priority in public health research. Preventive measures should be taken to reduce the risk of injury or illness to participants.
- Ethical approval: Before commencing research, ethical approval must be obtained from relevant ethics committees or institutions. Ethical approval ensures that the research complies with applicable ethical standards and safeguards the rights as well as well-being of research participants.

Respecting these ethical considerations in public health research is essential to maintain research integrity, public trust, and participant protection. By adhering to ethical principles, public health research can produce meaningful and beneficial results for the health and well-being of society as a whole.

4. Results and Discussion

Health data from a hospital in Indonesia reveal important information about the health profiles of patients treated at the hospital facility. These data include various variables such as a patient's age, gender, diagnosed diseases, laboratory test results, and treatment history. The data description results show a diverse age distribution of patients, ranging from infants to the elderly, highlighting the importance of age-appropriate care for specific population groups. The health data also depict a comparison of the number of male and female patients, potentially providing insights into health conditions that may affect these gender groups differently. The most common diagnosed diseases recorded in the health data provide an overview of the disease burden faced by the hospital and the prevalent health conditions in the community in that area. The laboratory test results indicate the monitoring and in-depth evaluation of the patient's health conditions, aiding the medical team in accurate diagnoses and appropriate treatments. Furthermore, patients' treatment histories record medical procedures performed, medications given, and health developments during treatment.

The results of this health data description hold significant value in enhancing the understanding of the public health profile in the North Sumatra region. These data can be used to plan more effective health interventions, identify emerging health trends, and support deeper public health research. Moreover, the data contribute to making informed clinical decisions and provide a strong foundation for evidence-based health policy formulation. Through analysing and understanding the results of this health data description, the hospital and relevant stakeholders can improve the quality of healthcare services and the well-being of the community in the North Sumatra region. Figure 7 shows the results of a hospital patient data analysis based on disease or clinic room visit for 2018. The results of the patient data analysis based on disease types in a hospital provide a comprehensive overview of the most common disease patterns in the area. Through this analysis, the most dominant types of diseases, their prevalence rates, and the age distribution of affected patients can be identified. Additionally, the data analysis can reveal disease trends over time, enabling the identification of changes in disease patterns in the past and future.

Information about the most common diseases and their prevalence is crucial for healthcare service planning and management. Hospitals and relevant stakeholders can use these data to allocate resources more efficiently and optimise patient care. The analysis results can also help formulate more effective prevention programmes and direct efforts to reduce the burden of specific diseases on the community. Figure 8 shows the data from the hospital's analysis of patients based on the most frequently treated disease types in 2019. The 2018 data show a significant increase in patient visits to the hospital in the early months, from January to September.

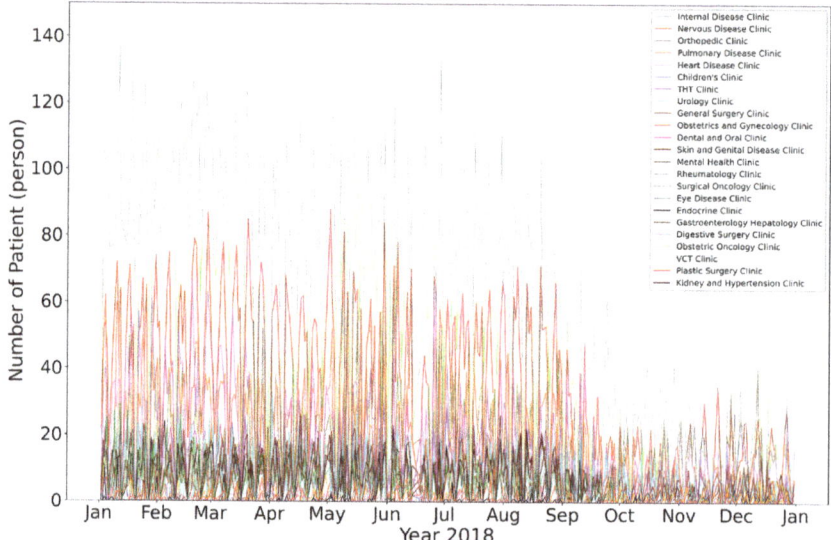

Figure 7. Results of the patient data in an analysis for 2018.

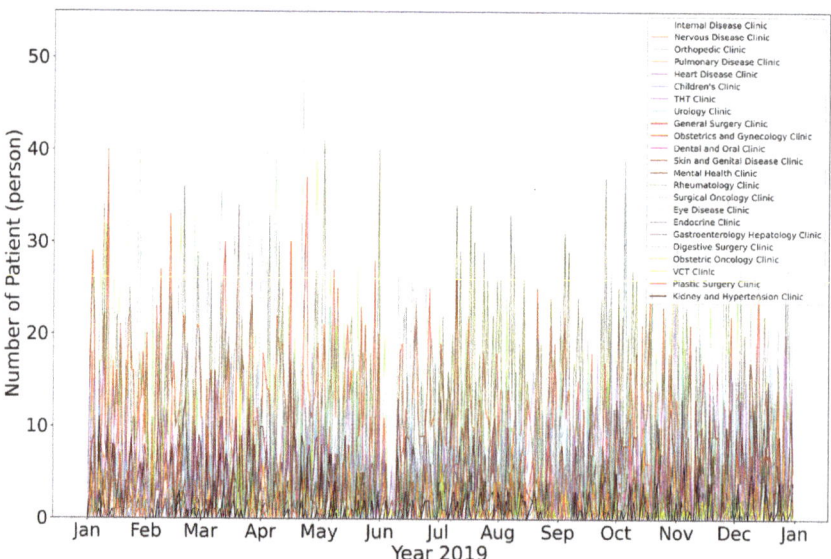

Figure 8. Results of the patient data in an analysis for 2019.

Furthermore, a patient data analysis based on disease types can serve as a foundation for further research on health. These data can be a valuable source of information for researchers to identify disease risk factors, test the effectiveness of therapies and interventions, and gain a deeper understanding of health determinants. Leveraging the results of a patient data analysis based on disease types, hospitals and other relevant stakeholders can take strategic steps to improve the quality of healthcare services, implement more targeted prevention efforts, and enhance their overall understanding of public health. The more accurate and detailed the data analysis conducted, the greater the benefits for decision making and overall public health improvement.

The data shown in Figure 9 indicate the number of patients who visited for disease analysis and consultation, which generally was not high and slightly decreased compared with the 2019 data, with an average of 20–30 people per day. This condition was influenced by the impact of the COVID-19 pandemic, which imposed travel restrictions and limitations on mobility, unlike the previous year. Figure 10 shows results in a graph of patient data in the hospital for 2021.

Overall, a patient data analysis based on disease types is an essential tool in managing and improving healthcare services at the hospital. Using these data, hospitals can provide more effective and targeted healthcare services to meet the needs of the community. Further research based on the results of this data analysis can provide deeper insights into the risk factors and determinants of health that influence disease patterns, thereby aiding in the development of more comprehensive and effective public health strategies. Figure 11 shows the data analysis results from 2022; however, the collected data of the patients in 2022 were limited to June because of a hospital system change and upgrade to another new computerisation system, as indicated by the six months of patient data increasing compared with the previous year.

Figure 12 shows the data analysis results from 2018 to 2022. The conditions were still those of the COVID-19 pandemic in 2019–2022, resulting in minimal changes compared with 2018, when human mobility was freer.

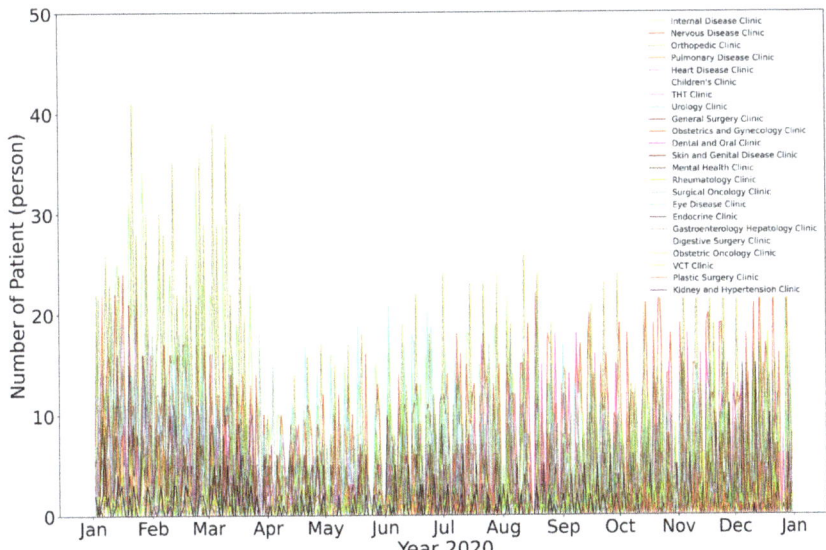

Figure 9. Results of the patient data in an analysis for 2020.

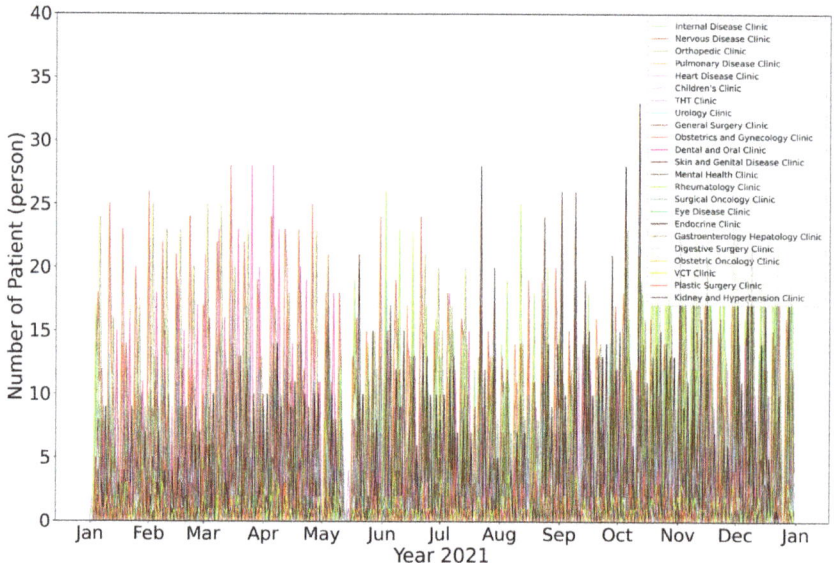

Figure 10. Results of the patient data in an analysis for 2021.

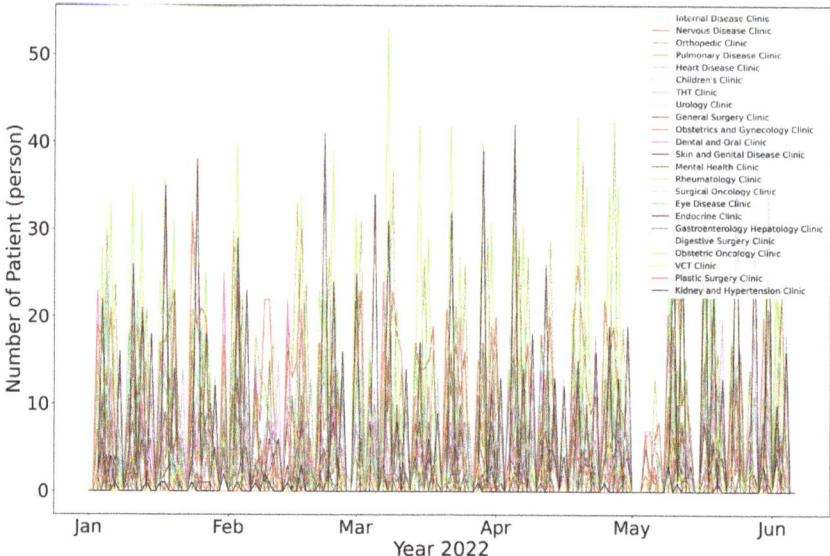

Figure 11. Results of the patient data in an analysis for 2022.

An analysis based on regional residence also provides information about variations in public health across different areas. Graphs and images have illustrated different disease patterns among specific regions (Figure 13). These results help identify areas with higher disease burdens and vulnerability, enabling relevant stakeholders to prioritise healthcare resources and interventions for these regions. An analysis based on gender also sheds light on differences in disease patterns between males and females. These results aid in designing gender-specific health programmes that align with the unique characteristics of each gender. For example, if certain diseases are more common in one gender, screening and health promotion programmes can be specifically directed towards preventing and managing these diseases in the vulnerable gender group.

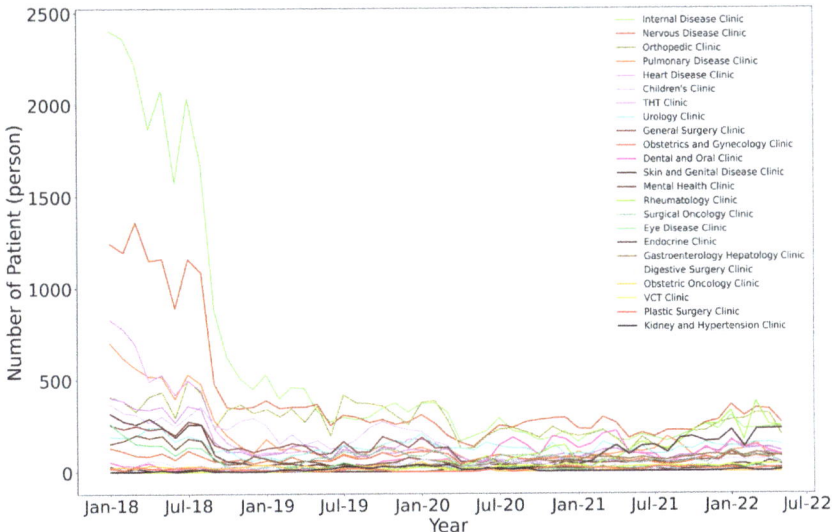

Figure 12. Results of the patient data disease analysis for 2018–2022.

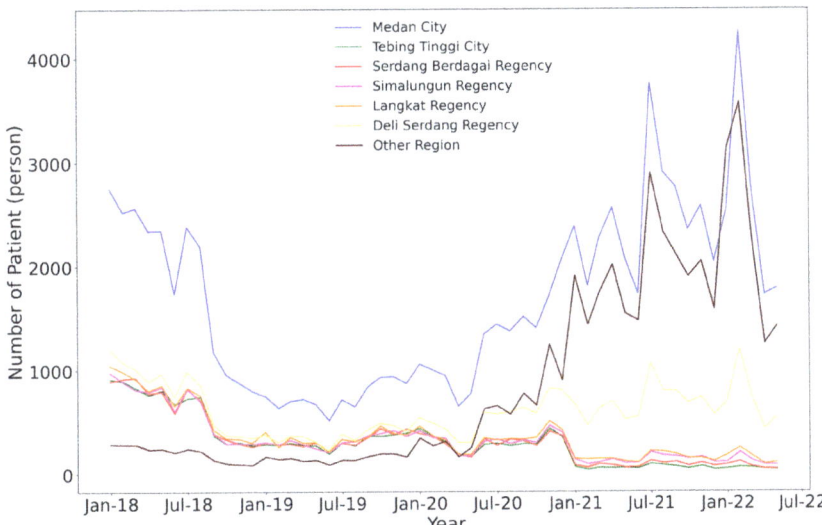

Figure 13. Results of patients based on a region of living analysis for 2018–2022.

An analysis based on age provides an understanding of variations in disease patterns at different stages of life, as shown in Figure 12 for 2018–2022, which was used in the prediction for 2023 for the rate based on the residents of stay-in districts. Graphs have identified specific age groups that are more vulnerable to certain types of diseases. These findings can be utilised to develop more responsive and age-specific public health programmes that cater to the health needs of various age groups. Overall, the data analysis from the graphs has a positive impact on public health. These findings serve as a foundation for formulating effective prevention strategies, health promotion efforts, and targeted healthcare for various population groups. The results of this research also serve as a reference for hospitals and relevant stakeholders to improve the quality of healthcare services and design more holistic as well as inclusive policies to enhance the overall well-being of the community. Figure 14 shows the patient data referring to age for the 2018–2022 results, with 2018 having a high number of patients. This decreased in the intervening years and returned in 2022 due to human mobility being free in many locations.

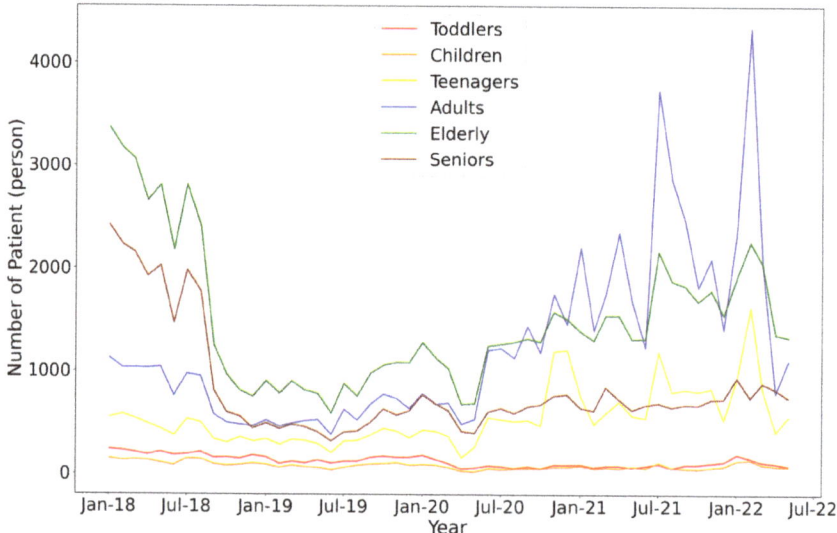

Figure 14. Results of patient data based on an age analysis for 2018–2022.

The hospital health prediction data from 2018 to 2022 for the forecast years 2022 to 2024 have been processed and presented in terms of disease classified and, in particular, medical treatment centre, as shown in Figure 15, to provide an overview of potential health trends in the future. These graphs utilise historical data from previous years to identify patterns and trends emerging in the number of disease cases and disease distribution based on age, gender, and regional residence. The predictive data offer valuable insights for the hospital and stakeholders in planning and allocating healthcare resources more efficiently and effectively. By understanding the projected number of patients and types of diseases that may be encountered in the upcoming period, the hospital can anticipate the need for more targeted healthcare services. Overall, no significant increase in patients occurred in 2022–2024.

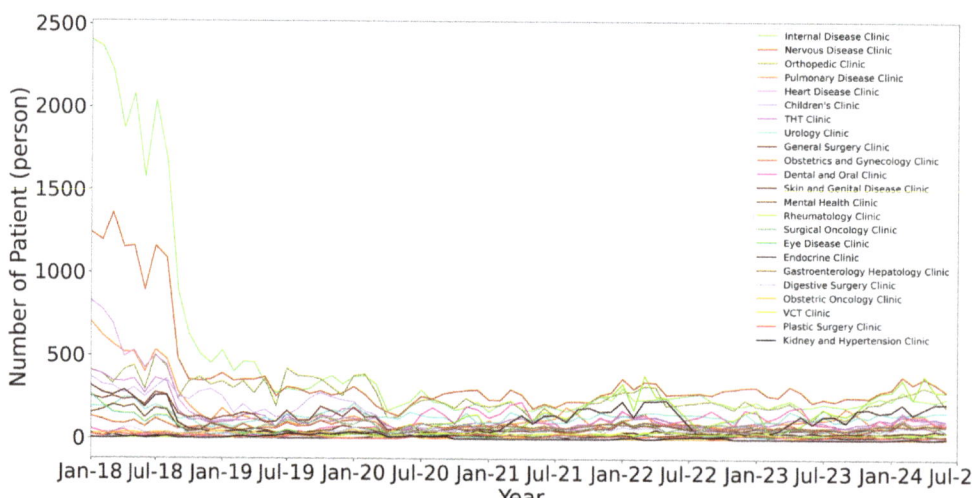

Figure 15. Prediction of patients up to 2024 as plotted.

Images such as the prediction graphs also aid in identifying changes in epidemiology that may occur from year to year. An increase or decrease in the number of specific disease cases can serve as an indicator of specific health issues that need to be addressed more seriously and continuously. Furthermore, these health prediction data provide a foundation for formulating prevention programmes and health promotion initiatives that focus on high-risk groups and vulnerable regions. When specific age groups or genders that may be more susceptible to a particular disease are identified, preventive measures and health education can be targeted specifically towards them. In the overall patient prediction data, an increasing trend is observed towards the end of 2023, particularly from August to September 2023 well into 2024. The highest number of patients is in March, as shown in Figure 16 for the overall patient data in a hospital.

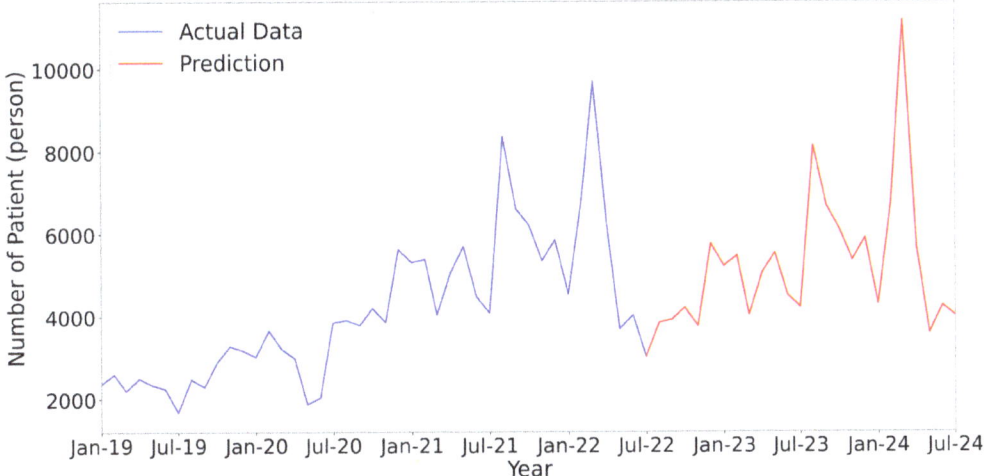

Figure 16. Prediction of overall patient data up to 2024.

In an analysis that involves predicting from a dataset, there is a level of uncertainty that needs to be acknowledged. Health prediction data are estimations based on historical data and certain assumptions. Factors such as lifestyle changes, environmental influences, or unforeseen events can impact actual outcomes in the future. Therefore, predictions should be used as a reference, and precautionary measures in decision making and management need to be carefully considered. As a result, prediction graphs should be interpreted cautiously and supplemented with more in-depth data analysis and ongoing monitoring to update and correct predictions over time. Ultimately, all data and analyses are essential for providing an overview, and some results indicate a relatively low level of error, making them useful as references for more effective decision making in organisational management. The full collected and analysis data can refer to the supplementary materials attached.

The work of patient data analyses with real cases at a hospital in Indonesia, predicting the number of potential cases of disease for future years, is presented as results. The method used, deep learning with the LSTM algorithm, has limitations due to the small amount of data collected and then the amount of data affected by the result, because the method refers to the data learning for the previous years. High numbers and longer spans of data collected for previous time periods contribute to the accuracy in decision making. Data analyses use machine learning, and test datasets require a large number of patient data followed by good decisions for predictions with high accuracy. In some cases, the small amount of data collected from the direct analysis to plot the graph and check the trend may assist in the decision. The results may be a good recommendation and plotted into a similar trend to the previous data collected from the hospital.

5. Conclusions

The final patient data analysis in a hospital in the city of Medan, Indonesia, provides a deeper understanding of the public health situation in the North Sumatra region, Indonesia. Gaining insights from these data, we hope that public health efforts can be more targeted, effective, and sustainable in improving the overall quality of life and well-being of the community. Through collaboration between healthcare professionals, hospital management, and local government, the implications and conclusions from this data analysis can serve as a strong foundation for achieving better public health goals in the North Sumatra region. Despite some weaknesses, a patient data analysis in hospitals still provides valuable contributions to understanding public health and helps in formulating more targeted policies and interventions. Acknowledging these weaknesses allows for the improvement and enhancement of health studies in the future to make a more optimal contribution to the health and well-being of a community.

Based on the results of a patient data analysis in hospitals in the city of Medan, we make several recommendations to be considered for the future in an attempt to improve healthcare services in the region. First, health data sources must be enhanced and diversified. By integrating data from various hospitals and healthcare facilities in the region, we can have a more comprehensive and representative picture of public health. Additionally, the second recommendation is to involve healthcare professionals and researchers from various disciplines in the process of data analysis and interpretation. Collaboration across disciplines will bring together different perspectives and enrich the understanding of public health conditions, providing insights for more holistic healthcare system improvements. Furthermore, efforts are needed to improve the accuracy and quality of collected data. Training for healthcare personnel in proper documentation and data collection will minimise errors and potential biases. Future work advises integration not only in North Sumatra but also in larger areas covering all hospitals in Sumatra or Indonesia to obtain high-accuracy data analyses. The method proposed and used in this work can be used with any patient data from other hospitals or health centres, either in Indonesia or other countries. Analyses and scenarios with which to visualise results with abnormality concerns and make predictions for future years are the main objectives in checking disease trends before, during, and after the COVD-19 pandemic.

Supplementary Materials: The following supporting information can be downloaded at: https://www.mdpi.com/article/10.3390/info15010041/s1.

Author Contributions: Idea concept and writing—original draft preparation, L.D.P.; supervising, administration, funding, and conceptual, E.G.; facilities of project administration and funding, I.N.E.L.; methodology and review as well as software, H.T.K.; formal analysis, methodology, and software, E.A.K.; data collection and analysis, S.L.R. All authors have read and agreed to the published version of the manuscript.

Funding: This research and work were funded internally by the Universitas Prima Indonesia for the 2023 fiscal year, and were supported by collaborators for the facilities and labour.

Informed Consent Statement: In this research, there is no direct interaction or conflict of interest to the patient in hospital.

Data Availability Statement: Data are contained within the article.

Acknowledgments: This work was supported by Universitas Prima Indonesia in collaboration with the Universitas Islam Riau of Indonesia and Harvard University under university collaboration programmes.

Conflicts of Interest: All of the authors declare no conflicts of interest for this manuscript.

References

1. Hospital PI. *Hospital Patient Data in South Sumatra*; Hospital PI: Medan, India, 2022.
2. Stoto, M.A. Population Health Measurement: Applying Performance Measurement Concepts in Population Health Settings. *Public Health Syst. Serv. Res.* **2014**, *2*, 1–27. [CrossRef] [PubMed]

3. Hirani, R.; Noruzi, K.; Iqbal, A.; Hussaini, A.S.; Khan, R.A.; Harutyunyan, A.; Etienne, M.; Tiwari, R.K. A Review of the Past, Present, and Future of the Monkeypox Virus: Challenges, Opportunities, and Lessons from COVID-19 for Global Health Security. *Microorganisms* **2023**, *11*, 2713. [CrossRef] [PubMed]
4. Connerton, P.; Vicente de Assunção, J.; Maura de Miranda, R.; Dorothée Slovic, A.; José Pérez-Martínez, P.; Ribeiro, H. Air Quality during COVID-19 in Four Megacities: Lessons and Challenges for Public Health. *Int. J. Environ. Res. Public Health* **2020**, *17*, 5067. [CrossRef] [PubMed]
5. Zhou, Y.; Chen, T.; Wang, J.; Xu, X. Analyzing the Factors Driving the Changes of Ecosystem Service Value in the Liangzi Lake Basin—A GeoDetector-Based Application. *Sustainability* **2023**, *15*, 15763. [CrossRef]
6. Salamah, Y.; Asyifa, R.D.; Afifah, T.Y.; Maulana, F.; Asfarian, A. Thymun: Smart Mobile Health Platform for the Autoimmune Community to Improve the Health and Well-Being of Autoimmune Sufferers in Indonesia. In Proceedings of the 2020 8th International Conference on Information and Communication Technology (ICoICT), Yogyakarta, Indonesia, 24–26 June 2020; pp. 1–6.
7. Bernasconi, A.; Grandi, S. A Conceptual Model for Geo-Online Exploratory Data Visualization: The Case of the COVID-19 Pandemic. *Information* **2021**, *12*, 69. [CrossRef]
8. Monlezun, D.J. Percutaneous Coronary Intervention Mortality, Cost, Complications, and Disparities after Radiation Therapy: Artificial Intelligence-Augmented, Cost Effectiveness, and Computational Ethical Analysis. *J. Cardiovasc. Dev. Dis.* **2023**, *10*, 445. [CrossRef]
9. Vazanic, D.; Kurtovic, B.; Balija, S.; Milosevic, M.; Brborovic, O. Predictors, Prevalence, and Clinical Outcomes of Out-of-Hospital Cardiac Arrests in Croatia: A Nationwide Study. *Healthcare* **2023**, *11*, 2729. [CrossRef]
10. Montuori, P.; Gentile, I.; Fiorilla, C.; Sorrentino, M.; Schiavone, B.; Fattore, V.; Coscetta, F.; Riccardi, A.; Villani, A.; Trama, U.; et al. Understanding Factors Contributing to Vaccine Hesitancy in a Large Metropolitan Area. *Vaccines* **2023**, *11*, 1558. [CrossRef]
11. Dalapati, T.; Nick, S.E.; Chari, T.A.; George, I.A.; Hunter Aitchison, A.; MacEachern, M.P.; O'Sullivan, A.N.; Taber, K.A.; Muzyk, A. Interprofessional Climate Change Curriculum in Health Professional Programs: A Scoping Review. *Educ. Sci.* **2023**, *13*, 945. [CrossRef]
12. De Vito, A.; Moi, G.; Saderi, L.; Puci, M.V.; Colpani, A.; Firino, L.; Puggioni, A.; Uzzau, S.; Babudieri, S.; Sotgiu, G.; et al. Vaccination and Antiviral Treatment Reduce the Time to Negative SARS-CoV-2 Swab: A Real-Life Study. *Viruses* **2023**, *15*, 2180. [CrossRef]
13. Tanumihardjo, J.P.; Davis, H.; Zhu, M.; On, H.; Guillory, K.K.; Christensen, J. Enhancing Chronic-Disease Education through Integrated Medical and Social Care: Exploring the Beneficial Role of a Community Teaching Kitchen in Oregon. *Nutrients* **2023**, *15*, 4368. [CrossRef] [PubMed]
14. Swaney, R.; Jokomo-Nyakabau, R.; Nguyen, A.A.N.; Kenny, D.; Millner, P.G.; Selim, M.; Destache, C.J.; Velagapudi, M. Diagnosis and Outcomes of Fungal Co-Infections in COVID-19 Infections: A Retrospective Study. *Microorganisms* **2023**, *11*, 2326. [CrossRef] [PubMed]
15. Khatri, S.; al-Sulbi, K.; Attaallah, A.; Ansari, M.T.; Agrawal, A.; Kumar, R. Enhancing Healthcare Management during COVID-19: A Patient-Centric Architectural Framework Enabled by Hyperledger Fabric Blockchain. *Information* **2023**, *14*, 425. [CrossRef]
16. Sekiyama, M.; Roosita, K.; Ohtsuka, R. Locally Sustainable School Lunch Intervention Improves Hemoglobin andHematocrit Levels andBody Mass Index among Elementary Schoolchildren in Rural West Java, Indonesia. *Nutrients* **2017**, *9*, 868. [CrossRef] [PubMed]
17. Abdul Kadir, E.; Listia Rosa, S.; Syukur, A.; Othman, M.; Daud, H. Forest fire spreading and carbon concentration identification in tropical region Indonesia. *Alex. Eng. J.* **2022**, *61*, 1551–1561. [CrossRef]
18. Huang, L. Developing Place-Based Health during the COVID-19 Pandemic: A Case Study of Taipei City's Jiuzhuang Community Garden. *Sustainability* **2023**, *15*, 12422. [CrossRef]
19. Gan, D.R.Y.; Cheng, G.H.-L.; Ng, T.P.; Gwee, X.; Soh, C.Y.; Fung, J.C.; Cho, I.S. Neighborhood Makes or Breaks Active Ageing? Findings from Cross-Sectional Path Analysis. *Int. J. Environ. Res. Public Health* **2022**, *19*, 3695. [CrossRef]
20. Gunawan, H.; Abdul Kadir, E. Integration protocol student academic information to campus RFID gate pass system. In Proceedings of the International Conference on Electrical Engineering, Computer Science and Informatics (EECSI), Yogyakarta, Indonesia, 19–21 September 2017.
21. Kadir, E.A.; Shamsuddin, S.M.; Rahman, T.A.; Samad Ismail, A. Big Data Network Architecture and Monitoring Use Wireless 5G Technology. *Int. J. Adv. Soft Comput. Appl.* **2015**, *7*, 1–14.
22. Chae, K.; Kim, M.; Kim, B.O.; Jung, C.Y.; Kang, H.-J.; Oh, D.-J.; Jeon, D.W.; Chung, W.Y.; Choi, C.U.; Han, K.R.; et al. Public Reporting on the Quality of Care in Patients with Acute Myocardial Infarction: The Korean Experience. *Int. J. Environ. Res. Public Health* **2022**, *19*, 3169. [CrossRef]
23. Ramirez-Alcocer, U.M.; Tello-Leal, E.; Romero, G.; Macías-Hernández, B.A. A Deep Learning Approach for Predictive Healthcare Process Monitoring. *Information* **2023**, *14*, 508. [CrossRef]
24. Kadir, E.A.; Siswanto, A.; Yulian, A. Home Monitoring System Based on Cloud Computing Technology and Object Sensor. In Proceedings of the Second International Conference on the Future of ASEAN (ICoFA) 2017, Kangar, Malaysia, 15–16 August 2017; Volume 2.
25. Zeng, H.; Deng, S.; Zhou, Z.; Qiu, X.; Jia, X.; Li, Z.; Wang, J.; Duan, H.; Tu, L. Diagnostic value of combined nucleic acid and antibody detection in suspected COVID-19 cases. *Public Health* **2020**, *186*, 1–5. [CrossRef] [PubMed]

26. Kadir, E.A. Development of information and communication technology (ICT) in container terminal for speed up clearance process. *J. Commun.* **2017**, *12*, 207–213. [CrossRef]
27. Kadir, E.A.; Kung, H.T.; AlMansor, A.A.; Irie, H.; Rosa, S.L.; Fauzi, S.S. Wildfire Hotspots Forecasting and Mapping for Environmental Monitoring Based on the Long Short-Term Memory Networks Deep Learning Algorithm. *Environments* **2023**, *10*, 124. [CrossRef]
28. Shaikh, M.A. Prevalence and Correlates of Intimate Partner Violence against Women in Liberia: Findings from 2019–2020 Demographic and Health Survey. *Int. J. Environ. Res. Public Health* **2022**, *19*, 3519. [CrossRef]
29. Taniguchi, Y.; Yamazaki, S.; Nakayama, S.F.; Sekiyama, M.; Michikawa, T.; Isobe, T.; Iwai-Shimada, M.; Kobayashi, Y.; Takagi, M.; Kamijima, M.; et al. Baseline Complete Blood Count and Chemistry Panel Profile from the Japan Environment and Children's Study (JECS). *Int. J. Environ. Res. Public Health* **2022**, *19*, 3277. [CrossRef]
30. Dierbach, C. Python as a First Programming Language. *J. Comput. Sci. Coll.* **2014**, *29*, 73.
31. Sherstinsky, A. Fundamentals of Recurrent Neural Network (RNN) and Long Short-Term Memory (LSTM) network. *Phys. D Nonlinear Phenom.* **2020**, *404*, 132306. [CrossRef]
32. Kadir, E.A.; Kung, H.T.; Rosa, S.L.; Sabot, A.; Othman, M.; Ting, M. Forecasting of Fires Hotspot in Tropical Region Using LSTM Algorithm Based on Satellite Data. In Proceedings of the 2022 IEEE Region 10 Symposium (TENSYMP), Mumbai, India, 1–3 July 2022; pp. 1–7.
33. Wang, K.; Niu, D.; Sun, L.; Zhen, H.; Liu, J.; De, G.; Xu, X. Wind Power Short-Term Forecasting Hybrid Model Based on CEEMD-SE Method. *Processes* **2019**, *7*, 843. [CrossRef]
34. Hochreiter, S.; Schmidhuber, J. Long Short-Term Memory. *Neural Comput.* **1997**, *9*, 1735–1780. [CrossRef]
35. Ding, W.; Qie, X. Prediction of Air Pollutant Concentrations via RANDOM Forest Regressor Coupled with Uncertainty Analysis—A Case Study in Ningxia. *Atmosphere* **2022**, *13*, 960. [CrossRef]
36. Liu, Y.; Wu, R.; Yang, A. Research on Medical Problems Based on Mathematical Models. *Mathematics* **2023**, *11*, 2842. [CrossRef]
37. Bishop, C.M. *Neural Networks for Pattern Recognition*; Oxford University Press: New York, NY, USA, 1995; 504p.

Disclaimer/Publisher's Note: The statements, opinions and data contained in all publications are solely those of the individual author(s) and contributor(s) and not of MDPI and/or the editor(s). MDPI and/or the editor(s) disclaim responsibility for any injury to people or property resulting from any ideas, methods, instructions or products referred to in the content.

MDPI
St. Alban-Anlage 66
4052 Basel
Switzerland
www.mdpi.com

Information Editorial Office
E-mail: information@mdpi.com
www.mdpi.com/journal/information

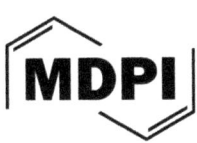

Disclaimer/Publisher's Note: The statements, opinions and data contained in all publications are solely those of the individual author(s) and contributor(s) and not of MDPI and/or the editor(s). MDPI and/or the editor(s) disclaim responsibility for any injury to people or property resulting from any ideas, methods, instructions or products referred to in the content.